MEDICAL FEES in the UNITED STATES

Nationwide Charges for Medicine, Surgery, Laboratory, Radiology and Allied Health Services

2002

PMIC

CPT™ is a registered trademark of the American Medical Association. CPT codes and descriptors are copyright 2002 by the American Medical Association. All rights reserved. Applicable FARS/DFARS apply. This book is published under a license agreement with the American Medical Association.

ISBN 1-57066-233-9

Practice Management Information Corporation (PMIC)
4727 Wilshire Boulevard
Los Angeles, California 90010

Printed in the United States of America

FOREWORD

Fee strategies are becoming more and more important as the very structure of healthcare delivery changes. It is absolutely critical to the success of your medical practice for you to carefully review, analyze and adjust your fees frequently. This comprehensive publication is designed to help you accomplish this formidable task accurately, quickly, and easily.

Medical Fees in the United States 2002, our ninth annual edition, is a listing of medical procedure codes, descriptions, UCR fees at the 50th, 75th and 90th percentiles, Medicare fees and Medicare relative value units. The UCR fees listed in this publication are derived from an analysis of over 400 million actual charges. The CPT codes and short descriptions are from the official CPT 2002 as published by the American Medical Association. The Medicare fees and RVUs are taken from the *Medicare Physician Fee Schedule for Calendar Year 2002* as published in the *Federal Register*.

James B. Davis, Publisher

DISCLAIMER

This publication is designed to offer basic information regarding fee schedule management. The information presented is based upon extensive databases and the experience and interpretations of the authors. Though all of the information has been carefully researched and checked for accuracy and completeness, neither the authors nor the publisher accepts any responsibility or liability with regard to errors, omissions, misuse or misinterpretation.

CONTRIBUTORS

Medical Fees in the United States 2002 is the result of a publishing collaboration between ADP/Context and Practice Management Information Corporation.

ADP/CONTEXT SOFTWARE SYSTEMS, INC.

ADP/Context is a leading developer of reimbursement products for the healthcare industry. Perhaps best known for its CodeLink, Claims Editor and ICD-9-CM software programs, the firm also markets numerous fee, coding and regulatory database products. ADP/Context products are used by thousands of healthcare organizations, from solo physician practices to Fortune 500 companies.

PRACTICE MANAGEMENT INFORMATION CORPORATION

PMIC is the nation's leading independent publisher and distributor of coding, reimbursement and practice management books and software. The company is known for its innovative, high quality products and excellent customer service. Over 100,000 physicians, hospitals, insurance carriers, and other healthcare professionals regularly choose PMIC as their complete medical book resource. The company was listed twice in the Inc. Magazine list of the 500 fastest growing privately held companies in America. PMIC maintains its corporate office in Los Angeles and its sales office in the metropolitan Chicago area.

CONTENTS

FOREWORD iii

CONTRIBUTORS v

TERMINOLOGY xi

INTRODUCTION 1
    Key Points Regarding Setting Fees 1
    Practice Management Applications 2
    Sources Of The Data 3
    How We Estimated Fees For Codes New to CPT 2002 4
    A Short Course In Statistics 5
    How To Review Your Fee Schedule 7
    Determining Fees For New Procedures 13
    Computerized Fee Schedules 14
    Multiple Fee Schedules 14
    Expanded Application of the Medicare Fee Schedule 15
    How To Implement Your New Fee Schedule 16
    Discussing Fees With Your Patients 17
    Strategic Pricing Concepts 20
    Options to Increasing Fees 21

MEDICAL FEES 23
    Format of the Listings 23

EVALUATION & MANAGEMENT 27
    Office or Other Outpatient Services 27
    Hospital Observation Services 27
    Hospital Inpatient Services 27
    Consultations 28
    Emergency Department Services 29
    Patient Transport 29
    Critical Care Services 29
    Neonatal Intensive Care Services 29
    Nursing Facility Services 29
    Domiciliary, Rest Home or Custodial Care Services 30
    Home Services 30
    Prolonged Services 30
    Case Management Services 31

CONTENTS

Care Plan Oversight Services 31
Preventive Medicine Services 31
Newborn Care 32
Special E/M Services 32

SURGERY 33
General 33
Integumentary System 33
Musculoskeletal System 49
Respiratory System 109
Cardiovascular System 121
Hemic and Lymphatic Systems 143
Mediastinum And Diaphragm 147
Digestive System 149
Urinary System 181
Male Genital System 193
Female Genital System 201
Maternity Care And Delivery 209
Endocrine System 213
Nervous System 215
Eye And Ocular Adnexa 233
Auditory System 245

RADIOLOGY 251
Diagnostic Radiology 251
Diagnostic Ultrasound 283
Radiation Oncology 289
Nuclear Medicine 295

PATHOLOGY AND LABORATORY 307
Organ or Disease Oriented Panels 307
Drug Testing 308
Therapeutic Drug Assays 308
Evocative/Suppression Testing 310
Consultations (Clinical Pathology) 312
Urinalysis 312
Chemistry 313
Hematology and Coagulation 345

CONTENTS

Immunology 353
Transfusion Medicine 366
Microbiology 369
Anatomic Pathology 382
Cytopathology 382
Cytogenic Studies 385
Surgical Pathology 387
Other Procedures 389

MEDICINE SERVICES 393
Immune Globulins 393
Immunization Administration for Vaccines, Toxoids 393
Vaccines, Toxoids 394
Therapeutic or Diagnostic Infusions 396
Therapeutic, Prophylactic or Diagnostic Injections 396
Psychiatry 396
Biofeedback 398
Dialysis 398
Gastroenterology 399
Ophthalmology 400
Special Otorhinolaryngologic Services 403
Cardiovascular Services 406
Non-Invasive Vascular Diagnostic Services 415
Pulmonary Services 417
Allergy and Clinical Immunology Services 419
Neurology and Neuromuscular Procedures 421
Health and Behavior Assessments Intervention 426
Chemotherapy Administration 426
Photodyanmic Therapy 427
Special Dermatological Procedures 427
Physical Medicine and Rehabilitation 427
Medical Nutrition Therapy 429
Osteopathic Manipulative Treatment 429
Chiropractic Manipulative Treatment 430
Special Services, Procedures and Reports 430
Qualifying Circumstances for Anesthesia 431
Sedation With or Without Analgesia Conscious Sedation 431
Other Services and Procedures 431

GEOGRAPHIC ADJUSTMENTS 433
Geographic Variability of Medical Fees 433
The Geographic Adjustment Factor 433
How to Use The GAF to Adjust Medical Fees 435
Geographic Adjustment Factors by State or Territory 436

INDEX 443

TERMINOLOGY

Managing the medical fee schedule and reimbursement process requires a fundamental working knowledge of the words and acronyms used by healthcare professionals, government agencies, health insurance companies and third party payers to describe services, benefits and reimbursement policies. While glossaries are most often found in the back of books, we feel that readers should have an opportunity to review and learn new terminology before they encounter it within the text.

Adjusted Historical Payment Basis (AHPB): The average historical Medicare payment in a specific locality for a specific service.

Allowed Charge: The maximum charge allowed by Medicare or other health insurance company or third party payer for a specific service or procedure.

Capitation: A census-driven reimbursement system wherein a health plan provides medical services for a fixed monthly fee. Contracting providers may be reimbursed in the same way.

Center for Medicare and Medicaid Services (CMS): The U.S. Government agency with responsibility for managing the Medicare and Medicaid programs, formerly known as the Health Care Financing Administration, or more commonly, HCFA.

Charge reduction [Medicare]: The percentage difference between a provider's billed charge and the Medicare allowed charge.

Conversion factor: The multiplicative factor applied to a relative value scale to produce a fee schedule for medical services and procedures.

Cost of practice index [Medicare]: A measurement of the differences across geographic areas of the cost of operating a medical practice.

CPT: Current procedural terminology. A system of procedure codes and descriptions published annually by the American Medical Association. This procedure coding system is accepted by virtually all commercial health insurance companies and third party payers and required by Medicare and Medicaid.

Customary charge: One of the factors used by commercial health insurance companies and third party payers to set payment limits for services and procedures. The health insurance company or third party payer typically sets the customary charge for a specific service at the 75th to 90th percentile of all charges for the service within a specific geographic area.

EM [E/M]: Evaluation and management services.

EOB: Explanation of benefits. A form included with a check from an health insurance company or third party payer which explains the benefits that were paid and/or reasons for reduction or denial of unpaid services.

EOMB: Explanation of Medicare benefits. See EOB.

Evaluation and management services: Nontechnical services provided by most physicians and other healthcare professionals for the purpose of diagnosing and/or treating diseases including counseling and evaluating patients.

Fee-for-service: Refers to paying healthcare providers for individual services rendered. UCR and fee schedules are examples of fee-for-service systems.

Fee schedule: A list of predetermined payments for medical services and procedures.

Fee schedule payment areas: Geographic areas within which payment under the Medicare Fee Schedule will be equal. See Geographic adjustment factor.

FFS: Fee-for-service.

GAF: Geographic adjustment factor.

Gaming: Gaining advantage by using improper means to evade the letter or intent or a rule, policy or system.

Geographic adjustment factor: The adjustment made to a Medicare fee to determine the correct payment amount in a specific fee schedule payment area. The geographic adjustment factor for a specific service is determined by combining three separate adjustment factors: physician work, practice expense and malpractice expense.

Geographic practice cost index: An index summarizing the adjustments to pricing of healthcare services in a specific geographic area relative to national average prices.

GPCI: Geographic practice cost index.

HCFA: See Center for Medicare and Medicaid Services.

HCPCS: Health care common procedure coding system. A coding system based upon a combination of CPT supplemented by CMS assigned national codes and carrier assigned local codes for procedures and services not listed in CPT.

HCFA1500: A universal health insurance claim form required for Medicare and accepted by virtually all commercial health insurance companies and third party payers.

ICD-9-CM: International Classification of Diseases, 9th Revision, Clinical Modification. A system of codes and descriptions for injuries, illnesses, signs, symptoms and ill-defined conditions. Required by Medicare and accepted by virtually all commercial health insurance companies and third party payers.

Managed care: The use of a planned and coordinated approach to providing healthcare with the goal of providing quality care at a lower cost.

Maximum fee schedule: A payment arrangement in which a participating physician agrees to accept a pre-established amount as his/her total fee for a covered service.

Medicare Fee Schedule: The fee schedule used by Medicare to pay for physician services. The fee schedule is based upon resource costs, and composed of factors representing physician work, practice expense, and malpractice expense.

MFS: Medicare Fee Schedule.

Modifiers: Codes used with CPT and/or HCPCS to indicate that a basic service or procedure was changed in some way.

Participating physician: A physician who signs a participation agreement, agreeing to accept assignment on all Medicare claims for a period of one year. Frequently referred to as PAR.

Percentile: A value on a scale of one hundred that indicates the percent of a distribution that is equal to or below it. For example, 50th percentile would indicate that 50 percent of all recorded values are equal to or below the value listed as 50th percentile.

Practice expense: The cost of nonphysician resources incurred by the physician in order to provide physician services. Examples are salaries and benefits received by nurses, physician assistants, and administrative staff employed by the physician and the expense associated with the purchase of equipment and supplies required in the physician's office.

Professional component: The part of the relative value or fee for a service or procedure that represents the physician work and excludes costs for materials and/or facilities.

RBRVS: Resource based relative value system. A government mandated relative value system, based on a study conducted by William Hsiao, ph.D. at Harvard University that was the basis for the Medicare Fee Schedule.

Reasonable charge: Generally defined as the lesser of the billed fee, the usual fee, or is otherwise justifiable due to special circumstances.

Relative value scale: An index that assigns specific numeric values to medical services and procedures. Multiplying the relative value by a conversion factor results in a fee.

RVS: Relative Value Scale.

RVU: Relative Value Unit.

Schedule of allowances: A list of specific amounts which a health insurance company or third party payer will pay toward the costs of medical services provided.

Specialty differential: The difference in the relative value or amount paid for the same service when performed by different medical specialists.

Technical component: The part of the relative value or fee for a service or procedure that represents the costs of doing the procedure excluding physician work.

UCR: Usual, customary and reasonable.

Usual fee: The fee charged by a healthcare professional most of the time for the majority of patients for a specific service or procedure.

INTRODUCTION

Setting fees for medical services involves a lot more than simply deciding the dollar amount associated with a particular service or procedure. Setting fees requires a knowledge of how health insurance companies and third party payers process and pay health insurance claims, a method for determining the value of your procedures and services, an awareness of the going rates in your medical community, a comprehensive knowledge of Medicare, Medicaid, and Worker's Compensation laws, and non-governmental health insurance company and third party payer billing rules and regulations.

In today's competitive market environment, it is important to understand that your fees are part of your marketing strategy. Fees must be reviewed and adjusted periodically. The adjustment is usually in the form of raising fees; however, fee decreases are sometimes appropriate and may become more common as competition increases. The objective of fee schedule management is to set a fair price for your procedures and services, and to be paid that price most of the time. However, neither setting your fees or getting paid is as simple as that.

KEY POINTS REGARDING SETTING FEES

- It is difficult to obtain fee information, profiles, relative values, or conversion factors from most non-governmental health insurance companies and/or third party payers. In addition, professional medical associations are prevented by Federal antitrust legislation from disclosing the results of fee surveys.

- A variation of the Medicare Fee Schedule (MFS) based on the Resource Based Relative Value Scale (RBRVS) will likely become the method used for reimbursement by all health insurance companies and third party payers in the future.

- Charging a fee that is less than an insurance carrier will pay benefits the insurance carrier, not you or your patient.

- Health insurance companies and third party payers may be paying you 25-50% less than they are paying your peers for exactly the same service, simply because you have been careless in maintaining your provider profile.

- Essentially all medical fees are ultimately negotiated or discounted, either voluntarily or involuntarily.

- Fee schedule management puts you in control of the reimbursement process.

PRACTICE MANAGEMENT APPLICATIONS

FEE SCHEDULE REVIEW

The primary application of the information contained in this publication is to review your fees in comparison to the report in order to determine where your fees rank on a national basis. Your fees may then be adjusted, if appropriate, based upon the results of your review and analysis.

BARGAINING WITH HEALTH INSURANCE COMPANIES AND THIRD PARTY PAYERS

It is important to your patients and your practice that health insurance companies and third party payers are paying you and/or your patients based upon current, and accurate, UCR data for your geographic area and specialty. Theoretically, the percentile distribution of fees for a specific procedure or service performed in a given geographic area should be identical for all health insurance companies and third party payers. However, in reality these numbers vary considerably and are also affected by the payment policies of specific health insurance companies and third party payers.

Remember that under the usual, customary and reasonable concept, the health insurance company and/or third party payer will gladly pay you less than their allowable or customary amount if that's what you billed them. In addition, you can't increase your fees retroactively. However, if health insurance companies and third party payers allowables or customary amounts are significantly below your fees, resulting in low payments to you and/or your patients, then you should compare the codes that appear to be underpaid with the data in this publication. If you find that the published data supports a higher reimbursement, then you should appeal the payment to the health insurance company and/or third party payer.

We strongly suggest that you support your appeal letter by attaching a photocopy of the front cover of this book and the page(s) that include the codes and fees that you are basing your appeal on. We don't guarantee that this will work every time; however, our customers have informed us that this does indeed work most of the time.

COST BENEFIT ANALYSIS

This publication can be used to perform cost benefit analyses for both equipment and human resources. For example, suppose your group practice is considering installing its own automated laboratory equipment or x-ray equipment. A careful review of the RADIOLOGY and/or LABORATORY sections of this publication will provide you with the fee data you need to perform a cost/benefit analysis for the equipment. You would need to supply the estimated frequency for each service and the acquisition cost of the equipment to complete the analysis.

Likewise, you can perform a similar calculation based upon human resources. For example, suppose you are considering adding an associate to your practice. A careful review of EVALUATION & MANAGEMENT and appropriate specialty sections of the publication will provide you with the fee data you need to perform a cost/benefit analysis for the associate. As above you would need to provide the estimated frequency for each service and the cost of maintaining the human resource. In either of these examples, you would also have to adjust the forecast total charges by your average collection ratios to achieve an accurate forecast of revenues.

SOURCES OF THE DATA

The usual, customary and reasonable (UCR) fees listed in this book were developed over a period of several years. More than 400 million actual physician charges provides the basis for listed fees. Service bureaus, group practices, clinics, universities, and practice management system vendors are among the many types of organizations that supplied the claims data utilized for fee schedule development.

Although the creation of a fee schedule may seem rather straightforward, the process is actually quite complex. For example, many of the codes listed in CPT are performed infrequently. Thus, even with the largest of fee databases, there may be so few instances of a particular code's usage that it is difficult to establish reliable percentile ranges. As another example, some services listed in CPT are considered variable in performance. That is, when one physician reports the code, he/she may include items or services that another physician does not provide. Clearly, this can significantly impact UCR fee levels.

RELATIONSHIP TO PAYER ALLOWABLES

Contrary to widespread belief, there is no "secret" list of fees that health insurance companies and third party payers use to determine the appropriateness of your charges. Many different firms, including ADP/Context, sell fee databases to payers. Payers in turn may utilize one or more of these databases, as well as relative value systems, during the payment adjudication process. This is especially true for rarely performed services for which reliable payment guidelines are lacking. Additionally, different payers set payment limits at different levels. For example, one health insurance company and/or third party payer may reimburse at the 90th percentile, another at the 75th percentile, and yet another at the 80th percentile. Health maintenance organizations and other managed care groups typically negotiate fees that are closer to the 50th percentile for a given area.

HOW WE ESTIMATED FEES FOR CODES NEW TO CPT 2002

When new CPT codes are introduced at the beginning of each year, it takes several months before healthcare providers begin routinely submitting them on health insurance claims, before payers begin establishing payment criteria, and before enough claims data becomes available to establish UCR fees and percentiles. Thus, the UCR fees for codes new to *CPT 2002* book presented in this publication are estimates, and should be viewed as such.

Two methods were used in preparing these estimates. First, for new codes for which Medicare has assigned 2002 RBRVS values, estimates were created by scaling the Medicare RBRVS values to a level consistent with related procedure codes for which UCR fees already exist. As an example, if a new code's RBRVS value is 10, and if the RBRVS offset for procedures related to the new code is 2.6, then the scaled value for the new code will be 26. This scaled value is then used to calculate estimated 2002 fees and percentiles.

Second, in instances where Medicare has not assigned RBRVS values, Medicare Fee Schedule data was used. For example, most laboratory services covered by Medicare are under a non-RBRVS schedule. To estimate fees and values for the new lab codes, Medicare's 2002 laboratory fee schedule data was scaled to UCR levels using methods similar to those discussed above. In the case where no data existed that could be used to estimate the UCR percentiles for new codes no fee data is listed.

The reader is reminded that all UCR fees listed for new codes are *estimates*. Even though the estimates have been created on a logical basis by using relative value data, there is no way to determine the validity or accuracy of the estimates until data from actual claims has been obtained. At the same time, we feel strongly that setting your fees for these new codes somewhere between the 75th and 90th percentiles is justified based uponthe logic used to create the estimates.

GEOGRAPHIC VARIABILITY AND ADJUSTMENT

The 50th, 75th and 90th percentile fees provided in this text are based on national averages and are generally reflective of payer allowables. However, medical fees vary substantially by geographic area. In rural and smaller urban areas the payer allowables may be significantly lower than the percentiles presented in this text. Conversely, in large urban areas the payers may allow fees that are much higher than the average fees shown.

The last chapter of this book includes a list of geographic adjustment factors for cities, counties, areas, regions and states which may be used to "fine tune" the data in this report. The Geographic Adjustment Factors (GAF) listed are calculated using a weighted average of the work, practice expense and malpractice expense components of the GPCIs. The

GAFs can be used to make reasonably reliable geographic adjustments of the UCR fees and Medicare fees.

A SHORT COURSE IN STATISTICS

The usual, customary and reasonable fees in this publication are presented as percentiles. Other publications use fee ranges or average fees instead of percentiles. The use of percentiles is much better than using fee ranges or averages. Presenting a fee range of lowest to highest is only of use to find out if you are lower than the lowest or higher than the highest. It really doesn't help you determine where you should be within the range. In addition, the ranges tend to be so great that any fee would fit within them, which again does not serve the intend purpose of helping you determine where you are and where you should be.

A **percentile** is defined as a value on a scale of one hundred that indicates the percent of a distribution that is equal to or below it. The easiest way to understand percentile distribution is by showing it as a curve. The chart below illustrates the distribution curve for CPT code 99213, Office or other outpatient visit for the evaluation and management of an established patient.

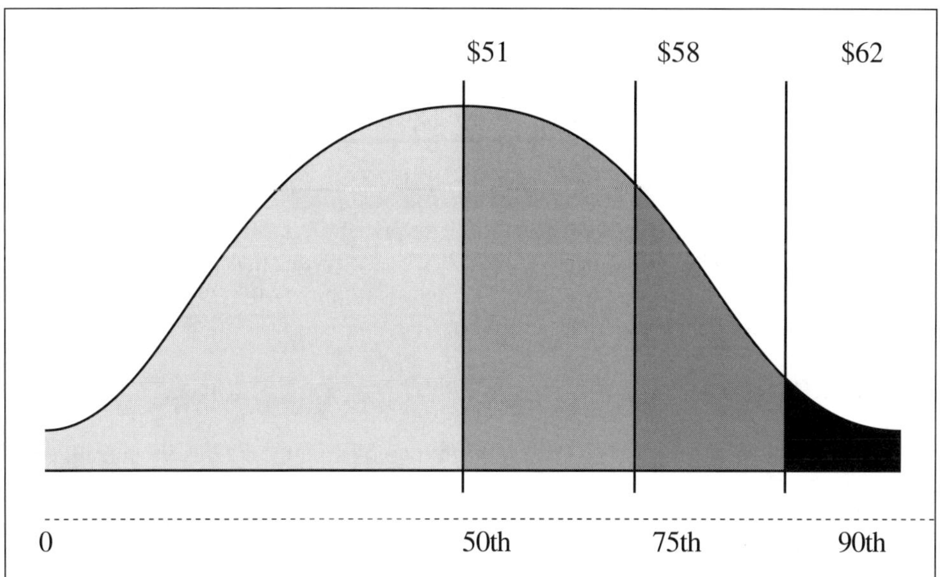

50TH PERCENTILE

In the preceding illustration, the 50th percentile means that 50 percent of all fees for CPT code 99213 fall <u>at or below</u> $66.00. It also means that 50 percent of all fees for CPT code 99213 fall <u>at or above</u> $66.00. You definitely do not want your fees to be on the left side of the curve because that means that a) you are charging less than over half of all providers for the service and b) you are not getting the reimbursement you deserve.

The 50th percentile is also known as the **median**. The 50th percentile or median is not the same as the average or mean. To illustrate this concept more clearly, lets presume that we have a series of 11 fees for a specific service or procedure that represent 11 different providers. The first step is to rank the fees in ascending order by dollar amount. Then we find the 50th percentile or median by counting down to the middle of the list.

Fee 1	$56	
Fee 2	$58	
Fee 3	$60	
Fee 4	$62	
Fee 5	$64	
Fee 6	**$66**	<------- 50th percentile or median
Fee 7	$68	
Fee 8	$70	
Fee 9	$72	
Fee 10	$74	
Fee 11	$76	

75TH PERCENTILE

In the curve shown on the previous page, the 75th percentile means that 75 percent of all fees for CPT code 99213 fall <u>at or below</u> $75.00. It also means that 25 percent of all fees for CPT code 99213 fall <u>at or above</u> $75.00. Being within the 50th-75th percentile range is better than being below the 50th percentile.

90TH PERCENTILE

In the curve shown on the previous page, the 90th percentile means that 90 percent of all fees for CPT code 99213 fall <u>at or below</u> $88.00. It also means that 10 percent of all fees for CPT code 99213 fall <u>at or above</u> $88.00. Being within the 75th-90th percentile range is better than being in the 50th-75th percentile range, *unless market forces dictate otherwise*. For example, for services that are frequently shopped by patients on price, such as total obstetrical care, it would be better to position your fee for this particular service closer to the 50th percentile in order to be competitive.

If your fee is above the 90th percentile, you are charging more than 90 percent of all other providers performing the same service or procedure. In most cases this would indicate that your fee is too high; however, there are some exceptions. The exceptions are usually based upon specialty differentials, i.e. the traditional thinking that a service performed by a specialist is worth more than the same service performed by a non-specialist.

WHERE YOU WANT TO BE

The objective of your fee schedule management program should be to keep your fees at the high end of the distribution while still considering other factors, such as local customs and market considerations, which may require an occasional exception. If you find that your fee for a specific service or procedure is lower than the 50th percentile fee, that means that more than 50 percent of all healthcare providers charge more than you do for this service. It also means your fee is too low and you should raise it.

Likewise, if you find that your fee is higher than the 90th percentile fee, then you are charging more than 90 percent of all healthcare providers for this service. It may also mean that your fee is too high, but not necessarily. You may simply have done a better job at fee schedule management for a long enough time to get your fees up to a maximum level. You may also be a member of a select group of super specialists who have traditionally charged higher fees for certain procedures and consultations in particular.

HOW TO REVIEW YOUR FEE SCHEDULE

The process of fee review includes gathering resource materials, reviewing the procedure and diagnostic codes you use, reviewing the fees charged for each procedure, making decisions regarding fee adjustments, and making sure that the resulting decisions are implemented and followed.

RESOURCE MATERIALS

Current Code Books

Your fees for medical services and procedures are linked by both common business practice and legislation to CPT, HCPCS and ICD-9-CM codes. There are still a few medical practices that still use pegboard systems or ledger cards with designations like "OV" for office visits and "HV" for hospital visits. But most medical practices converted to standard coding systems long ago. For commercial health insurance companies and third party payers, the various code systems define what you did and why you did it, plus their usual, customary and reasonable statistics are maintained by procedure code. For Medicare, the codes are an integral part of the Medicare Fee Schedule used to define the relative values of each procedure. CPT, HCPCS and ICD-9-CM code books may be obtained from many sources, including your local medical bookstore.

Instructions regarding CPT, HCPCS and ICD-9-CM coding are beyond the scope of this book. For specific training materials on these topics the reader is referred to the *Reimbursement Manual for the Medical Office*, Fourth Edition, or *CPT and HCPCS Coding Made Easy!*, Fifth Edition, both published by PMIC.

Relative Value Data

The relative value reflects the complexity of a service or procedure from a medical point of view. The most widely used source of relative value data is from the Resource Based Relative Value Scale (RBRVS), a component of the annual Medicare Physician Fee Schedule published by the Center for Medicare and Medicaid Services (CMS). RBRVS was originally developed for Medicare but is now widely used by commercial insurance plans and other government payers. RBRVS originally included only those CPT codes likely to be used by providers when treating Medicare patients, but has been expanded to include most CPT codes.

CMS depends heavily on the recommendations of the Relative Value Update Committee (RUC) of the American Medical Association. The RUC consists of physicians representing various specialty societies, geographic areas, and practice settings. The committee performs a major review of the relative values every five years, but every year the relative values are updated for all new or changed CPT codes. The specialty society advisors determine relative values based on time, mental effort and judgement, technical skill, physical effort and stress due to patient risk required to perform each service or procedure. The Specialty Society makes recommendations to the RUC which in turn makes a proposal to CMS. About 95% of the RUC recommendations are accepted by CMS each year. CMS publishes the relative values for the next calendar year in the Federal Register, usually in late November or early December.

Medicare Fee Schedule

The revised Medicare Fee Schedule is published in the *Federal Register* in late November or early December each year. You may obtain a copy of the Medicare Fee Schedule from your local Medicare carrier, the U.S. government Printing Office, or from private publishers.

Geographic Cost of Practice Indexes

The Geographic Cost of Practice Indexes (GPCIs) are an integral part of the Medicare Fee Schedule. GPCIs are used to make geographic adjustments to the fees calculated using the fee schedule. Current GPCIs are available from your local Medicare carrier, the U.S. government printing office, and private publishers.

Insurance carrier Explanation of Benefits (EOBs)

You should collect sample copies of Explanation of Benefits (EOBs) from commercial health insurance companies and third party payers for at least three months prior to your planned fee schedule review. Typically this would be in the last quarter of each calendar year. You don't need a copy of every EOB you receive but you should keep copies of those which include payment for your most common procedures and services. Plus, you should keep copies from different commercial health insurance companies and third party payers even when they are paying for the same procedures or services.

REVIEW PROCEDURE AND SERVICE CODES IN CPT 2002

Review each of the procedure codes from your code listing or superbill in CPT 2002. Pay particular attention to codes that have been added, changed or deleted. Your first step should be to review APPENDIX B of the CPT book. APPENDIX B is a summary of all additions, deletions and revisions in the current CPT. This is a quick way for your to first cross-reference the codes that you use frequently, then refer to the full text for make your changes.

- All CPT codes in the 2002 edition with a small black circle to the left of the code are NEW codes. Review all new codes carefully to see if any of them can be used instead of UNLISTED procedure codes or as replacements for HCPCS codes.

- All CPT codes in the 2002 edition with a small black triangle to the left of the code are CHANGED codes. Review the description of all changed codes carefully to make sure that your superbills and insurance forms have the same descriptions. Not only will this improve your reimbursement, it will also protect you from audit liability.

() Next look for codes that have been deleted. These are indicated by parenthesis. CPT includes a referral to a replacement code for all codes that are deleted. Make sure you substitute the replacement codes on your superbills and coding lists.

Review All Sections CPT 2002

Evaluation and Management	Review this section carefully each year for changes in office, hospital, consultation, and other location visit codes.
Surgery	Review all portions of this section of CPT which may be appropriate to your medical practice. Non-surgical practices should review the sections on wound repair, trauma related codes, and any other

procedures commonly performed. Pay particular attention to starred (*) procedures, add-on (+) procedures, and procedures classified as (separate) procedures.

Radiology   Practices which are providing and/or billing for radiology procedures should review this section of CPT carefully. This section includes procedures that are typically performed on a high volume basis, such as chest x-rays, where a small increase in an individual fee can result in a significant increase in total reimbursement.

Laboratory   Practices which provide and/or bill for laboratory procedures need to review this section of CPT carefully. This section typically includes procedures that are performed on a high volume basis, such blood counts, urinalysis, etc., where a small increase in an individual fee can result in a significant increase in total reimbursement.

Medicine   Review this entire section to update injections, specialty procedures and diagnostic procedures.

REVIEW HCPCS 2002 CODES

Review *HCPCS 2002* code listings, particularly the sections covering supplies, materials and injections. CMS revises these codes on an annual basis and most Medicare carriers make continual revisions which are published in the form of newsletters. Use of the proper HCPCS codes can make a significant difference in your reimbursement. You need to obtain a copy of the revised codes each year and review it carefully for any changes which may affect your practice.

Remember that while the HCPCS National Level 2 codes are uniform throughout the United States, the method of billing the codes properly varies from one Medicare carrier to another. In addition, each Medicare carrier maintains and publishes their own HCPCS Local Level 3 codes. Check with your local Medicare carrier for proper billing instructions.

REVIEW ICD-9-CM 2002 CODES

It is important that you are using the most current diagnosis codes from the International Classification of Diseases, 9th Revision (ICD-9-CM). This book is revised and published annually by PMIC and other publishers. You should purchase a new copy each year and review it carefully for any code changes which may affect your coding and billing. Keep track of the frequency of your ICD-9-CM code usage. Add frequently used codes to your reference listings and superbills.

REVIEW ALL YOUR FEES

Review and compare each of your procedures carefully to determine if fees need to be increased due to increased costs or to maintain your profile, or decreased in response to changing market conditions or decreased costs. Pay particular attention to the volume of procedures. Small increases in frequently performed procedures and large increases in infrequently performed procedures can usually be implemented without negative results.

COMPLETE A RELATIVE VALUE ANALYSIS FOR YOUR MOST COMMON PROCEDURES AND SERVICES

Complete a relative value analysis to calculate a conversion factor for your practice. Then use the calculated conversion factor to determine the appropriate fee for each of your procedures. To perform a relative value analysis you need a current relative value publication; a list of your 25 most commonly performed procedure codes from the Medicine, Surgery, Radiology, and Pathology sections of CPT; and your fees for the procedures. Then complete the following six steps for each section.

1) List 25 codes and fees for each section.

2) Look up the relative value and add to your list.

3) Total all of the fees.

4) Total all of the relative values.

5) Divide the total relative values into the total fees.

6) The result is your AVERAGE CONVERSION FACTOR.

After you calculate your AVERAGE CONVERSION FACTOR, you then multiply the relative value for each listed procedure by the conversion factor to determine the fee. You will likely find services and procedures both under and over priced based on relative value analysis. Before raising your prices based on relative value analysis, consider that health insurance companies and third party payers have a maximum dollar value, based on customary fees, that they allow for a given procedure. However, the use of relative values gives you a strong argument in a review of a disputed or underpaid claim.

SAMPLE RELATIVE VALUE ANALYSIS—SELECTED OB/GYN PROCEDURES

On the following page you will find an analysis that was performed using 25 commonly reported OB/GYN procedures. In addition to the CPT code and description you will find the 75th percentile fee and relative value from this publication. The conversion factor is calculated by dividing the total relative values into the total charges. Obviously a conversion factor calculated using fees at the 50th percentile would be lower and a conversion factor using fees at the 90th percentile would be higher.

SAMPLE RELATIVE VALUE ANALYSIS

CODE	DESCRIPTION	FEE	RVU
56420	Drainage of gland abscess	$ 272	4.02
56630	Extensive vulva surgery	$ 3,179	21.52
57061	Destruction vagina lesion(s)	$ 228	3.75
57170	Fitting of diaphragm/cap	$ 109	2.46
57180	Treat vaginal bleeding	$ 360	4.11
57265	Extensive repair vagina	$ 2,847	19.70
57500	Biopsy of cervix	$ 215	3.36
58120	Dilation and curettage (D & C)	$ 1,047	7.61
58150	Total hysterectomy	$ 3,578	24.67
58200	Extensive hysterectomy	$ 5,361	33.36
58300	Insert intrauterine device	$ 253	2.53
58301	Remove intrauterine device	$ 141	3.02
58400	Suspension of uterus	$ 1,745	11.15
58600	Division of fallopian tube	$ 1,746	9.50
58800	Drainage of ovarian cyst(s)	$ 1,076	8.93
58820	Drainage of ovarian abscess	$ 1,352	7.89
58940	Removal of ovary(s)	$ 1,857	17.89
59000	Amniocentesis	$ 421	3.58
59015	Chorion biopsy	$ 556	4.24
59120	Treat ectopic pregnancy	$ 2,589	19.90
59400	Obstetrical care	$ 3,342	42.61
59510	Cesarean delivery	$ 4,029	48.53
59610	VBAC delivery	$ 3,758	45.32
59812	Treatment of miscarriage	$ 973	8.34
59840	Abortion by D & C	$ 762	7.56
TOTALS		**$41,766**	**367.63**
CONVERSION FACTOR			**$113.61**

REVIEW AND REVISE YOUR SUPERBILLS AND FEE SCHEDULES

After you have reviewed all CPT, HCPCS, and ICD-9-CM codes and descriptions and made any necessary revisions to your fees, you need to carefully review all of your superbills and any other documents that may have codes, descriptions or fees printed on them. Make the required changes and then make sure that the revisions are made and the documents printed.

We strongly recommend that you limit the quantity of superbills printed to no more than a six month supply. Inevitably you will change procedure codes, diagnosis codes and/or fees during a six month period and you want to reserve the ability to reprint your superbills without throwing too many away. We also recommend that you do not print fees on your superbills. While it is easier than looking up fees at the cashier's or receptionist's desk, it also causes potential billing errors for interim fee changes.

Distribute copies of the revised superbills and/or fee schedules to all staff members. Consider that not only billing personnel are involved with codes and fees. The person who answers the telephone in response to fee inquiries from potential patients needs to be well informed about your current fee schedules.

STAND BY YOUR FEES

Once your fees are set, stand by them. Make few exceptions to your standard fees and always document exceptions by posting full charges followed by an adjustment. This makes billing easier for everyone and provides an accurate record of how much you are discounting.

DETERMINING FEES FOR NEW PROCEDURES

If you perform a service or procedure for the first time and need to determine a fee, the first place to look would be your relative value reference. If the procedure is listed and has a numeric value, then simply multiply the relative value by your conversion factor to determine the appropriate fee. However, if the procedure or service is unlisted, then you can not calculate a fee by this method. The best alternative is to use a comparative procedure as the basis for first determining approximate relative value and then to calculate the proper fee. Review some of the more common procedures you perform and try to find one that requires similar skills, about the same amount of time, and has the same level of complexity and risk as the new procedure.

Use the relative value of the common procedure as a basis for calculating the fee for the new procedure. Watch insurance carrier EOBs carefully to see how much they are allowing for the new procedure and adjust your fee accordingly. You can also request the prevailing charge for the procedure from your local Medicare intermediary.

COMPUTERIZED FEE SCHEDULES

Several companies maintain, publish or distribute computerized fee schedules. The stated intent of these fee schedules is to make fee schedule review much easier by letting the computer do all the work. The usefulness of any of these products depends mostly on the quality of the database used to prepare the data and the degree to which the databases can be manipulated in terms of geographic location and medical specialty. The database used to prepare this publication is from ADP/Context Software Systems, Inc.

MULTIPLE FEE SCHEDULES

It is essential to have multiple fee schedules in the well managed medical practice. The argument can certainly be made that any service or procedure is worth the same, based on relative value calculations. However, all of your potential payers do not use the same method to pay you or to calculate the value of the services and procedures you perform.

Fees charged for services provided to Medicare patients are highly regulated by Federal law. Fees charged for services provided to Medicaid beneficiaries and Worker's Compensation Carriers are generally based on fixed fee schedules published by state agencies. Many HMOs and PPOs also reimburse based on fee schedules.

None of these rules and regulations or fee schedules applies to services provided to patients paying cash, services rendered to patients in personal injury cases, or for services covered by private health insurance companies and third party payers. A medical practice with a typical patient mix including Medicare, Medicaid, worker's compensation and private insurance patients would need to use a minimum of two or three different fee schedules for proper billing.

MEDICARE FEE SCHEDULE

Practices which are NON-PARTICIPATING must use the Medicare billing limits when billing for services provided to Medicare patients. Practices which are PARTICIPATING may charge their regular fees for services provided to Medicare patients.

REGULAR FEE SCHEDULE

This is your standard fee schedule representing the fees that you charge for cash patients, private insurance patients, Medicaid patients, and, if you are PARTICIPATING, to Medicare patients also.

WORKER'S COMPENSATION

This fee schedule is used to bill for services related to treating illnesses and injuries related to employment. The fee schedules are generally maintained and published by the state agency responsible for worker's compensation cases.

CONTRACT FEE SCHEDULES

You may have additional fee schedules, based on participating agreements with HMOs, PPOs, etc. that must be used to bill for services provided to beneficiaries of these plans.

EXPANDED APPLICATION OF THE MEDICARE FEE SCHEDULE

The traditional development path in the areas of coding and billing is that policies and procedures mandated by Medicare are implemented shortly thereafter by Medicaid, followed by private health insurance companies and third party payers. However, there are significant issues which must be dealt with before private health insurance companies and third party payers can implement a fee schedule.

Private health insurance companies and third party payers have expressed interest in revising their methods of physician payment. Many support the objectives of Medicare payment reform but have yet to determine the extent to which physician markets will permit changes in relative values. Although few plan to adopt the Medicare Fee Schedule in total, many are contemplating at least marginal changes in relative values to reflect the direction of Medicare changes. Private health insurance companies and third party payers face limits to the magnitude of change they can institute. Insurers offering indemnity policies are concerned that balance billing for technical procedures will increase. Carriers that contract with physicians are concerned about whether specialists would agree to participate in sufficient numbers if their fees would fall.

More extensive or more rapid changes by private health insurance companies and third party payers will require public regulation of their payment policies. Under an all-payer system, the Medicare relative value scale could be used by each of the payers. A public body would determine payment rates for the various physician services. While the conversion factors used by different payers need not be the same, the entity that determines rates would have a deliberate policy concerning how they would differ. Conversion factors could be updated through volume performance standards or a similar mechanism. Balance billing would be limited, but again, the limits could differ by class of payer. The entity making these decisions (presumably the U.S. Government) would (try to) balance the interests of physicians, private payers, public payers, and patients.

HOW TO IMPLEMENT YOUR NEW FEE SCHEDULE

Regardless of how carefully you review and set your fees, you will still have complaints from patients. While studies have continued to indicate that most patients do not choose providers of medical care based on fees, it is important to keep in mind that many malpractice cases start out as fee disputes. Fee related complaints tend to fall under the five general categories.

FEE COMPARISON

Patients compare fees among each other. In addition, many patients shop fees for elective procedures or routine care. Patients may be well informed regarding the going rates for specific procedures and may ask why your fee is higher than that of other providers. Be prepared to explain your fees for common procedures.

FEE CONSISTENCY

Patients may question what appears to be inconsistencies in your fees from one visit to the next. Patients are not aware of the various levels of service defined by CPT and the fact that some services are packaged or bundled and others are not. Make sure the patient understands exactly what is included in bundled procedures, and is made aware of the levels of care if he/she questions your fees for visits.

TIME SPENT (WITH THE PATIENT)

Patients frequently consider the value of your services to be directly proportional to the time you spent with them. This is logical thinking on the patient's part, as many professional services tend to be rendered and billed based on units of time. Prior to publication of the 1992 edition of CPT, there were very few services or procedures that included time components. Therefore, you could explain simply to the patient that your fees are not based on the amount of time spent but rather the complexity of the situation and the level of care required.

With publication of the 1992 CPT, time became part of the definition of the new Evaluation and Management services. As the definition and understanding of the new coding system becomes widespread among the patient population, you may expect some patients to time your services and compare their time with the time associated with particular Evaluation and Management codes.

RELATIVE VALUE

Due to the lack of knowledge and understanding regarding anatomy, physiology and the difficulties involved in various medical procedures, patients make inappropriate comparisons of procedures. They may not understand why a repair of a hip fracture costs more than life-saving treatment for an acute myocardial infarction. Patients are not aware of the traditional discrepancy between the value of cognitive procedures versus technical procedures. Of interest is the fact that the patients do not recognize any differences in value between cognitive and technical services.

This subjective attitude of the patient population is verified in part by the findings of the Harvard study of Resource Based Relative Values. One of the objectives of the Medicare Fee Schedule is to legislate away the discrepancy by creating a reimbursement system based upon measurable work and cost of practice indexes. If patients question this issue, be prepared to explain how fees for technical services are calculated. Expect Medicare patients to be knowledgeable of Medicare Fee Schedule rules, regulations, and formulas.

ABILITY TO PAY

In the past it was quite common for healthcare providers to charge patients based on ability to pay. Therefore, some patients were charged a little more, some a little less, and some nothing at all. It was sort of a private Medicaid system. Now with most patients covered by insurance plans and, more importantly, generally aware of basic fees for the most common procedures and services, the situation is different. If patients perceive that you are charging them more because they can pay more, they will probably not come back. Make sure that your discussion of fees includes assurances that your fees are not based on the patient's ability to pay, but rather on the specific services provided.

DISCUSSING FEES WITH YOUR PATIENTS

DISCUSSING FEES AT THE TIME OF APPOINTMENT SCHEDULING

Some practices discuss fees in advance with patients who call to make an appointment. While this may occasionally cause problems when the bill turns out to be higher than quoted on the phone, the major benefit is that the patient has been informed that there will be a charge, and that they are expected to pay. Any statements regarding fees or amounts made during telephone conversations should be noted on the appointment schedule.

SMALL FEES CAN BE STATED AFTER SERVICES HAVE BEEN RENDERED

Services such as office visits, injections and minor procedures can generally be provided without advance discussion of fees. The provider can fill out the charge slip or superbill including fees and instruct the patient to give it to the receptionist, or the provider can leave the fees blank to be filled out by the receptionist.

When the charge slip is totalled and presented to the patient for payment, the patient has the opportunity to ask questions regarding the services provided and the fees charged.

Even if the patient does not pay at the time of service, this presentation of the itemized charge slip makes the patient aware of the fees, which will correspond to the bill received.

DISCUSS LARGER FEES BEFORE PROVIDING SERVICE

Numerous studies have confirmed that when patients are about to undergo major procedures that their first concern is outcome, and their second concern is how much it is going to cost and how are they going to pay for it. Unfortunately, most patients will never express this concern voluntarily.

Most medical professionals discuss their findings, treatment plans and the probable outcome(s) of treatment with their patients; however, many neglect any discussion of fees or payment methods. In addition to appreciating the information, discussing the potential cost gives the patient the ability to make an informed decision regarding the service. In order to gain a little perspective on this issue, ask yourself the following questions:

- Would you order a meal in an expensive restaurant from a menu without prices?

- Would you allow a mechanic to perform major service on your car without an estimate of what it was going to cost?

- Would you allow a contractor to begin construction on your new kitchen or bathroom without a bid?

While you most likely answered "no" to each of the above questions, consider that many medical and surgical procedures have fees that are far in excess of repairing cars or adding additions to a house. Yet many medical practices routinely expect the patient to receive (and pay for) services without any advance knowledge of their cost. None of this has anything to do with ethics. It is simply a matter of providing professional services with the expectation of being paid for those services. You always have the option to provide services at no charge if that is what you want to do.

HOW TO INITIATE FEE DISCUSSIONS

Not everyone is comfortable in discussing fees or money with patients. Many medical professionals absolutely refuse to engage in such discussions. It is not necessary for the medical professional to have this fee discussion with the patient, although patient surveys consistently reveal that the patient prefers to discuss fees directly with the medical professional. But it is important that someone representing the practice, the office manager, insurance manager, or the financial counselor, have a discussion with the patient regarding the fees before major services are rendered.

It is important to make the patient aware that your fees are within the going rates for the community, that the fees to this patient are the same as that for every patient, and, for bundled procedures, that your fee includes specific services and procedures. The following statements represent some of the more successful approaches to this subject:

- *My (our, the doctor's) usual charge for this service is....*

  This lets the patient know what the charge will be and that they are being charged the same as everyone else.

- *The going rate for this service (around here, in the community)....*

  This opening gives you two options. Either it assures the patient that your fees are in line with those of your colleagues, or it gives you the opportunity to explain why your fees are higher.

- *My (our, the doctor's) fee covers....*

  This approach is often used when discussing fees that are global in nature, primarily surgical procedures which include a standard amount of routine follow-up care. Another example would be prenatal care, uncomplicated vaginal delivery and the post-partum visit. This lets the patient know that a single fee covers all of the service.

  It is better to state your usual charge first and then explain that any insurance proceeds will be applied against it. By mentioning insurance first, you risk the patient assuming that you will scale your charges based upon insurance payment.

- *Don't worry. We'll take your insurance as full payment....*

  What if the patient isn't covered, but doesn't know it? What about deductibles and coinsurance? What about pre-existing conditions and exclusions? You can be sued by the patient for breach of contract if you make the above statement and then attempt to collect from the patient any unpaid balance after insurance, even if the insurance pays you nothing!

Many health insurance companies and third party payers are helping you to protect yourself by requiring precertification before covering services and providing benefits. Many insurance contracts now require preauthorization for non-emergency hospitalization as well as for certain "abused" procedures such as Total Abdominal Hysterectomy. Failure to obtain preauthorization can result in outright denial of claims and/or benefit reductions of up to 50 percent with no appeal! In most cases, the patient does not even know that these requirements exist.

STRATEGIC PRICING CONCEPTS

In today's competitive environment the successful practice will learn how to keep its existing patients, attract new patients, and increase its profitability by raising some fees, lowering others, and maintaining enough flexibility to adjust specific fees in response to new opportunities. This process is known as STRATEGIC PRICING and incorporates the following concepts:

MARKET DRIVEN PROCEDURES

Some procedures are price sensitive and patients do call to ask prices of some procedures or services, such as total obstetrical care. It is important that fees for such services be kept comparatively low. On the other hand, consumers know that some procedures are absolutely necessary for them to maintain and they don't shop around for these procedures.

In addition, if your practice provides services that are market driven you want to make sure that the person handling these telephone inquiries is a good salesperson. Ideally, the prospective patient would be "sold" on how good the practice, doctor and/or service is before the requested fee is quoted. This simple technique can significantly increase your new patient volume.

RELATIONSHIP BUILDING

Successful practices are dependent on long-term relationships with patients and/or referral sources. Part of your pricing strategy should be based on attracting new relationships with patients or referral sources and on maintaining and develop existing relationships. How much you charge, whether you charge, and how you bill are all considerations that may impact a relationship.

An example of this component of strategic pricing is the "free" consultation that most pediatricians provide to parents who are interviewing potential physicians for their new (or about to be born) babies. An investment of 30 to 45 minutes late in an afternoon can result in a patient relationship lasting for 20 years! More and more medical professionals are making themselves available for patient interviews.

PRICE SENSITIVITY

Patients are consumers and they expect prices to increase, including yours. However, they do not react positively to sudden or large increases in fees. This happens most often when the practice has held down fees for a long time and then increases fees suddenly, and by large amounts. This is easy to avoid by using more frequent, small increases.

VOLUME CONSIDERATION

Pay particular attention to volume when considering fee increases. A large increase in a fee that is infrequently performed or rarely repeated on the same patient will likely go unnoticed. A small increase in fees for frequent procedures is expected by most patients.

PROMOTIONAL PRICING

Fees for certain services and procedures may be used to attract new patients to your practice. Many practices offer "free" screenings, or reduced fees for physical exams, pap smears, and other preventive services. In today's more health conscious society, patients are very receptive to these new marketing techniques. In addition, you or your practice may have particular services, skills, methods, or special office hours, that are not offered elsewhere or close by. Patients do place special value on special services and abilities and are usually willing to pay more for them.

OPTIONS TO INCREASING YOUR FEES

INCREASE PRACTICE PRODUCTIVITY

This doesn't necessarily mean you have to work more, harder or longer. It means simply that you need to look at how you work in order to make sure you are using your time in the most profitable manner. You may need to implement a more formal scheduling and record keeping system for out-of-the-office services in order to keep track of your time better, and to make sure you are billing for all your services.

Maybe its time to bring in an associate to take care of those referrals you have been turning down. Or maybe you are considering extended office hours one evening during the week and Saturday mornings to meet the increasing demands of your patients for more convenient (to them) hours.

Make sure that the time you spend with each patient is appropriate for the level of care you need to provide. This means that you have to provide exactly the right amount of your time, from your perspective, in order to keep your schedule, and, the right amount of your time, from the patient's perspective, to provide the perception of value received.

REDUCE YOUR DISCOUNT BUSINESS

In spite of the continuous national furor over medical fees, the truth is, that with few exceptions, all medical practices are operated as discount businesses. Typical discounts include:

- Giving a discount for cash payment at the time of service

- Discounting your services as a professional courtesy

- Accepting insurance payment as payment in full

- Accepting payments on account without interest charges

- Referring accounts to a collection agency

- Writing off an account as a bad debt

- Accepting a capitation or discounted payment from an HMO, IPA or PPO

- Participating in Medicare

- Providing services to Medicaid patients

You must take the time to review your practice by revenue sources in order to determine if the types of patients you are attracting and the associations you have with payers are profitable. This review process should include answering the following questions:

- Is Medicare participation in the best interest of my practice?

- Should I implement payment at the time of service?

- Are the contracts I have with HMOs and PPOs profitable?

- Do I have too many Medicaid patients?

- If I reduce my nonprofitable patient categories, can I replace them with profitable ones?

Finding the right answers to these questions for your practice requires an in depth evaluation of your practice economics, patient demographics, the potential patient pool, patient attitudes, and the attitudes, practices and standards of your medical community.

MEDICAL FEES

FORMAT OF THE LISTINGS

The medical fees listings are presented in six sections, which correspond to the six sections of CPT 2002. Within each section are subsections with anatomic, procedural, condition or descriptor subheadings. The procedures and services are listed in numeric order with exception of the EVALUATION AND MANAGEMENT section. The EVALUATION AND MANAGEMENT section has been placed at the beginning of the medical fees listings, because these CPT codes are used by most physicians in reporting a significant portion of their services.

Each entry includes the CPT code, a short description of the procedure or service, UCR fees at the 50th, 75th and 90th percentiles, the national average Medicare fee and the Medicare RVU. Some CPT codes are listed twice. The second listing includes the modifier -26 to indicate that the listing is for the "professional component" of the procedure only.

CPT PROCEDURE CODE (CODE)

All procedure codes listed in this publication are CPT 2002 codes. CPT codes are revised and published annually by the American Medical Association (AMA). Procedures that are new to the 2002 edition of CPT are noted by a black dot (•) to the left of the procedure code.

MODIFIER -26

Certain medical procedures are a combination of a physician, or professional, component and a technical component. When the physician performs and reports both parts of the service, the service is reported *without* modifier -26. When the physician performs and reports only the professional component, the modifier -26 is added to the basic procedure and the fee reduced accordingly. The technical component is usually reported by the hospital.

SHORT DESCRIPTION

The descriptions listed in this publication are short descriptions of 35 characters or less. These descriptions are from a database of CPT codes and short descriptions maintained by PMIC. The primary source of the CPT codes and short descriptions is the Physician Fee Schedule revised and published each year in the Federal Register by CMS. Whenever possible, errors from the original source are corrected and some of the descriptions have been edited to improve understanding. The short descriptions in this publication are provided for reference only. If you have any questions regarding the complete description for any procedure listed in this publication, you should consult a complete copy of *CPT 2002*.

50TH PERCENTILE (50%)

The amount listed in this column represents the 50th percentile of usual, customary, and reasonable fees for the specific service or procedure. The 50th percentile is that point where 50 percent of fees for a given procedure are at or below the amount listed and 50 percent are higher than the amount listed. A zero in this column means that the procedure is an unlisted procedure or there is no data with which to make the calculation or insufficient data to calculate the amount.

75TH PERCENTILE (75%)

The amount listed in this column represents the 75th percentile of usual, customary, and reasonable fees for the specific service or procedure. The 75th percentile is that point where 75 percent of fees for a given procedure are at or below the amount listed and 25 percent are higher than the amount listed. A zero in this column means that the procedure is an unlisted procedure or there is no data with which to make the calculation or insufficient data to calculate the amount.

90TH PERCENTILE (90%)

The amount listed in this column represents the 90th percentile of usual, customary, and reasonable fees for the specific service or procedure. The 90th percentile is that point where 90 percent of fees for a given procedure are at or below the amount listed and 10 percent are higher than the amount listed. A zero in this column means that the procedure is an unlisted procedure or there is no data with which to make the calculation or insufficient data to calculate the amount.

MEDICARE FEE SCHEDULE (MFS)

The amount listed in this column was calculated by multiplying the total Medicare relative value units from the Medicare Fee Schedule times the proper conversion factor for the code. This amount is listed as a reference so that you can see the relative differences between the UCR and Medicare Fee Schedule amounts for a particular service.

RELATIVE VALUE UNITS (RVU)

The number listed in this column is the relative value unit from the Resource Based Relative Value Scale (RBRVS), a component of the annual Medicare Physician Fee Schedule published by the Center for Medicare and Medicaid Services (CMS). The relative value reflects the complexity of the procedure from a medical point of view. CPT codes for "unlisted" or "by report" services do not have assigned relative values in RBRVS for obvious reasons. Other services or procedures may be provided too infrequently for CMS to establish a relative value. For the latter codes, the relative values in this book have been supplied by Relative Value Studies, Inc., a well-known medical fee research organization.

EVALUATION & MANAGEMENT

CPT	SHORT DESCRIPTION	50th	75th	90th	MFS	RVU
OFFICE OR OTHER OUTPATIENT SERVICES						
99201	Office visit, new	59	68	81	34	.94
99202	Office visit, new	80	94	111	62	1.70
99203	Office visit, new	110	128	152	92	2.54
99204	Office visit, new	161	187	222	131	3.61
99205	Office visit, new	206	240	285	166	4.59
99211	Office visit, established	33	38	44	20	.56
99212	Office visit, established	49	56	66	36	1.00
99213	Office visit, established	66	75	88	50	1.39
99214	Office visit, established	98	112	131	79	2.18
99215	Office visit, established	151	173	202	116	3.20
HOSPITAL OBSERVATION SERVICES						
99217	Observation care discharge	104	123	146	64	1.78
99218	Observation care	125	147	175	64	1.78
99219	Observation care	177	208	247	108	2.97
99220	Observation care	229	269	319	151	4.16
HOSPITAL INPATIENT SERVICES						
99221	Initial hospital care	139	163	196	65	1.80
99222	Initial hospital care	188	222	266	108	2.99
99223	Initial hospital care	243	286	343	151	4.17
99231	Subsequent hospital care	71	85	107	33	.90
99232	Subsequent hospital care	99	118	148	54	1.48

CPT	SHORT DESCRIPTION	50th	75th	90th	MFS	RVU
99233	Subsequent hospital care	153	182	228	76	2.11
99234	Observe/hosp same date	188	224	281	130	3.60
99235	Observe/hosp same date	257	306	384	172	4.76
99236	Observe/hosp same date	323	384	483	215	5.93
99238	Hospital discharge day	108	130	161	66	1.83
99239	Hospital discharge day	156	188	234	91	2.51

CONSULTATIONS

CPT	SHORT DESCRIPTION	50th	75th	90th	MFS	RVU
99241	Office consultation	99	115	135	47	1.30
99242	Office consultation	136	159	186	87	2.41
99243	Office consultation	178	207	242	116	3.20
99244	Office consultation	234	273	319	164	4.54
99245	Office consultation	305	356	416	213	5.88
99251	Initial inpatient consult	115	134	156	35	.96
99252	Initial inpatient consult	152	177	206	70	1.93
99253	Initial inpatient consult	191	222	259	95	2.63
99254	Initial inpatient consult	241	281	327	137	3.78
99255	Initial inpatient consult	314	365	425	189	5.21
99261	Follow-up inpatient consult	65	78	98	22	.60
99262	Follow-up inpatient consult	99	119	150	43	1.20
99263	Follow-up inpatient consult	139	168	211	65	1.79
99271	Confirmatory consultation	103	125	151	42	1.15
99272	Confirmatory consultation	129	157	190	65	1.79
99273	Confirmatory consultation	178	216	262	87	2.39
99274	Confirmatory consultation	227	275	334	117	3.23
99275	Confirmatory consultation	316	384	465	148	4.09

NEW CODE CPT 2002 •

CPT	SHORT DESCRIPTION	50th	75th	90th	MFS	RVU
EMERGENCY DEPARTMENT SERVICES						
99281	Emergency department visit	60	69	80	16	.44
99282	Emergency department visit	94	108	126	26	.73
99283	Emergency department visit	155	179	209	59	1.64
99284	Emergency department visit	236	272	317	93	2.56
99285	Emergency department visit	348	402	468	145	4.00
99288	Direct advanced life support	153	176	205	0	.00
PATIENT TRANSPORT						
• **99289**	Patient transport, 30-74 min	0	0	0	0	.00
• **99290**	Patient transport, +30 min	0	0	0	0	.00
CRITICAL CARE SERVICES						
99291	Critical care, first hour	373	439	584	209	5.77
99292	Critical care, +30 min	196	230	306	108	2.99
NEONATAL INTENSIVE CARE						
99295	Neonatal critical care	1568	1846	2455	769	21.23
99296	Neonatal critical care	979	1153	1533	391	10.81
99297	Neonatal critical care	720	848	1127	197	5.44
99298	Neonatal critical care	334	392	522	138	3.82
NURSING FACILITY SERVICE						
99301	Nursing facility care	84	105	118	70	1.94
99302	Nursing facility care	115	144	162	96	2.64
99303	Nursing facility care	160	200	224	119	3.28
99311	Nursing fac care, subseq	53	63	74	40	1.11
99312	Nursing fac care, subseq	76	91	107	62	1.71
99313	Nursing fac care, subseq	99	118	139	84	2.33

CPT	SHORT DESCRIPTION	50th	75th	90th	MFS	RVU
99315	Nursing fac discharge day	94	112	132	69	1.91
99316	Nursing fac discharge day	124	147	173	90	2.50

DOMICILIARY, REST HOME OR CUSTODIAL CARE SERVICES

CPT	SHORT DESCRIPTION	50th	75th	90th	MFS	RVU
99321	Rest home visit, new patient	60	80	91	44	1.22
99322	Rest home visit, new patient	82	109	125	63	1.74
99323	Rest home visit, new patient	120	159	182	81	2.25
99331	Rest home visit, established	55	67	79	39	1.09
99332	Rest home visit, established	68	82	97	51	1.42
99333	Rest home visit, established	70	84	100	64	1.76

HOME SERVICES

CPT	SHORT DESCRIPTION	50th	75th	90th	MFS	RVU
99341	Home visit, new patient	64	77	92	59	1.62
99342	Home visit, new patient	95	114	141	88	2.44
99343	Home visit, new patient	142	170	210	131	3.63
99344	Home visit, new patient	184	221	272	170	4.70
99345	Home visit, new patient	227	272	334	209	5.77
99347	Home visit, established	50	60	74	46	1.28
99348	Home visit, established	63	92	119	74	2.04
99349	Home visit, established	124	148	182	114	3.16
99350	Home visit, established	181	217	267	167	4.60

PROLONGED SERVICES

CPT	SHORT DESCRIPTION	50th	75th	90th	MFS	RVU
99354	Prolonged service, office	154	191	229	119	3.29
99355	Prolonged service, office	112	139	166	111	3.07
99356	Prolonged service, inpatient	203	252	302	86	2.38
99357	Prolonged service, inpatient	133	165	197	87	2.40
99358	Prolonged service, w/o contact	140	174	208	0	.00

NEW CODE CPT 2002 •

CPT	SHORT DESCRIPTION	50th	75th	90th	MFS	RVU
99359	Prolonged service, w/o contact	78	97	116	0	.00
99360	Physician standby services	167	207	248	0	.00

CASE MANAGEMENT SERVICES

CPT	SHORT DESCRIPTION	50th	75th	90th	MFS	RVU
99361	Physician/team conference	93	116	139	0	.00
99362	Physician/team conference	127	158	189	0	.00
99371	Physician phone consultation	16	20	24	0	.00
99372	Physician phone consultation	32	40	47	0	.00
99373	Physician phone consultation	80	100	120	0	.00

CARE PLAN OVERSIGHT SERVICES

CPT	SHORT DESCRIPTION	50th	75th	90th	MFS	RVU
99374	Home health care supervision	105	130	156	94	2.61
99375	Home health care supervision	334	415	497	0	.00
99377	Hospice care supervision	110	137	164	94	2.61
99378	Hospice care supervision	117	145	174	0	.00
99379	Nursing fac care supervision	110	137	164	94	2.60
99380	Nursing fac care supervision	192	239	286	127	3.50

PREVENTIVE MEDICINE SERVICES

CPT	SHORT DESCRIPTION	50th	75th	90th	MFS	RVU
99381	Prev visit, new, infant	103	128	152	99	2.73
99382	Prev visit, new, age 1-4	110	137	163	106	2.94
99383	Prev visit, new, age 5-11	108	134	160	104	2.88
99384	Prev visit, new, age 12-17	121	150	179	113	3.13
99385	Prev visit, new, age 18-39	149	185	221	113	3.13
99386	Prev visit, new, age 40-64	162	201	241	133	3.68
99387	Prev visit, new, 65 & over	172	214	256	144	3.99
99391	Prev visit, established, infant	78	97	117	75	2.07
99392	Prev visit, established, age 1-4	84	104	125	84	2.32

CPT	SHORT DESCRIPTION	50th	75th	90th	MFS	RVU
99393	Prev visit, established, age 5-11	89	111	133	83	2.29
99394	Prev visit, established, age 12-17	97	121	145	92	2.55
99395	Prev visit, established, age 18-39	121	150	180	93	2.58
99396	Prev visit, established, age 40-64	133	165	198	103	2.85
99397	Prev visit, established, 65 & over	153	190	227	113	3.13
99401	Preventive counseling, individual	108	127	152	40	1.11
99402	Preventive counseling, individual	68	80	96	67	1.86
99403	Preventive counseling, individual	103	122	145	94	2.59
99404	Preventive counseling, individual	127	150	179	121	3.34
99411	Preventive counseling, group	37	43	52	12	.34
99412	Preventive counseling, group	39	46	55	18	.50
99420	Health risk assessment test	406	480	571	0	.00
99429	Unlisted preventive service	0	0	0	0	.00

NEWBORN CARE SERVICES

CPT	SHORT DESCRIPTION	50th	75th	90th	MFS	RVU
99431	Initial care, normal newborn	157	186	222	58	1.60
99432	Newborn care, not in hospital	121	143	171	88	2.44
99433	Normal newborn care/hospital	77	91	108	31	.85
99435	Newborn discharge day hospital	187	222	264	76	2.09
99436	Attendance, birth	302	357	425	74	2.05
99440	Newborn resuscitation	369	437	520	152	4.21

SPECIAL E/M SERVICES

CPT	SHORT DESCRIPTION	50th	75th	90th	MFS	RVU
99450	Life/disability evaluation	0	0	0	0	.00
99455	Disability examination	0	0	0	0	.00
99456	Disability examination	0	0	0	0	.00
99499	Unlisted E/M service	0	0	0	0	.00

NEW CODE CPT 2002 •

CPT	SHORT DESCRIPTION	50th	75th	90th	MFS	RVU

GENERAL

CPT	SHORT DESCRIPTION	50th	75th	90th	MFS	RVU
• 10021	FNA w/o image	98	121	152	87	2.39
• 10022	FNA w/image	101	124	156	89	2.46

INTEGUMENTARY SYSTEM

SKIN, SUBCUTANEOUS AND ACCESSORY STRUCTURES

CPT	SHORT DESCRIPTION	50th	75th	90th	MFS	RVU
10040	Acne surgery	85	104	131	81	2.23
10060	Drain skin abscess	108	132	167	100	2.76
10061	Drain skin abscess	203	250	315	161	4.45
10080	Drain pilonidal cyst	150	184	232	125	3.44
10081	Drain pilonidal cyst	312	384	485	205	5.66
10120	Remove foreign body	125	154	194	103	2.84
10121	Remove foreign body	302	371	468	215	5.93
10140	Drain hematoma/fluid	131	161	203	117	3.22
10160	Puncture drain lesion	105	129	163	74	2.05
10180	Complex drain wound	307	378	477	145	4.01
11000	Debride infected skin	80	108	158	47	1.31
11001	Debride infected skin add-on	51	69	100	25	.69
11010	Debride skin, fx	698	944	1377	260	7.18
11011	Debride skin/muscle, fx	931	1259	1836	340	9.38
11012	Debride skin/muscle/bone, fx	1305	1764	2574	481	13.29
11040	Debride skin partial	73	99	145	40	1.10
11041	Debride skin, full	106	143	208	58	1.59
11042	Debride skin/tissue	190	257	375	82	2.27
11043	Debride tissue/muscle	474	640	934	193	5.34

CPT	SHORT DESCRIPTION	50th	75th	90th	MFS	RVU
11044	Debride tissue/muscle/bone	698	943	1376	243	6.70
11055	Trim skin lesion	48	64	84	35	.97
11056	Trim skin lesions, 2 to 4	52	69	90	45	1.23
11057	Trim skin lesions, over 4	55	74	96	54	1.49
11100	Biopsy skin lesion	106	131	163	85	2.34
11101	Biopsy skin add-on	63	77	96	41	1.14
11200	Remove skin tags	92	114	142	73	2.01
11201	Remove skin tags add-on	47	58	73	30	.84
11300	Shave skin lesion	92	114	144	58	1.59
11301	Shave skin lesion	116	144	182	73	2.01
11302	Shave skin lesion	146	181	229	84	2.31
11303	Shave skin lesion	190	236	298	96	2.66
11305	Shave skin lesion	97	121	153	54	1.48
11306	Shave skin lesion	124	154	195	75	2.06
11307	Shave skin lesion	154	191	242	85	2.34
11308	Shave skin lesion	206	256	323	100	2.77
11310	Shave skin lesion	117	145	183	70	1.92
11311	Shave skin lesion	138	171	217	85	2.34
11312	Shave skin lesion	174	215	272	93	2.58
11313	Shave skin lesion	217	269	340	121	3.34
11400	Remove skin lesion	129	160	202	96	2.65
11401	Remove skin lesion	162	200	253	117	3.24
11402	Remove skin lesion	205	254	321	157	4.34
11403	Remove skin lesion	265	329	416	178	4.92
11404	Remove skin lesion	334	415	524	195	5.40
11406	Remove skin lesion	486	603	761	230	6.34

     NEW CODE CPT 2002 •

CPT	SHORT DESCRIPTION	50th	75th	90th	MFS	RVU
11420	Remove skin lesion	136	169	213	96	2.66
11421	Remove skin lesion	181	225	284	126	3.48
11422	Remove skin lesion	229	284	359	163	4.50
11423	Remove skin lesion	305	379	479	194	5.36
11424	Remove skin lesion	373	463	585	218	6.03
11426	Remove skin lesion	532	660	834	287	7.93
11440	Remove skin lesion	167	207	261	126	3.49
11441	Remove skin lesion	215	266	337	152	4.20
11442	Remove skin lesion	272	338	427	178	4.92
11443	Remove skin lesion	355	441	557	220	6.08
11444	Remove skin lesion	472	585	739	275	7.59
11446	Remove skin lesion	611	759	959	332	9.16
11450	Remove sweat gland lesion	710	881	1113	260	7.19
11451	Remove sweat gland lesion	784	973	1230	346	9.57
11462	Remove sweat gland lesion	576	715	903	256	7.06
11463	Remove sweat gland lesion	642	796	1006	363	10.02
11470	Remove sweat gland lesion	538	668	844	308	8.52
11471	Remove sweat gland lesion	675	837	1058	375	10.35
11600	Remove skin lesion	201	254	326	144	3.98
11601	Remove skin lesion	251	317	407	165	4.57
11602	Remove skin lesion	300	378	486	177	4.88
11603	Remove skin lesion	366	461	592	197	5.44
11604	Remove skin lesion	445	562	722	218	6.03
11606	Remove skin lesion	606	764	982	275	7.59
11620	Remove skin lesion	235	296	380	141	3.90
11621	Remove skin lesion	304	384	493	168	4.65

CPT	SHORT DESCRIPTION	50th	75th	90th	MFS	RVU
11622	Remove skin lesion	369	465	597	194	5.36
11623	Remove skin lesion	440	555	713	233	6.43
11624	Remove skin lesion	526	663	852	268	7.40
11626	Remove skin lesion	749	945	1213	330	9.13
11640	Remove skin lesion	301	379	487	150	4.14
11641	Remove skin lesion	381	481	617	200	5.53
11642	Remove skin lesion	458	578	742	235	6.48
11643	Remove skin lesion	552	696	894	274	7.57
11644	Remove skin lesion	655	827	1061	351	9.69
11646	Remove skin lesion	875	1104	1418	438	12.09

NAILS

CPT	SHORT DESCRIPTION	50th	75th	90th	MFS	RVU
11719	Trim nail(s)	31	38	48	16	.43
11720	Debride nail, 1-5	43	53	67	25	.68
11721	Debride nail, 6 or more	60	74	93	37	1.02
11730	Remove nail plate	106	132	166	74	2.05
11732	Remove nail plate, add-on	54	67	85	33	.92
11740	Drain blood from under nail	72	89	112	44	1.21
11750	Remove nail bed	339	420	530	136	3.77
11752	Remove nail bed/finger tip	353	437	552	188	5.20
11755	Biopsy nail unit	161	200	252	89	2.47
11760	Repair nail bed	290	359	453	129	3.55
11762	Reconstruct nail bed	440	544	688	199	5.49
11765	Excision nail fold, toe	119	148	187	68	1.88
11770	Remove pilonidal lesion	601	744	940	216	5.96
11771	Remove pilonidal lesion	1008	1248	1578	438	12.10
11772	Remove pilonidal lesion	1259	1559	1970	529	14.61

    NEW CODE CPT 2002 •

CPT	SHORT DESCRIPTION	50th	75th	90th	MFS	RVU
11900	Inject into skin lesions	64	84	104	47	1.31
11901	Added skin lesions inject	100	132	163	62	1.72
11920	Correct skin color defects	445	584	724	146	4.03
11921	Correct skin color defects	990	1299	1610	178	4.92
11922	Correct skin color defects	234	307	380	34	.94
11950	Therapy for contour defects	196	258	319	77	2.13
11951	Therapy for contour defects	206	270	334	100	2.76
11952	Therapy for contour defects	226	296	367	127	3.51
11954	Therapy for contour defects	271	356	441	169	4.66
11960	Insert tissue expander(s)	1220	1601	1984	778	21.50
11970	Replace tissue expander	2550	3345	4146	470	12.98
11971	Remove tissue expander(s)	369	484	599	306	8.44
11975	Insert contraceptive cap	255	334	414	116	3.20
11976	Remove contraceptive cap	248	325	403	133	3.67
11977	Remove/reinsert contra cap	313	410	508	214	5.92
11980	Implant hormone pellet(s)	158	208	257	98	2.72
• **11981**	Insert drug implant device	169	222	275	116	3.20
• **11982**	Remove drug implant device	193	253	313	132	3.65
• **11983**	Remove/insert drug implant	313	410	508	214	5.92

REPAIR (CLOSURE)

CPT	SHORT DESCRIPTION	50th	75th	90th	MFS	RVU
12001	Repair superficial wound(s)	170	199	225	143	3.96
12002	Repair superficial wound(s)	211	246	278	153	4.22
12004	Repair superficial wound(s)	271	316	357	177	4.88
12005	Repair superficial wound(s)	344	401	454	222	6.13
12006	Repair superficial wound(s)	353	412	466	274	7.57
12007	Repair superficial wound(s)	511	597	675	317	8.75

CPT	SHORT DESCRIPTION	50th	75th	90th	MFS	RVU
12011	Repair superficial wound(s)	202	236	267	152	4.20
12013	Repair superficial wound(s)	249	290	328	167	4.60
12014	Repair superficial wound(s)	296	346	391	194	5.36
12015	Repair superficial wound(s)	394	460	520	247	6.81
12016	Repair superficial wound(s)	395	461	521	295	8.14
12017	Repair superficial wound(s)	818	954	1080	254	7.03
12018	Repair superficial wound(s)	735	857	970	296	8.17
12020	Close split wound	251	293	332	194	5.37
12021	Close split wound	215	251	284	133	3.68
12031	Layer close wound(s)	211	257	317	163	4.51
12032	Layer close wound(s)	267	325	401	198	5.46
12034	Layer close wound(s)	366	446	549	226	6.25
12035	Layer close wound(s)	473	577	711	251	6.93
12036	Layer close wound(s)	494	602	742	354	9.79
12037	Layer close wound(s)	617	752	927	388	10.73
12041	Layer close wound(s)	233	284	350	179	4.95
12042	Layer close wound(s)	292	356	439	215	5.94
12044	Layer close wound(s)	358	437	538	239	6.60
12045	Layer close wound(s)	433	527	650	272	7.52
12046	Layer close wound(s)	559	681	839	394	10.89
12047	Layer close wound(s)	645	786	968	444	12.27
12051	Layer close wound(s)	289	352	434	208	5.74
12052	Layer close wound(s)	346	422	520	215	5.94
12053	Layer close wound(s)	423	516	635	236	6.52
12054	Layer close wound(s)	543	662	815	262	7.23
12055	Layer close wound(s)	748	912	1123	336	9.27

NEW CODE CPT 2002 •

CPT	SHORT DESCRIPTION	50th	75th	90th	MFS	RVU
12056	Layer close wound(s)	848	1034	1274	470	12.98
12057	Layer close wound(s)	782	953	1174	462	12.77
13100	Repair wound or lesion	335	433	574	243	6.72
13101	Repair wound or lesion	462	596	791	280	7.73
13102	Repair wound/lesion add-on	208	268	356	76	2.09
13120	Repair wound or lesion	424	547	726	254	7.01
13121	Repair wound or lesion	597	771	1023	305	8.42
13122	Repair wound/lesion add-on	230	297	394	89	2.45
13131	Repair wound or lesion	530	684	907	282	7.79
13132	Repair wound or lesion	824	1063	1410	392	10.84
13133	Repair wound/lesion add-on	297	383	508	130	3.59
13150	Repair wound or lesion	493	637	844	336	9.29
13151	Repair wound or lesion	645	833	1105	355	9.80
13152	Repair wound or lesion	1020	1317	1747	452	12.49
13153	Repair wound/lesion add-on	389	503	667	143	3.94
13160	Late close wound	1084	1400	1856	657	18.14
14000	Skin tissue rearrangement	884	1124	1413	504	13.93
14001	Skin tissue rearrangement	1198	1523	1916	646	17.84
14020	Skin tissue rearrangement	1070	1360	1711	548	15.14
14021	Skin tissue rearrangement	1450	1842	2317	725	20.04
14040	Skin tissue rearrangement	1285	1634	2055	601	16.59
14041	Skin tissue rearrangement	1584	2013	2532	799	22.07
14060	Skin tissue rearrangement	1591	2022	2543	642	17.73
14061	Skin tissue rearrangement	1801	2289	2879	865	23.89
14300	Skin tissue rearrangement	2644	3361	4227	824	22.75
14350	Skin tissue rearrangement	990	1258	1582	622	17.18

CPT	SHORT DESCRIPTION	50th	75th	90th	MFS	RVU
15000	Skin graft	665	841	1101	249	6.88
15001	Skin graft add-on	217	275	359	63	1.75
15050	Skin pinch graft	604	763	998	353	9.74
15100	Skin split graft	1397	1767	2311	589	16.26
15101	Skin split graft add-on	549	695	909	119	3.30
15120	Skin split graft	1853	2342	3064	699	19.32
15121	Skin split graft add-on	714	903	1181	173	4.77
15200	Skin full graft	839	1061	1388	675	18.66
15201	Skin full graft add-on	370	467	611	89	2.46
15220	Skin full graft	992	1254	1640	649	17.93
15221	Skin full graft add-on	456	577	755	81	2.23
15240	Skin full graft	1579	1996	2612	681	18.82
15241	Skin full graft add-on	593	749	980	127	3.50
15260	Skin full graft	1574	1991	2604	713	19.70
15261	Skin full graft add-on	683	863	1129	144	3.99
15342	Cultured skin graft, 25 cm	247	312	409	118	3.27
15343	Cultured skin graft, +25 cm	43	54	70	25	.69
15350	Skin homograft	636	804	1051	442	12.20
15351	Skin homograft add-on	187	237	309	71	1.96
15400	Skin heterograft	523	662	865	336	9.29
15401	Skin heterograft add-on	155	196	257	98	2.70
15570	Form skin pedicle flap	1443	1825	2387	650	17.97
15572	Form skin pedicle flap	1390	1757	2298	662	18.28
15574	Form skin pedicle flap	1727	2184	2857	703	19.41
15576	Form skin pedicle flap	1718	2172	2841	662	18.30
15600	Skin graft	703	889	1164	317	8.76

     NEW CODE CPT 2002 •

CPT	SHORT DESCRIPTION	50th	75th	90th	MFS	RVU
15610	Skin graft	765	967	1265	310	8.57
15620	Skin graft	932	1179	1542	371	10.26
15630	Skin graft	991	1253	1639	349	9.64
15650	Transfer skin pedicle flap	985	1245	1629	363	10.02
15732	Muscle-skin graft head/neck	2785	3522	4607	1121	30.97
15734	Muscle-skin graft trunk	4171	5274	6900	1129	31.19
15736	Muscle-skin graft arm	2869	3627	4745	1057	29.19
15738	Muscle-skin graft leg	2951	3731	4881	1134	31.34
15740	Island pedicle flap graft	1832	2316	3030	710	19.61
15750	Neurovascular pedicle graft	2183	2761	3612	759	20.98
15756	Free muscle flap, microvasc	4170	5273	6897	2202	60.84
15757	Free skin flap, microvasc	6008	7597	9938	2213	61.14
15758	Free fascial flap, microvasc	6352	8032	10507	2222	61.37
15760	Composite skin graft	1704	2155	2819	678	18.73
15770	Derma-fat-fascia graft	1676	2119	2772	523	14.44
15775	Hair transplant punch grafts	738	933	1221	272	7.51
15776	Hair transplant punch grafts	700	885	1158	366	10.11
15780	Abrasion treatment skin	1509	2095	2838	511	14.11
15781	Abrasion treatment skin	555	771	1045	372	10.29
15782	Abrasion treatment skin	530	736	997	322	8.90
15783	Abrasion treatment skin	560	778	1054	346	9.57
15786	Abrasion lesion, single	295	409	555	140	3.87
15787	Abrasion lesions, add-on	47	65	88	27	.74
15788	Chemical peel face, epiderm	407	566	767	194	5.35
15789	Chemical peel face, dermal	1501	2085	2825	392	10.84
15792	Chemical peel nonfacial	368	511	692	175	4.83

CPT	SHORT DESCRIPTION	50th	75th	90th	MFS	RVU
15793	Chemical peel, nonfacial	438	608	823	279	7.72
15810	Salabrasion	1110	1542	2089	333	9.20
15811	Salabrasion	1625	2257	3058	426	11.76
15819	Plastic surgery neck	1163	1614	2188	593	16.39
15820	Revise lower eyelid	853	1185	1606	572	15.79
15821	Revise lower eyelid	1079	1498	2030	648	17.90
15822	Revise upper eyelid	1000	1389	1882	552	15.25
15823	Revise upper eyelid	1280	1778	2409	679	18.75
15824	Remove forehead wrinkles	1520	2111	2860	0	.00
15825	Remove neck wrinkles	1821	2529	3426	0	.00
15826	Remove brow wrinkles	1519	2110	2858	0	.00
15828	Remove face wrinkles	4068	5649	7654	0	.00
15829	Remove skin wrinkles	4462	6197	8397	0	.00
15831	Excise excessive skin tissue	3309	4595	6227	791	21.84
15832	Excise excessive skin tissue	1587	2203	2986	754	20.84
15833	Excise excessive skin tissue	1541	2140	2900	693	19.15
15834	Excise excessive skin tissue	1498	2080	2818	710	19.62
15835	Excise excessive skin tissue	1579	2193	2971	751	20.74
15836	Excise excessive skin tissue	1617	2245	3042	608	16.80
15837	Excise excessive skin tissue	1112	1544	2092	598	16.51
15838	Excise excessive skin tissue	1021	1418	1921	485	13.41
15839	Excise excessive skin tissue	1607	2002	2527	648	17.90
15840	Graft for face nerve palsy	2524	3506	4750	887	24.51
15841	Graft for face nerve palsy	3090	4292	5815	1469	40.59
15842	Flap for face nerve palsy	3768	5233	7090	2344	64.76
15845	Skin and muscle repair face	2791	3876	5252	803	22.18

　　NEW CODE CPT 2002 •

CPT	SHORT DESCRIPTION	50th	75th	90th	MFS	RVU
15850	Remove sutures	171	238	322	81	2.25
15851	Remove sutures	194	269	365	92	2.55
15852	Dressing change,not for burn	140	195	264	104	2.86
15860	Test for blood flow in graft	231	320	434	124	3.43
15876	Suction assisted lipectomy	621	863	1169	0	.00
15877	Suction assisted lipectomy	1110	1541	2088	0	.00
15878	Suction assisted lipectomy	621	863	1169	0	.00
15879	Suction assisted lipectomy	1110	1541	2088	0	.00
15920	Remove tail bone ulcer	976	1195	1481	531	14.68
15922	Remove tail bone ulcer	1282	1569	1945	678	18.74
15931	Remove sacrum pressure sore	916	1121	1390	582	16.08
15933	Remove sacrum pressure sore	1182	1447	1794	735	20.31
15934	Remove sacrum pressure sore	1344	1645	2039	815	22.52
15935	Remove sacrum pressure sore	1617	1979	2453	950	26.25
15936	Remove sacrum pressure sore	1012	1238	1535	815	22.51
15937	Remove sacrum pressure sore	1184	1449	1796	958	26.47
15940	Remove hip pressure sore	948	1160	1438	597	16.49
15941	Remove hip pressure sore	1123	1374	1704	836	23.10
15944	Remove hip pressure sore	1301	1592	1974	776	21.44
15945	Remove hip pressure sore	1465	1793	2224	862	23.80
15946	Remove hip pressure sore	1498	1834	2274	1395	38.54
15950	Remove thigh pressure sore	931	1139	1412	498	13.77
15951	Remove thigh pressure sore	1184	1449	1796	721	19.93
15952	Remove thigh pressure sore	1206	1476	1830	740	20.44
15953	Remove thigh pressure sore	1648	2017	2500	842	23.25
15956	Remove thigh pressure sore	1134	1388	1721	1009	27.87

CPT	SHORT DESCRIPTION	50th	75th	90th	MFS	RVU
15958	Remove thigh pressure sore	1305	1597	1980	1026	28.34
15999	Remove pressure sore	0	0	0	0	.00
16000	Initial treat burn(s)	87	106	132	74	2.04
16010	Treat burn(s)	102	125	154	78	2.15
16015	Treat burn(s)	367	449	556	166	4.58
16020	Treat burn(s)	87	107	132	75	2.06
16025	Treat burn(s)	157	192	238	143	3.95
16030	Treat burn(s)	231	283	351	203	5.62
16035	Incise burn scab, initial	477	583	723	205	5.67
16036	Incise burn scab, addl incision	141	173	215	81	2.23

DESTRUCTION

CPT	SHORT DESCRIPTION	50th	75th	90th	MFS	RVU
17000	Destroy benign/premal lesion	78	94	120	63	1.73
17003	Destroy lesions, 2-14	26	32	40	14	.40
17004	Destroy lesions, 15 or more	307	370	470	198	5.47
17106	Destroy skin lesions	397	479	608	353	9.75
17107	Destroy skin lesions	746	900	1143	601	16.61
17108	Destroy skin lesions	1235	1489	1892	831	22.96
17110	Destroy lesion, 1-14	81	98	124	65	1.80
17111	Destroy lesion, 15 or more	124	150	190	76	2.09
17250	Chemical cautery tissue	64	77	97	47	1.30
17260	Destroy skin lesions	159	191	243	84	2.32
17261	Destroy skin lesions	188	226	287	98	2.70
17262	Destroy skin lesions	235	283	359	121	3.34
17263	Destroy skin lesions	294	354	450	133	3.67
17264	Destroy skin lesions	342	413	524	141	3.89
17266	Destroy skin lesions	245	296	376	164	4.53

NEW CODE CPT 2002 •

CPT	SHORT DESCRIPTION	50th	75th	90th	MFS	RVU
17270	Destroy skin lesions	185	223	283	107	2.95
17271	Destroy skin lesions	219	264	335	116	3.20
17272	Destroy skin lesions	263	318	403	131	3.63
17273	Destroy skin lesions	348	419	533	147	4.07
17274	Destroy skin lesions	244	295	374	178	4.91
17276	Destroy skin lesions	292	352	447	212	5.87
17280	Destroy skin lesions	207	250	317	95	2.63
17281	Destroy skin lesions	255	307	390	129	3.56
17282	Destroy skin lesions	302	364	462	147	4.06
17283	Destroy skin lesions	401	484	615	180	4.98
17284	Destroy skin lesions	292	352	447	212	5.87
17286	Destroy skin lesions	309	372	473	286	7.89
17304	Chemosurgery skin lesion	835	1040	1316	567	15.67
17305	2nd stage chemosurgery	428	533	674	238	6.57
17306	3rd stage chemosurgery	389	485	613	239	6.61
17307	Followup skin lesion therapy	336	418	530	239	6.59
17310	Extensive skin chemosurgery	228	284	359	92	2.54
17340	Cryotherapy skin	64	77	91	43	1.19
17360	Skin peel therapy	227	272	322	107	2.95
17380	Hair remove by electrolysis	58	70	83	0	.00
17999	Skin tissue procedure	0	0	0	0	.00

BREAST

CPT	SHORT DESCRIPTION	50th	75th	90th	MFS	RVU
19000	Drain breast lesion	129	163	216	79	2.18
19001	Drain breast lesion add-on	70	89	117	47	1.31
19020	Incision breast lesion	490	620	819	400	11.05
19030	Inject for breast x-ray	204	258	341	192	5.30

CPT	SHORT DESCRIPTION	50th	75th	90th	MFS	RVU
19100	Biopsy breast percut w/o image	210	266	355	104	2.87
19101	Biopsy breast, open	599	757	1010	313	8.65
19102	Biopsy breast percut w/image	405	512	683	263	7.26
19103	Biopsy breast percut w/device	910	1150	1535	601	16.59
19110	Nipple exploration	781	987	1317	526	14.53
19112	Excise breast duct fistula	662	838	1118	542	14.96
19120	Remove breast lesion	833	1054	1407	409	11.30
19125	Excise breast lesion	965	1220	1629	435	12.03
19126	Excise addl breast lesion	520	658	878	155	4.29
19140	Remove breast tissue	1174	1485	1982	576	15.92
19160	Remove breast tissue	1285	1625	2169	406	11.22
19162	Remove breast tissue, nodes	2492	3151	4206	832	22.98
19180	Remove breast	1638	2072	2765	570	15.76
19182	Remove breast	1511	1910	2549	492	13.58
19200	Remove breast	1813	2293	3061	953	26.33
19220	Remove breast	1930	2441	3258	970	26.80
19240	Remove breast	2692	3404	4544	961	26.56
19260	Remove chest wall lesion	1868	2362	3152	948	26.20
19271	Revise chest wall	2898	3664	4890	1169	32.30
19272	Extensive chest wall surgery	2776	3510	4685	1319	36.45
19290	Place needle wire breast	201	254	339	155	4.28
19291	Place needle wire breast	112	141	188	87	2.40
19295	Place breast clip percut	159	201	269	103	2.84
19316	Suspend breast	2659	3426	4289	718	19.84
19318	Reduce large breast	3261	4202	5261	1012	27.95
19324	Enlarge breast	1232	1587	1987	394	10.89

NEW CODE CPT 2002 •

CPT	SHORT DESCRIPTION	50th	75th	90th	MFS	RVU
19325	Enlarge breast with implant	1635	2106	2638	592	16.35
19328	Remove breast implant	736	948	1187	399	11.02
19330	Remove implant material	1090	1404	1758	500	13.81
19340	Immediate breast prosthesis	1163	1499	1876	373	10.31
19342	Delayed breast prosthesis	2733	3521	4409	744	20.56
19350	Breast reconstruct	2013	2593	3247	884	24.42
19355	Correct inverted nipple(s)	2464	3174	3974	753	20.79
19357	Breast reconstruct	3982	5131	6424	1250	34.52
19361	Breast reconstruct	4549	5860	7338	1223	33.79
19364	Breast reconstruct	4626	5961	7463	2547	70.36
19366	Breast reconstruct	2590	3337	4179	1288	35.57
19367	Breast reconstruct	7075	9115	11413	1603	44.28
19368	Breast reconstruct	6737	8680	10868	1990	54.97
19369	Breast reconstruct	6626	8536	10688	1859	51.35
19370	Surgery breast capsule	1729	2227	2789	554	15.30
19371	Remove breast capsule	2091	2694	3374	645	17.82
19380	Revise breast reconstruct	2049	2639	3305	632	17.47
19396	Design custom breast implant	1123	1447	1812	343	9.48
19499	Breast surgery procedure	0	0	0	0	.00

CPT	SHORT DESCRIPTION	50th	75th	90th	MFS	RVU

NEW CODE CPT 2002 •

CPT	SHORT DESCRIPTION	50th	75th	90th	MFS	RVU

MUSCULOSKELETAL SYSTEM

GENERAL

CPT	SHORT DESCRIPTION	50th	75th	90th	MFS	RVU
20000	Incise abscess	172	211	269	164	4.52
20005	Incise deep abscess	564	692	882	247	6.83
20100	Explore wound neck	1051	1288	1642	636	17.56
20101	Explore wound chest	1553	1904	2428	235	6.49
20102	Explore wound abdomen	1274	1562	1992	279	7.72
20103	Explore wound extremity	845	1035	1320	372	10.28
20150	Excise epiphyseal bar	1458	1788	2279	882	24.37
20200	Muscle biopsy	227	278	355	121	3.35
20205	Deep muscle biopsy	534	655	835	240	6.62
20206	Needle biopsy muscle	228	280	356	156	4.32
20220	Bone biopsy, trocar/needle	258	316	403	228	6.29
20225	Bone biopsy, trocar/needle	541	663	845	233	6.45
20240	Bone biopsy, exciseal	411	504	643	279	7.71
20245	Bone biopsy, exciseal	708	868	1107	548	15.13
20250	Open bone biopsy	1463	1793	2286	358	9.90
20251	Open bone biopsy	1427	1749	2230	406	11.21
20500	Inject sinus tract	399	489	624	241	6.67
20501	Inject sinus tract for x-ray	164	201	256	149	4.11
20520	Remove foreign body	457	561	715	277	7.64
20525	Remove foreign body	640	785	1001	404	11.16
• 20526	Ther inject carpal tunnel	102	125	159	62	1.70
20550	Inject tendon/ligament/cyst	93	115	146	64	1.77
• 20551	Inject tendon origin/insert	102	125	159	62	1.70

CPT	SHORT DESCRIPTION	50th	75th	90th	MFS	RVU
• 20552	Inject trigger point, 1 or 2	102	125	159	62	1.70
• 20553	Inject trigger points, > 3	102	125	159	62	1.70
20600	Drain/inject joint/bursa	84	103	132	50	1.39
20605	Drain/inject joint/bursa	93	114	146	55	1.52
20610	Drain/inject joint/bursa	108	132	168	66	1.83
20615	Treat bone cyst	290	355	453	266	7.36
20650	Insert and remove bone pin	289	354	452	274	7.57
20660	Apply,remove fixation device	700	858	1094	162	4.48
20661	Apply head brace	751	921	1174	454	12.55
20662	Apply pelvis brace	610	747	953	434	12.00
20663	Apply thigh brace	538	660	841	403	11.14
20664	Halo brace apply	1187	1455	1855	655	18.10
20665	Remove fixation device	228	280	356	138	3.81
20670	Remove support implant	282	345	440	279	7.70
20680	Remove support implant	760	932	1188	320	8.85
20690	Apply bone fixation device	902	1105	1409	214	5.90
20692	Apply bone fixation device	1160	1422	1813	383	10.58
20693	Adjust bone fixation device	1178	1444	1841	713	19.69
20694	Remove bone fixation device	698	856	1091	496	13.69
20802	Replant arm, complete	4738	5809	7406	2748	75.91
20805	Replant forearm, complete	6316	7743	9872	3355	92.67
20808	Replant hand, complete	7452	9136	11648	4509	124.55
20816	Replant digit, complete	4993	6122	7804	3021	83.45
20822	Replant digit, complete	4401	5396	6879	2702	74.63
20824	Replant thumb, complete	4750	5823	7424	3023	83.52
20827	Replant thumb, complete	4504	5522	7039	2725	75.27

NEW CODE CPT 2002 •

CPT	SHORT DESCRIPTION	50th	75th	90th	MFS	RVU
20838	Replant foot, complete	4776	5855	7465	2645	73.08
20900	Remove bone for graft	765	938	1196	446	12.32
20902	Remove bone for graft	1263	1548	1974	634	17.52
20910	Remove cartilage for graft	696	853	1087	540	14.93
20912	Remove cartilage for graft	783	960	1223	528	14.58
20920	Remove fascia for graft	536	657	838	409	11.29
20922	Remove fascia for graft	737	903	1151	579	15.99
20924	Remove tendon for graft	977	1198	1527	519	14.33
20926	Remove tissue for graft	800	981	1250	463	12.80
20930	Spinal bone allograft	436	535	682	0	.00
20931	Spinal bone allograft	463	567	723	113	3.13
20936	Spinal bone autograft	585	717	914	0	.00
20937	Spinal bone autograft	786	964	1229	172	4.76
20938	Spinal bone autograft	869	1065	1358	188	5.18
20950	Fluid pressure, muscle	160	196	250	129	3.57
20955	Fibula bone graft, microvasc	2855	3501	4463	2682	74.08
20956	Iliac bone graft, microvasc	2789	3419	4359	2651	73.22
20957	Mt bone graft, microvasc	2731	3348	4268	2465	68.10
20962	Other bone graft, microvasc	2776	3404	4339	2643	73.00
20969	Bone/skin graft, microvasc	4067	4986	6357	2953	81.57
20970	Bone/skin graft, iliac crest	3947	4839	6169	2816	77.78
20972	Bone/skin graft, metatarsal	3606	4421	5636	2436	67.29
20973	Bone/skin graft, great toe	3832	4698	5989	2930	80.93
20974	Electrical bone stimulation	504	619	789	43	1.18
20975	Electrical bone stimulation	852	1045	1332	161	4.44
20979	Us bone stimulation	310	380	484	45	1.24

CPT	SHORT DESCRIPTION	50th	75th	90th	MFS	RVU
20999	Musculoskeletal surgery	0	0	0	0	.00

HEAD

CPT	SHORT DESCRIPTION	50th	75th	90th	MFS	RVU
21010	Incise jaw joint	2359	3399	4592	649	17.92
21015	Resection facial tumor	875	1261	1704	477	13.19
21025	Excise bone lower jaw	1585	2283	3085	661	18.25
21026	Excise facial bone(s)	1706	2459	3322	379	10.48
21029	Contour face bone lesion	1909	2750	3716	566	15.63
21030	Remove face bone lesion	1087	1566	2116	454	12.53
21031	Remove exostosis mandible	410	591	799	250	6.91
21032	Remove exostosis maxilla	583	840	1134	249	6.89
21034	Remove face bone lesion	1939	2795	3776	1018	28.13
21040	Remove jaw bone lesion	532	767	1036	193	5.33
21041	Remove jaw bone lesion	1080	1556	2103	469	12.95
21044	Remove jaw bone lesion	1924	2773	3746	762	21.06
21045	Extensive jaw surgery	3468	4998	6753	1014	28.00
21050	Remove jaw joint	2797	4030	5445	852	23.54
21060	Remove jaw joint cartilage	3073	4428	5982	796	21.98
21070	Remove coronoid process	2242	3231	4365	551	15.23
21076	Prepare face/oral prosthesis	1930	2781	3757	892	24.65
21077	Prepare face/oral prosthesis	4491	6471	8743	2245	62.01
21079	Prepare face/oral prosthesis	3044	4386	5926	1502	41.48
21080	Prepare face/oral prosthesis	3473	5004	6761	1715	47.37
21081	Prepare face/oral prosthesis	3134	4515	6101	1546	42.72
21082	Prepare face/oral prosthesis	2950	4251	5743	1364	37.68
21083	Prepare face/oral prosthesis	2670	3848	5199	1318	36.42
21084	Prepare face/oral prosthesis	3064	4416	5966	1512	41.76

NEW CODE CPT 2002 •

CPT	SHORT DESCRIPTION	50th	75th	90th	MFS	RVU
21085	Prepare face/oral prosthesis	1061	1529	2066	589	16.27
21086	Prepare face/oral prosthesis	3402	4902	6623	1678	46.36
21087	Prepare face/oral prosthesis	3560	5130	6931	1646	45.47
21088	Prepare face/oral prosthesis	1099	1583	2139	0	.00
21089	Prepare face/oral prosthesis	0	0	0	0	.00
21100	Maxillofacial fixation	788	1135	1533	364	10.06
21110	Interdental fixation	746	1074	1451	389	10.74
21116	Inject jaw joint x-ray	684	986	1332	316	8.74
21120	Reconstruct chin	1674	2412	3259	477	13.18
21121	Reconstruct chin	1994	2873	3882	575	15.88
21122	Reconstruct chin	2560	3688	4983	618	17.06
21123	Reconstruct chin	2916	4202	5678	724	20.00
21125	Augment lower jaw bone	1758	2534	3423	757	20.90
21127	Augment lower jaw bone	2549	3673	4962	816	22.54
21137	Reduce forehead	2224	3204	4329	671	18.55
21138	Reduce forehead	2819	4061	5487	814	22.48
21139	Reduce forehead	3570	5145	6951	864	23.86
21141	Reconstruct midface, Lefort	4034	5813	7854	1101	30.42
21142	Reconstruct midface, Lefort	4533	6532	8826	1222	33.77
21143	Reconstruct midface, Lefort	4625	6665	9005	1147	31.69
21145	Reconstruct midface, Lefort	4824	6951	9391	1221	33.72
21146	Reconstruct midface, Lefort	5024	7239	9781	1247	34.45
21147	Reconstruct midface, Lefort	5232	7539	10186	1280	35.36
21150	Reconstruct midface, Lefort	5358	7721	10431	1576	43.53
21151	Reconstruct midface, Lefort	6271	9036	12209	1869	51.63
21154	Reconstruct midface, Lefort	6639	9566	12924	2042	56.41

CPT	SHORT DESCRIPTION	50th	75th	90th	MFS	RVU
21155	Reconstruct midface, Lefort	7641	11010	14876	2285	63.13
21159	Reconstruct midface, Lefort	9304	13406	18114	2564	70.84
21160	Reconstruct midface, Lefort	5452	7856	10615	2940	81.22
21172	Reconstruct orbit/forehead	4071	5867	7926	1669	46.10
21175	Reconstruct orbit/forehead	6485	9345	12625	2104	58.12
21179	Reconstruct entire forehead	5437	7835	10586	1581	43.67
21180	Reconstruct entire forehead	5873	8463	11434	1653	45.67
21181	Contour cranial bone lesion	2123	3059	4133	700	19.33
21182	Reconstruct cranial bone	6978	10054	13585	2052	56.69
21183	Reconstruct cranial bone	7565	10901	14728	2208	60.99
21184	Reconstruct cranial bone	7960	11470	15497	2241	61.90
21188	Reconstruct midface	5104	7355	9937	1454	40.17
21193	Reconst lower jaw w/o graft	5068	7302	9866	1066	29.45
21194	Reconst lower jaw w/graft	5719	8241	11134	1219	33.67
21195	Reconst lower jaw w/o fixation	4936	7112	9609	1115	30.80
21196	Reconst lower jaw w/fixation	5306	7645	10329	1208	33.36
21198	Reconstr lower jaw segment	2544	3665	4952	996	27.51
21199	Reconstr lower jaw w/advance	1912	2755	3723	1018	28.11
21206	Reconstruct upper jaw bone	3733	5379	7267	887	24.50
21208	Augment facial bones	1960	2824	3815	728	20.10
21209	Reduce facial bones	1523	2194	2965	556	15.37
21210	Face bone graft	2503	3607	4874	721	19.93
21215	Lower jaw bone graft	2361	3402	4597	751	20.76
21230	Rib cartilage graft	2661	3834	5180	817	22.58
21235	Ear cartilage graft	1768	2548	3443	693	19.14
21240	Reconstruct jaw joint	3910	5634	7612	977	26.99

NEW CODE CPT 2002 •

CPT	SHORT DESCRIPTION	50th	75th	90th	MFS	RVU
21242	Reconstruct jaw joint	3938	5675	7668	912	25.20
21243	Reconstruct jaw joint	5515	7947	10738	1325	36.61
21244	Reconstruct lower jaw	3228	4651	6284	810	22.37
21245	Reconstruct jaw	4145	5973	8070	1361	37.59
21246	Reconstruct jaw	4483	6460	8729	864	23.88
21247	Reconstruct lower jaw bone	4600	6628	8955	1629	45.01
21248	Reconstruct jaw	3528	5084	6869	775	21.40
21249	Reconstruct jaw	4558	6569	8875	1099	30.35
21255	Reconstruct lower jaw bone	3735	5381	7271	1123	31.01
21256	Reconstruct orbit	5027	7243	9786	1126	31.10
21260	Revise eye sockets	4905	7067	9549	1133	31.31
21261	Revise eye sockets	6358	9161	12378	1945	53.73
21263	Revise eye sockets	8420	12133	16393	1653	45.67
21267	Revise eye sockets	8980	12940	17483	1267	35.00
21268	Revise eye sockets	2701	3893	5259	1463	40.42
21270	Augment cheek bone	2151	3099	4187	773	21.35
21275	Revise orbitofacial bones	5888	8484	11463	843	23.29
21280	Revise eyelid	1785	2571	3474	455	12.57
21282	Revise eyelid	1354	1952	2637	329	9.08
21295	Revise jaw muscle/bone	1187	1710	2311	217	6.00
21296	Revise jaw muscle/bone	2412	3475	4696	313	8.64
21299	Cranio/maxillofacial surgery	0	0	0	0	.00
21300	Treat skull fracture	410	500	640	130	3.58
21310	Treat nose fracture	143	174	223	121	3.33
21315	Treat nose fracture	366	446	571	185	5.12
21320	Treat nose fracture	708	863	1105	252	6.96

CPT	SHORT DESCRIPTION	50th	75th	90th	MFS	RVU
21325	Treat nose fracture	993	1211	1550	283	7.81
21330	Treat nose fracture	1788	2181	2792	417	11.53
21335	Treat nose fracture	2713	3309	4237	601	16.59
21336	Treat nasal septal fracture	1254	1530	1959	431	11.91
21337	Treat nasal septal fracture	752	918	1175	295	8.16
21338	Treat nasoethmoid fracture	1766	2154	2757	461	12.74
21339	Treat nasoethmoid fracture	1896	2313	2961	573	15.82
21340	Treat nose fracture	2500	3049	3904	738	20.40
21343	Treat sinus fracture	2474	3018	3864	850	23.49
21344	Treat sinus fracture	3714	4529	5799	1276	35.26
21345	Treat nose/jaw fracture	2416	2946	3772	692	19.12
21346	Treat nose/jaw fracture	3004	3664	4691	781	21.58
21347	Treat nose/jaw fracture	3666	4471	5724	851	23.51
21348	Treat nose/jaw fracture	3621	4416	5654	1077	29.76
21355	Treat cheek bone fracture	817	996	1276	288	7.95
21356	Treat cheek bone fracture	1268	1547	1980	283	7.82
21360	Treat cheek bone fracture	1650	2013	2577	460	12.72
21365	Treat cheek bone fracture	2983	3638	4658	1012	27.97
21366	Treat cheek bone fracture	3524	4298	5503	1211	33.46
21385	Treat eye socket fracture	1879	2292	2934	646	17.84
21386	Treat eye socket fracture	2189	2670	3418	664	18.35
21387	Treat eye socket fracture	2888	3523	4510	689	19.03
21390	Treat eye socket fracture	2790	3403	4357	708	19.56
21395	Treat eye socket fracture	2986	3642	4663	833	23.01
21400	Treat eye socket fracture	421	513	657	174	4.81
21401	Treat eye socket fracture	680	829	1061	287	7.94

  NEW CODE CPT 2002 •

CPT	SHORT DESCRIPTION	50th	75th	90th	MFS	RVU
21406	Treat eye socket fracture	1738	2120	2714	536	14.80
21407	Treat eye socket fracture	2127	2594	3321	625	17.27
21408	Treat eye socket fracture	2518	3071	3933	866	23.91
21421	Treat mouth roof fracture	1519	1853	2373	463	12.79
21422	Treat mouth roof fracture	2007	2448	3134	613	16.94
21423	Treat mouth roof fracture	2394	2920	3739	723	19.98
21431	Treat craniofacial fracture	1693	2064	2643	582	16.07
21432	Treat craniofacial fracture	2393	2919	3737	623	17.22
21433	Treat craniofacial fracture	4254	5189	6643	1633	45.10
21435	Treat craniofacial fracture	4325	5275	6754	1154	31.88
21436	Treat craniofacial fracture	5265	6422	8222	1679	46.38
21440	Treat dental ridge fracture	880	1074	1375	303	8.36
21445	Treat dental ridge fracture	1292	1576	2018	473	13.07
21450	Treat lower jaw fracture	897	1094	1400	349	9.65
21451	Treat lower jaw fracture	1705	2080	2663	424	11.72
21452	Treat lower jaw fracture	2315	2823	3615	563	15.56
21453	Treat lower jaw fracture	1677	2045	2618	483	13.35
21454	Treat lower jaw fracture	2078	2535	3245	461	12.73
21461	Treat lower jaw fracture	2194	2676	3426	623	17.22
21462	Treat lower jaw fracture	2586	3154	4038	748	20.65
21465	Treat lower jaw fracture	2992	3650	4673	766	21.17
21470	Treat lower jaw fracture	3410	4158	5324	978	27.01
21480	Reset dislocated jaw	245	299	383	83	2.28
21485	Reset dislocated jaw	622	758	971	294	8.12
21490	Repair dislocated jaw	2224	2712	3473	755	20.86
21493	Treat hyoid bone fracture	236	287	368	183	5.05

CPT	SHORT DESCRIPTION	50th	75th	90th	MFS	RVU
21494	Treat hyoid bone fracture	484	590	755	396	10.93
21495	Treat hyoid bone fracture	1709	2084	2668	412	11.38
21497	Interdental wiring	705	860	1101	320	8.85
21499	Head surgery procedure	0	0	0	0	.00

NECK (SOFT TISSUES) AND THORAX

CPT	SHORT DESCRIPTION	50th	75th	90th	MFS	RVU
21501	Drain neck/chest lesion	643	836	1123	314	8.67
21502	Drain chest lesion	764	994	1334	542	14.96
21510	Drain bone lesion	786	1022	1373	502	13.88
21550	Biopsy neck/chest	288	375	504	163	4.51
21555	Remove lesion neck/chest	562	731	981	326	9.01
21556	Remove lesion neck/chest	1054	1371	1840	339	9.37
21557	Remove tumor neck/chest	3007	3912	5251	637	17.60
21600	Partial remove rib	1054	1371	1841	561	15.50
21610	Partial remove rib	1765	2296	3083	1003	27.72
21615	Remove rib	2110	2745	3685	687	18.97
21616	Remove rib and nerves	2409	3134	4208	807	22.29
21620	Partial remove sternum	1925	2504	3362	568	15.69
21627	Sternal debridement	2071	2694	3617	716	19.79
21630	Extensive sternum surgery	3028	3940	5289	1208	33.36
21632	Extensive sternum surgery	4413	5741	7707	1182	32.65
21700	Revise neck muscle	1424	1852	2487	548	15.13
21705	Revise neck muscle/rib	1764	2295	3081	666	18.39
21720	Revise neck muscle	1179	1533	2059	550	15.19
21725	Revise neck muscle	1291	1679	2254	549	15.17
21740	Reconstruct sternum	2975	3870	5196	1136	31.38
21750	Repair sternum separation	1627	2117	2842	779	21.53

   NEW CODE CPT 2002 •

CPT	SHORT DESCRIPTION	50th	75th	90th	MFS	RVU
21800	Treat rib fracture	159	207	278	122	3.36
21805	Treat rib fracture	1203	1565	2100	258	7.12
21810	Treat rib fracture(s)	3748	4876	6546	541	14.95
21820	Treat sternum fracture	328	427	573	153	4.23
21825	Treat sternum fracture	1291	1680	2256	657	18.15
21899	Neck/chest surgery procedure	0	0	0	0	.00

BACK AND FLANK

CPT	SHORT DESCRIPTION	50th	75th	90th	MFS	RVU
21920	Biopsy soft tissue back	213	277	372	166	4.58
21925	Biopsy soft tissue back	658	856	1150	547	15.12
21930	Remove lesion back or flank	829	1078	1447	363	10.04
21935	Remove tumor back	2137	2780	3732	1208	33.36

SPINE (VERTEBRAL COLUMN)

CPT	SHORT DESCRIPTION	50th	75th	90th	MFS	RVU
22100	Remove part neck vertebra	1151	1497	2010	711	19.64
22101	Remove part thorax vertebra	1154	1501	2015	737	20.36
22102	Remove part lumbar vertebra	1104	1437	1929	740	20.45
22103	Remove extra spine segment	309	402	539	144	3.98
22110	Remove part neck vertebra	1479	1925	2584	941	26.00
22112	Remove part thorax vertebra	1490	1939	2603	931	25.72
22114	Remove part lumbar vertebra	1668	2170	2913	923	25.50
22116	Remove extra spine segment	422	549	737	144	3.98
22210	Revise neck spine	4001	5206	6988	1646	45.47
22212	Revise thorax spine	4105	5341	7170	1332	36.80
22214	Revise lumbar spine	4088	5318	7140	1359	37.55
22216	Revise extra spine segment	1298	1689	2267	374	10.33
22220	Revise neck spine	4487	5837	7836	1471	40.63

CPT	SHORT DESCRIPTION	50th	75th	90th	MFS	RVU
22222	Revise thorax spine	4198	5462	7332	1436	39.68
22224	Revise lumbar spine	4424	5755	7726	1463	40.42
22226	Revise extra spine segment	1302	1693	2273	372	10.27
22305	Treat spine process fracture	355	462	620	202	5.59
22310	Treat spine fracture	748	974	1307	281	7.75
22315	Treat spine fracture	1068	1389	1865	707	19.53
22318	Treat odontoid fracture w/o graft	2782	3620	4859	1476	40.78
22319	Treat odontoid fracture w/graft	3146	4093	5495	1672	46.18
22325	Treat spine fracture	2787	3625	4867	1298	35.85
22326	Treat neck spine fracture	3204	4169	5596	1405	38.80
22327	Treat thorax spine fracture	3062	3983	5347	1353	37.38
22328	Treat each add spine fracture	819	1066	1431	279	7.70
22505	Manipulate spine	293	382	512	243	6.72
22520	Percut vertebroplasty thor	949	1235	1658	509	14.05
22521	Percut vertebroplasty lumb	891	1159	1556	477	13.19
22522	Percut vertebroplasty addl	311	404	543	231	6.39
22548	Neck spine fusion	5163	6370	8172	1769	48.88
22554	Neck spine fusion	4821	5947	7630	1306	36.07
22556	Thorax spine fusion	5226	6447	8271	1594	44.04
22558	Lumbar spine fusion	5027	6201	7955	1474	40.73
22585	Additional spinal fusion	1330	1640	2104	342	9.45
22590	Spine & skull spinal fusion	5689	7018	9003	1444	39.88
22595	Neck spinal fusion	5396	6657	8540	1361	37.59
22600	Neck spine fusion	4732	5838	7489	1147	31.69
22610	Thorax spine fusion	4489	5538	7104	1146	31.66
22612	Lumbar spine fusion	4851	5985	7678	1449	40.03

     NEW CODE CPT 2002 •

CPT	SHORT DESCRIPTION	50th	75th	90th	MFS	RVU
22614	Spine fusion, extra segment	1444	1782	2286	399	11.02
22630	Lumbar spine fusion	4832	5961	7647	1471	40.64
22632	Spine fusion, extra segment	1617	1995	2559	321	8.88
22800	Fusion spine	5388	6647	8527	1276	35.26
22802	Fusion spine	6957	8583	11011	2070	57.18
22804	Fusion spine	8360	10313	13230	2388	65.98
22808	Fusion spine	5645	6964	8934	1770	48.90
22810	Fusion spine	6810	8401	10778	1969	54.39
22812	Fusion spine	7581	9352	11998	2145	59.26
22818	Kyphectomy, 1-2 segments	4214	5199	6669	2119	58.53
22819	Kyphectomy, 3 or more	4536	5595	7178	2311	63.83
22830	Exploration spinal fusion	5926	7310	9379	819	22.63
22840	Insert spine fixation device	3249	4008	5142	775	21.41
22841	Insert spine fixation device	0	0	0	0	.00
22842	Insert spine fixation device	4558	5623	7214	776	21.45
22843	Insert spine fixation device	4081	5035	6459	831	22.95
22844	Insert spine fixation device	4297	5301	6801	1018	28.12
22845	Insert spine fixation device	4043	4988	6399	744	20.56
22846	Insert spine fixation device	3970	4898	6283	774	21.38
22847	Insert spine fixation device	4253	5246	6730	841	23.24
22848	Insert pelvic fixation device	839	1035	1327	371	10.26
22849	Reinsert spinal fixation	3279	4046	5190	1289	35.60
22850	Remove spine fixation device	2269	2799	3591	721	19.92
22851	Apply spine prosth device	1759	2169	2783	411	11.36
22852	Remove spine fixation device	2284	2818	3615	688	19.01
22855	Remove spine fixation device	4063	5012	6430	1069	29.54

CPT	SHORT DESCRIPTION	50th	75th	90th	MFS	RVU
22899	Spine surgery procedure	0	0	0	0	.00
22900	Remove abdominal wall lesion	1024	1263	1620	391	10.80
22999	Abdomen surgery procedure	0	0	0	0	.00

SHOULDER

CPT	SHORT DESCRIPTION	50th	75th	90th	MFS	RVU
23000	Remove calcium deposits	712	886	1240	503	13.90
23020	Release shoulder joint	1551	1929	2700	749	20.69
23030	Drain shoulder lesion	503	625	875	371	10.25
23031	Drain shoulder bursa	500	621	870	321	8.87
23035	Drain shoulder bone lesion	1092	1359	1902	939	25.93
23040	Exploratory shoulder surgery	1419	1765	2470	803	22.19
23044	Exploratory shoulder surgery	848	1054	1476	681	18.82
23065	Biopsy shoulder tissues	376	468	655	182	5.02
23066	Biopsy shoulder tissues	510	635	888	471	13.00
23075	Remove shoulder lesion	477	594	831	291	8.04
23076	Remove shoulder lesion	1037	1290	1806	610	16.86
23077	Remove tumor shoulder	3587	4462	6244	1170	32.31
23100	Biopsy shoulder joint	1190	1480	2072	564	15.57
23101	Shoulder joint surgery	1252	1558	2180	542	14.98
23105	Remove shoulder joint lining	2045	2543	3560	707	19.54
23106	Incise collarbone joint	1430	1778	2489	581	16.05
23107	Explore treat shoulder joint	1591	1979	2770	732	20.22
23120	Partial remove collar bone	1351	1681	2352	639	17.65
23125	Remove collar bone	1836	2284	3196	776	21.44
23130	Remove shoulder bone, part	1531	1905	2666	667	18.43
23140	Remove bone lesion	864	1075	1505	580	16.02
23145	Remove bone lesion	1205	1500	2099	767	21.20

     NEW CODE CPT 2002 •

CPT	SHORT DESCRIPTION	50th	75th	90th	MFS	RVU
23146	Remove bone lesion	1022	1272	1780	711	19.64
23150	Remove humerus lesion	1504	1870	2618	715	19.76
23155	Remove humerus lesion	1790	2227	3117	864	23.88
23156	Remove humerus lesion	1560	1941	2716	735	20.31
23170	Remove collar bone lesion	1145	1424	1993	689	19.03
23172	Remove shoulder blade lesion	1421	1768	2475	631	17.44
23174	Remove humerus lesion	2292	2851	3990	816	22.55
23180	Remove collar bone lesion	1069	1330	1861	936	25.87
23182	Remove shoulder blade lesion	1101	1370	1917	920	25.41
23184	Remove humerus lesion	1621	2016	2821	979	27.05
23190	Partial remove scapula	909	1131	1583	614	16.95
23195	Remove head humerus	1902	2366	3312	768	21.22
23200	Remove collar bone	1505	1872	2620	1012	27.95
23210	Remove shoulder blade	2376	2955	4136	1016	28.06
23220	Partial remove humerus	2492	3100	4338	1164	32.16
23221	Partial remove humerus	2787	3466	4851	1346	37.18
23222	Partial remove humerus	3095	3850	5389	1736	47.95
23330	Remove shoulder foreign body	613	763	1067	296	8.18
23331	Remove shoulder foreign body	766	952	1333	655	18.10
23332	Remove shoulder foreign body	2622	3262	4565	918	25.36
23350	Inject for shoulder x-ray	620	771	1079	299	8.27
23395	Muscle transfer,shoulder/arm	2605	3240	4032	1203	33.23
23397	Muscle transfers	2261	2813	3500	1167	32.23
23400	Fixation shoulder blade	2594	3226	4015	1085	29.97
23405	Incise tendon & muscle	1243	1545	1923	693	19.15
23406	Incise tendon(s) & muscle(s)	1853	2305	2869	862	23.82

CPT	SHORT DESCRIPTION	50th	75th	90th	MFS	RVU
23410	Repair tendon(s)	2463	3063	3812	967	26.72
23412	Repair tendon(s)	2755	3426	4264	1022	28.22
23415	Release shoulder ligament	1654	2058	2561	781	21.58
23420	Repair shoulder	3241	4031	5017	1053	29.10
23430	Repair biceps tendon	1713	2130	2651	816	22.53
23440	Remove/transplant tendon	1494	1858	2312	850	23.49
23450	Repair shoulder capsule	2614	3251	4046	1024	28.28
23455	Repair shoulder capsule	3372	4194	5220	1086	30.00
23460	Repair shoulder capsule	2546	3166	3940	1149	31.75
23462	Repair shoulder capsule	2552	3175	3951	1127	31.14
23465	Repair shoulder capsule	2846	3539	4405	1156	31.93
23466	Repair shoulder capsule	3533	4395	5469	1081	29.85
23470	Reconstruct shoulder joint	2818	3505	4362	1256	34.71
23472	Reconstruct shoulder joint	4744	5901	7343	1479	40.87
23480	Revise collar bone	1334	1659	2065	893	24.68
23485	Revise collar bone	1887	2346	2920	1027	28.37
23490	Reinforce clavicle	1608	2000	2489	967	26.71
23491	Reinforce shoulder bones	1984	2468	3071	1077	29.75
23500	Treat clavicle fracture	347	421	512	225	6.21
23505	Treat clavicle fracture	440	533	649	368	10.17
23515	Treat clavicle fracture	1286	1558	1898	604	16.68
23520	Treat clavicle dislocation	365	442	538	229	6.33
23525	Treat clavicle dislocation	495	600	731	405	11.20
23530	Treat clavicle dislocation	1172	1419	1729	583	16.10
23532	Treat clavicle dislocation	1404	1701	2072	645	17.81
23540	Treat clavicle dislocation	292	354	431	254	7.03

NEW CODE CPT 2002 •

CPT	SHORT DESCRIPTION	50th	75th	90th	MFS	RVU
23545	Treat clavicle dislocation	378	458	558	312	8.63
23550	Treat clavicle dislocation	1886	2285	2783	596	16.47
23552	Treat clavicle dislocation	2118	2566	3126	668	18.45
23570	Treat shoulder blade fracture	382	463	564	230	6.36
23575	Treat shoulder blade fracture	467	565	689	391	10.81
23585	Treat scapula fracture	1691	2049	2496	707	19.52
23600	Treat humerus fracture	530	642	782	325	8.97
23605	Treat humerus fracture	747	905	1102	502	13.86
23615	Treat humerus fracture	1900	2302	2804	755	20.85
23616	Treat humerus fracture	2977	3607	4393	1466	40.51
23620	Treat humerus fracture	488	591	720	292	8.07
23625	Treat humerus fracture	529	641	780	428	11.81
23630	Treat humerus fracture	1336	1619	1972	600	16.58
23650	Treat shoulder dislocation	430	521	634	336	9.28
23655	Treat shoulder dislocation	630	764	930	343	9.48
23660	Treat shoulder dislocation	1472	1784	2172	607	16.77
23665	Treat dislocation/fracture	564	683	832	462	12.75
23670	Treat dislocation/fracture	1889	2288	2787	641	17.72
23675	Treat dislocation/fracture	813	985	1199	547	15.10
23680	Treat dislocation/fracture	2322	2813	3427	772	21.34
23700	Fixation shoulder	524	635	773	230	6.35
23800	Fuse shoulder joint	2164	2622	3193	1101	30.41
23802	Fuse shoulder joint	2784	3373	4108	1259	34.77
23900	Amputate arm & girdle	2999	3634	4426	1395	38.54
23920	Amputate at shoulder joint	2170	2629	3202	1094	30.23
23921	Amputate follow-up surgery	820	993	1209	468	12.94

CPT	SHORT DESCRIPTION	50th	75th	90th	MFS	RVU
23929	Shoulder surgery procedure	0	0	0	0	.00

HUMERUS (UPPER ARM) AND ELBOW

CPT	SHORT DESCRIPTION	50th	75th	90th	MFS	RVU
23930	Drain arm lesion	546	689	951	339	9.36
23931	Drain arm bursa	578	729	1006	281	7.76
23935	Drain arm/elbow bone lesion	1166	1472	2030	718	19.83
24000	Exploratory elbow surgery	1368	1726	2382	458	12.65
24006	Release elbow joint	1493	1885	2600	696	19.22
24065	Biopsy arm/elbow soft tissue	642	810	1117	279	7.72
24066	Biopsy arm/elbow soft tissue	635	801	1105	518	14.30
24075	Remove arm/elbow lesion	577	728	1004	440	12.15
24076	Remove arm/elbow lesion.	1058	1336	1842	521	14.39
24077	Remove tumor arm/elbow	2556	3226	4451	989	27.31
24100	Biopsy elbow joint lining	1079	1362	1878	412	11.38
24101	Explore/treat elbow joint	1351	1706	2353	499	13.79
24102	Remove elbow joint lining	1703	2150	2967	613	16.93
24105	Remove elbow bursa	870	1099	1516	339	9.36
24110	Remove humerus lesion	1547	1954	2695	656	18.13
24115	Remove/graft bone lesion	1793	2264	3123	781	21.58
24116	Remove/graft bone lesion	1660	2095	2890	929	25.67
24120	Remove elbow lesion	1244	1570	2166	524	14.48
24125	Remove/graft bone lesion	1657	2091	2885	559	15.44
24126	Remove/graft bone lesion	1648	2081	2871	615	17.00
24130	Remove head radius	1166	1472	2030	508	14.03
24134	Remove arm bone lesion	1689	2132	2941	997	27.54
24136	Remove radius bone lesion	1445	1824	2516	577	15.93
24138	Remove elbow bone lesion	1470	1856	2561	624	17.23

NEW CODE CPT 2002 •

CPT	SHORT DESCRIPTION	50th	75th	90th	MFS	RVU
24140	Partial remove arm bone	1663	2100	2897	980	27.08
24145	Partial remove radius	1220	1540	2124	725	20.02
24147	Partial remove elbow	1048	1323	1825	723	19.98
24149	Radical resection elbow	2215	2797	3858	991	27.38
24150	Extensive humerus surgery	2346	2962	4086	1086	30.00
24151	Extensive humerus surgery	2962	3739	5158	1246	34.41
24152	Extensive radius surgery	2738	3457	4769	768	21.21
24153	Extensive radius surgery	2972	3752	5176	714	19.73
24155	Remove elbow joint	1895	2392	3300	826	22.81
24160	Remove elbow joint implant	1406	1775	2448	603	16.67
24164	Remove radius head implant	1194	1508	2080	507	14.00
24200	Remove arm foreign body	641	809	1116	279	7.71
24201	Remove arm foreign body	606	765	1056	490	13.54
24220	Inject for elbow x-ray	1042	1315	1815	454	12.54
• 24300	Manipulate elbow w/anesth	808	1020	1408	352	9.73
24301	Muscle/tendon transfer	1713	2162	2983	746	20.61
24305	Arm tendon lengthening	845	1067	1472	584	16.13
24310	Revise arm tendon	650	821	1133	548	15.15
24320	Repair arm tendon	1923	2428	3349	827	22.85
24330	Revise arm muscles	1628	2056	2836	710	19.60
24331	Revise arm muscles	1904	2403	3315	771	21.31
• 24332	Tenolysis triceps	1118	1411	1946	487	13.45
24340	Repair biceps tendon	1389	1753	2418	605	16.71
24341	Repair arm tendon/muscle	1628	2056	2836	609	16.83
24342	Repair ruptured tendon	2242	2831	3905	777	21.47
• 24343	Repair elbow lat ligmnt w/tiss	1476	1864	2571	643	17.77

CPT	SHORT DESCRIPTION	50th	75th	90th	MFS	RVU
• 24344	Reconstruct elbow lat ligmnt	2228	2813	3881	971	26.82
• 24345	Repair elbow med ligmnt w/tiss	1476	1864	2571	643	17.77
• 24346	Reconstruct elbow med ligmnt	2228	2813	3881	971	26.82
24350	Repair tennis elbow	980	1238	1707	442	12.22
24351	Repair tennis elbow	1079	1362	1879	487	13.45
24352	Repair tennis elbow	1108	1399	1930	519	14.34
24354	Repair tennis elbow	1105	1396	1925	514	14.21
24356	Revise tennis elbow	1528	1930	2662	535	14.79
24360	Reconstruct elbow joint	2706	3416	4713	879	24.29
24361	Reconstruct elbow joint	2727	3443	4750	989	27.33
24362	Reconstruct elbow joint	2565	3238	4467	1021	28.21
24363	Replace elbow joint	3955	4993	6888	1260	34.81
24365	Reconstruct head radius	1167	1473	2033	632	17.46
24366	Reconstruct head radius	1536	1939	2674	684	18.89
24400	Revise humerus	1908	2409	3323	908	25.07
24410	Revise humerus	2091	2640	3642	1103	30.46
24420	Revise humerus	2041	2576	3554	1134	31.34
24430	Repair humerus	2284	2883	3978	995	27.49
24435	Repair humerus with graft	2579	3255	4491	1049	28.99
24470	Revise elbow joint	1898	2396	3305	599	16.56
24495	Decompression forearm	1609	2032	2803	701	19.37
24498	Reinforce humerus	2152	2717	3748	938	25.90
24500	Treat humerus fracture	526	658	819	315	8.71
24505	Treat humerus fracture	951	1190	1481	535	14.77
24515	Treat humerus fracture	1383	1731	2154	893	24.68
24516	Treat humerus fracture	1638	2049	2550	910	25.13

NEW CODE CPT 2002 •

CPT	SHORT DESCRIPTION	50th	75th	90th	MFS	RVU
24530	Treat humerus fracture	598	749	932	368	10.16
24535	Treat humerus fracture	762	954	1187	602	16.64
24538	Treat humerus fracture	1799	2251	2802	771	21.29
24545	Treat humerus fracture	1306	1634	2034	800	22.11
24546	Treat humerus fracture	1750	2189	2725	1142	31.56
24560	Treat humerus fracture	511	639	795	290	8.02
24565	Treat humerus fracture	833	1043	1298	521	14.39
24566	Treat humerus fracture	855	1070	1331	682	18.85
24575	Treat humerus fracture	1166	1459	1816	745	20.59
24576	Treat humerus fracture	507	635	790	285	7.86
24577	Treat humerus fracture	858	1074	1337	536	14.82
24579	Treat humerus fracture	1356	1697	2112	888	24.54
24582	Treat humerus fracture	922	1154	1436	732	20.21
24586	Treat elbow fracture	1654	2070	2576	1034	28.56
24587	Treat elbow fracture	2049	2563	3190	1029	28.43
24600	Treat elbow dislocation	670	1047	1625	418	11.54
24605	Treat elbow dislocation	648	811	1010	404	11.16
24615	Treat elbow dislocation	1081	1353	1684	676	18.67
24620	Treat elbow fracture	672	841	1046	525	14.51
24635	Treat elbow fracture	1436	1796	2236	1143	31.58
24640	Treat elbow dislocation	180	226	281	169	4.66
24650	Treat radius fracture	441	552	687	253	6.99
24655	Treat radius fracture	713	892	1111	446	12.31
24665	Treat radius fracture	1027	1285	1599	676	18.67
24666	Treat radius fracture	1241	1553	1933	760	20.99
24670	Treat ulnar fracture	431	539	671	266	7.36

CPT	SHORT DESCRIPTION	50th	75th	90th	MFS	RVU
24675	Treat ulnar fracture	748	936	1166	468	12.92
24685	Treat ulnar fracture	1696	2122	2641	717	19.82
24800	Fuse elbow joint	1350	1689	2102	815	22.51
24802	Fuse/graft elbow joint	1930	2415	3006	980	27.08
24900	Amputate upper arm	1020	1276	1588	802	22.15
24920	Amputate upper arm	1432	1792	2230	895	24.72
24925	Amputate follow-up surgery	1023	1280	1593	639	17.66
24930	Amputate follow-up surgery	1075	1345	1674	809	22.34
24931	Amputate upper arm & implant	1262	1579	1965	938	25.91
24935	Revise amputate	1458	1824	2270	1099	30.36
24940	Revise upper arm	1333	1668	2076	0	.00
24999	Upper arm/elbow surgery	0	0	0	0	.00

FOREARM AND WRIST

CPT	SHORT DESCRIPTION	50th	75th	90th	MFS	RVU
25000	Incise tendon sheath	893	1124	1535	410	11.32
• 25001	Incise flexor carpi radialis	646	813	1111	294	8.13
25020	Decompress forearm 1 space	898	1130	1544	657	18.16
25023	Decompress forearm 1 space	2540	3196	4367	1157	31.96
• 25024	Decompress forearm 2 spaces	1500	1887	2579	683	18.87
• 25025	Decompress forearm 2 spaces	2424	3050	4168	1104	30.50
25028	Drain forearm lesion	1276	1606	2195	581	16.06
25031	Drain forearm bursa	1182	1488	2033	539	14.88
25035	Treat forearm bone lesion	1048	1319	1802	888	24.52
25040	Explore/treat wrist joint	1087	1368	1869	635	17.54
25065	Biopsy forearm soft tissues	203	255	349	168	4.64
25066	Biopsy forearm soft tissues	517	650	888	471	13.02
25075	Remove forearm lesion subcut	564	709	969	408	11.27

     NEW CODE CPT 2002 •

CPT	SHORT DESCRIPTION	50th	75th	90th	MFS	RVU
25076	Remove forearm lesion deep	1065	1340	1831	658	18.19
25077	Remove tumor forearm/wrist	2189	2755	3764	960	26.52
25085	Incise wrist capsule	1391	1750	2391	633	17.50
25100	Biopsy wrist joint	973	1224	1673	449	12.39
25101	Explore/treat wrist joint	1081	1361	1860	472	13.04
25105	Remove wrist joint lining	1271	1600	2186	646	17.84
25107	Remove wrist joint cartilage	1483	1866	2550	675	18.66
25110	Remove wrist tendon lesion	536	674	921	483	13.34
25111	Remove wrist tendon lesion	858	1080	1476	380	10.51
25112	Reremove wrist tendon lesion	991	1247	1704	452	12.50
25115	Remove wrist/forearm lesion	1612	2029	2773	982	27.12
25116	Remove wrist/forearm lesion	1414	1780	2432	876	24.21
25118	Excise wrist tendon sheath	1069	1346	1839	465	12.85
25119	Partial remove ulna	1290	1623	2218	662	18.29
25120	Remove forearm lesion	1257	1582	2161	788	21.78
25125	Remove/graft forearm lesion	1434	1804	2465	891	24.61
25126	Remove/graft forearm lesion	1407	1771	2420	880	24.31
25130	Remove wrist lesion	1133	1426	1949	516	14.25
25135	Remove & graft wrist lesion	1333	1678	2293	607	16.78
25136	Remove & graft wrist lesion	1256	1581	2161	572	15.81
25145	Remove forearm bone lesion	1543	1942	2654	819	22.62
25150	Partial remove ulna	1221	1537	2100	726	20.05
25151	Partial remove radius	1165	1467	2004	888	24.54
25170	Extensive forearm surgery	1843	2319	3168	1092	30.17
25210	Remove wrist bone	946	1190	1626	557	15.39
25215	Remove wrist bones	1683	2118	2894	767	21.18

CPT	SHORT DESCRIPTION	50th	75th	90th	MFS	RVU
25230	Partial remove radius	876	1102	1506	511	14.12
25240	Partial remove ulna	979	1232	1684	602	16.64
25246	Inject for wrist x-ray	931	1172	1602	424	11.72
25248	Remove forearm foreign body	638	803	1098	591	16.34
25250	Remove wrist prosthesis	1299	1635	2234	592	16.35
25251	Remove wrist prosthesis	1847	2324	3176	841	23.24
• 25259	Manipulate wrist w/anesthes	765	962	1315	348	9.62
25260	Repair forearm tendon/muscle	1386	1744	2383	937	25.88
25263	Repair forearm tendon/muscle	1242	1563	2136	884	24.41
25265	Repair forearm tendon/muscle	1444	1817	2483	1020	28.18
25270	Repair forearm tendon/muscle	908	1143	1561	825	22.80
25272	Repair forearm tendon/muscle	990	1246	1703	884	24.43
25274	Repair forearm tendon/muscle	1319	1660	2269	985	27.22
• 25275	Repair forearm tendon sheath	1362	1714	2342	620	17.14
25280	Revise wrist/forearm tendon	979	1232	1684	866	23.93
25290	Incise wrist/forearm tendon	1917	2412	3296	873	24.12
25295	Release wrist/forearm tendon	916	1153	1576	816	22.55
25300	Fuse tendons at wrist	1580	1989	2718	720	19.89
25301	Fuse tendons at wrist	1462	1840	2513	711	19.63
25310	Transplant forearm tendon	1485	1870	2554	927	25.62
25312	Transplant forearm tendon	1654	2081	2843	1015	28.03
25315	Revise palsy hand tendon(s)	2067	2602	3555	1088	30.05
25316	Revise palsy hand tendon(s)	2381	2996	4094	1175	32.47
25320	Repair/revise wrist joint	2301	2896	3957	855	23.62
25332	Revise wrist joint	1968	2476	3383	896	24.76
25335	Realignment hand	2747	3457	4724	1019	28.14

NEW CODE CPT 2002 •

CPT	SHORT DESCRIPTION	50th	75th	90th	MFS	RVU
25337	Reconstruct ulna/radioulnar	2009	2528	3455	915	25.28
25350	Revise radius	1334	1679	2294	964	26.63
25355	Revise radius	1755	2208	3017	1042	28.78
25360	Revise ulna	1301	1638	2238	958	26.46
25365	Revise radius & ulna	1962	2470	3374	1188	32.81
25370	Revise radius or ulna	1833	2306	3152	1197	33.08
25375	Revise radius & ulna	2489	3132	4280	1134	31.32
25390	Shorten radius or ulna	1759	2214	3025	1056	29.16
25391	Lengthen radius or ulna	1807	2274	3107	1245	34.39
25392	Shorten radius & ulna	2126	2675	3655	1132	31.27
25393	Lengthen radius & ulna	2305	2901	3964	1428	39.46
• 25394	Repair carpal bone, shorten	1588	1998	2730	723	19.98
25400	Repair radius or ulna	1580	1989	2717	1100	30.40
25405	Repair/graft radius or ulna	1930	2428	3318	1329	36.71
25415	Repair radius & ulna	1811	2279	3114	1244	34.36
25420	Repair/graft radius & ulna	2130	2681	3663	1457	40.25
25425	Repair/graft radius or ulna	1775	2234	3053	1432	39.57
25426	Repair/graft radius & ulna	2068	2603	3556	1310	36.20
• 25430	Vasc graft into carpal bone	1401	1763	2409	638	17.63
• 25431	Repair nonunion carpal bone	1384	1742	2380	631	17.42
25440	Repair/graft wrist bone	1768	2225	3040	829	22.90
25441	Reconstruct wrist joint	2114	2660	3635	976	26.97
25442	Reconstruct wrist joint	1872	2355	3218	852	23.55
25443	Reconstruct wrist joint	1985	2498	3414	904	24.98
25444	Reconstruct wrist joint	2135	2687	3672	973	26.87
25445	Reconstruct wrist joint	2055	2586	3534	885	24.45

CPT	SHORT DESCRIPTION	50th	75th	90th	MFS	RVU
25446	Wrist replacement	2786	3507	4791	1202	33.20
25447	Repair wrist joint(s)	2351	2958	4042	832	22.98
25449	Remove wrist joint implant	1435	1806	2468	1175	32.46
25450	Revise wrist joint	1801	2266	3097	820	22.66
25455	Revise wrist joint	1228	1545	2111	933	25.78
25490	Reinforce radius	1400	1762	2407	993	27.43
25491	Reinforce ulna	1242	1563	2135	1026	28.35
25492	Reinforce radius and ulna	1590	2001	2734	1087	30.04
25500	Treat fracture radius	433	525	634	253	7.00
25505	Treat fracture radius	802	973	1176	498	13.77
25515	Treat fracture radius	1307	1585	1916	738	20.40
25520	Treat fracture radius	551	668	808	547	15.11
25525	Treat fracture radius	1450	1759	2127	926	25.57
25526	Treat fracture radius	1648	1999	2417	1078	29.79
25530	Treat fracture ulna	478	579	700	238	6.57
25535	Treat fracture ulna	606	735	889	491	13.56
25545	Treat fracture ulna	1286	1560	1887	724	20.01
25560	Treat fracture radius & ulna	530	643	777	253	6.99
25565	Treat fracture radius & ulna	1071	1299	1571	522	14.41
25574	Treat fracture radius & ulna	1603	1944	2350	604	16.69
25575	Treat fracture radius/ulna	2298	2787	3370	820	22.65
25600	Treat fracture radius/ulna	539	654	790	271	7.50
25605	Treat fracture radius/ulna	875	1061	1283	536	14.80
25611	Treat fracture radius/ulna	1429	1733	2096	684	18.89
25620	Treat fracture radius/ulna	1728	2096	2534	702	19.39
25622	Treat wrist bone fracture	537	651	787	269	7.42

NEW CODE CPT 2002 •

CPT	SHORT DESCRIPTION	50th	75th	90th	MFS	RVU
25624	Treat wrist bone fracture	561	681	823	454	12.54
25628	Treat wrist bone fracture	1233	1496	1809	697	19.25
25630	Treat wrist bone fracture	501	607	734	286	7.91
25635	Treat wrist bone fracture	542	657	794	443	12.23
25645	Treat wrist bone fracture	817	991	1198	642	17.74
25650	Treat wrist bone fracture	513	622	752	296	8.17
• 25651	Pin ulnar styloid fracture	739	896	1084	379	10.48
• 25652	Treat fracture ulnar styloid	1091	1323	1600	560	15.47
25660	Treat wrist dislocation	569	690	834	391	10.80
25670	Treat wrist dislocation	1183	1434	1735	671	18.53
• 25671	Pin radioulnar dislocation	900	1092	1321	462	12.77
25675	Treat wrist dislocation	903	1095	1324	464	12.81
25676	Treat wrist dislocation	870	1056	1277	675	18.66
25680	Treat wrist fracture	813	986	1192	472	13.05
25685	Treat wrist fracture	1497	1815	2195	769	21.23
25690	Treat wrist dislocation	735	891	1077	481	13.28
25695	Treat wrist dislocation	1346	1633	1974	691	19.09
25800	Fuse wrist joint	1448	1756	2123	794	21.93
25805	Fuse/graft wrist joint	1642	1992	2409	883	24.40
25810	Fuse/graft wrist joint	1875	2273	2749	842	23.27
25820	Fuse hand bones	1538	1865	2256	650	17.95
25825	Fuse hand bones with graft	2045	2481	3000	759	20.98
25830	Fuse radioulnar jnt/ulna	1984	2406	2909	1025	28.32
25900	Amputate forearm	1480	1795	2171	910	25.13
25905	Amputate forearm	1146	1389	1680	884	24.43
25907	Amputate follow-up surgery	1697	2058	2489	871	24.07

CPT	SHORT DESCRIPTION	50th	75th	90th	MFS	RVU
25909	Amputate follow-up surgery	1319	1600	1935	888	24.54
25915	Amputate forearm	1477	1791	2166	1252	34.60
25920	Amputate hand at wrist	1400	1698	2054	719	19.86
25922	Amputate hand at wrist	1123	1362	1647	577	15.93
25924	Amputate follow-up surgery	1390	1686	2039	714	19.72
25927	Amputate hand	1457	1767	2137	866	23.93
25929	Amputate follow-up surgery	1121	1360	1644	576	15.90
25931	Amputate follow-up surgery	1374	1666	2014	886	24.48
25999	Forearm or wrist surgery	0	0	0	0	.00

HAND AND FINGERS

CPT	SHORT DESCRIPTION	50th	75th	90th	MFS	RVU
26010	Drain finger abscess	476	633	956	250	6.92
26011	Drain finger abscess	391	520	785	359	9.92
26020	Drain hand tendon sheath	733	975	1473	665	18.36
26025	Drain palm bursa	758	1008	1522	676	18.68
26030	Drain palm bursa(s)	1552	2064	3118	748	20.67
26034	Treat hand bone lesion	893	1188	1794	791	21.86
26035	Decompress fingers/hand	1774	2360	3564	934	25.80
26037	Decompress fingers/hand	1430	1901	2872	753	20.79
26040	Release palm contracture	1145	1523	2300	603	16.65
26045	Release palm contracture	830	1103	1667	741	20.47
26055	Incise finger tendon sheath	838	1114	1683	404	11.17
26060	Incise finger tendon	738	981	1482	388	10.73
26070	Explore/treat hand joint	721	960	1449	569	15.73
26075	Explore/treat finger joint	772	1026	1550	603	16.66
26080	Explore/treat finger joint	850	1130	1707	646	17.85
26100	Biopsy hand joint lining	709	943	1424	454	12.55

NEW CODE CPT 2002 •

CPT	SHORT DESCRIPTION	50th	75th	90th	MFS	RVU
26105	Biopsy finger joint lining	653	869	1312	619	17.11
26110	Biopsy finger joint lining	1130	1503	2270	595	16.43
26115	Remove hand lesion subcut	659	877	1324	434	12.00
26116	Remove hand lesion deep	1051	1398	2111	729	20.13
26117	Remove tumor hand/finger	2362	3141	4744	904	24.97
26121	Release palm contracture	1717	2283	3449	879	24.28
26123	Release palm contracture	2306	3067	4633	984	27.19
26125	Release palm contracture	627	835	1260	282	7.78
26130	Remove wrist joint lining	1072	1425	2153	785	21.69
26135	Revise finger joint, each	1020	1356	2048	900	24.87
26140	Revise finger joint, each	930	1237	1868	842	23.26
26145	Tendon excise palm/finger	939	1249	1886	867	23.95
26160	Remove tendon sheath lesion	730	971	1467	415	11.47
26170	Remove palm tendon, each	595	792	1196	503	13.90
26180	Remove finger tendon	628	835	1261	543	15.01
26185	Remove finger bone	655	871	1315	531	14.68
26200	Remove hand bone lesion	822	1093	1651	731	20.19
26205	Remove/graft bone lesion	1027	1366	2064	869	24.00
26210	Remove finger lesion	1012	1346	2033	728	20.11
26215	Remove/graft finger lesion	952	1267	1913	824	22.76
26230	Partial remove hand bone	844	1122	1695	725	20.04
26235	Partial remove finger bone	820	1090	1647	707	19.53
26236	Partial remove finger bone	761	1013	1530	673	18.60
26250	Extensive hand surgery	1277	1698	2564	934	25.80
26255	Extensive hand surgery	1653	2199	3321	1166	32.22
26260	Extensive finger surgery	1230	1635	2470	878	24.25

CPT	SHORT DESCRIPTION	50th	75th	90th	MFS	RVU
26261	Extensive finger surgery	1430	1902	2873	942	26.03
26262	Partial remove finger	1169	1555	2349	767	21.18
26320	Remove implant from hand	1207	1605	2424	635	17.55
• 26340	Manipulate finger w/anesth	403	501	622	266	7.35
26350	Repair finger/hand tendon	1256	1561	1940	976	26.96
26352	Repair/graft hand tendon	1666	2070	2572	1026	28.35
26356	Repair finger/hand tendon	1949	2421	3008	1108	30.61
26357	Repair finger/hand tendon	2085	2591	3219	1119	30.90
26358	Repair/graft hand tendon	2334	2900	3604	1182	32.64
26370	Repair finger/hand tendon	1569	1950	2423	1036	28.62
26372	Repair/graft hand tendon	1660	2063	2563	1096	30.28
26373	Repair finger/hand tendon	1552	1928	2396	1149	31.75
26390	Revise hand/finger tendon	1492	1853	2303	985	27.21
26392	Repair/graft hand tendon	1895	2355	2926	1251	34.57
26410	Repair hand tendon	907	1127	1401	777	21.46
26412	Repair/graft hand tendon	1151	1430	1777	867	23.94
26415	Excise hand/finger tendon	1259	1564	1943	986	27.25
26416	Graft hand or finger tendon	1214	1509	1875	1069	29.52
26418	Repair finger tendon	949	1180	1466	763	21.09
26420	Repair/graft finger tendon	1205	1497	1861	924	25.52
26426	Repair finger/hand tendon	1314	1633	2029	868	23.97
26428	Repair/graft finger tendon	1736	2158	2681	872	24.10
26432	Repair finger tendon	666	827	1028	651	17.99
26433	Repair finger tendon	905	1124	1397	707	19.54
26434	Repair/graft finger tendon	1161	1443	1793	801	22.14
26437	Realignment tendons	983	1222	1518	750	20.72

     NEW CODE CPT 2002 •

CPT	SHORT DESCRIPTION	50th	75th	90th	MFS	RVU
26440	Release palm/finger tendon	1127	1401	1740	873	24.12
26442	Release palm & finger tendon	1161	1442	1792	1032	28.50
26445	Release hand/finger tendon	866	1076	1337	837	23.12
26449	Release forearm/hand tendon	1262	1568	1949	1014	28.00
26450	Incise palm tendon	687	854	1061	465	12.84
26455	Incise finger tendon	685	851	1057	452	12.49
26460	Incise hand/finger tendon	654	812	1009	433	11.96
26471	Fuse finger tendons	1201	1493	1855	738	20.39
26474	Fuse finger tendons	826	1026	1275	699	19.31
26476	Tendon lengthening	791	983	1221	670	18.52
26477	Tendon shortening	783	973	1209	705	19.48
26478	Lengthening hand tendon	991	1231	1530	771	21.30
26479	Shortening hand tendon	1012	1257	1562	732	20.21
26480	Transplant hand tendon	1281	1592	1978	983	27.16
26483	Transplant/graft hand tendon	1596	1983	2464	1054	29.11
26485	Transplant palm tendon	1647	2047	2543	1040	28.72
26489	Transplant/graft palm tendon	1952	2426	3015	1009	27.87
26490	Revise thumb tendon	1334	1658	2060	881	24.33
26492	Tendon transfer with graft	1726	2144	2664	965	26.65
26494	Hand tendon/muscle transfer	1817	2258	2806	837	23.12
26496	Revise thumb tendon	1943	2414	2999	952	26.29
26497	Finger tendon transfer	1682	2090	2597	983	27.16
26498	Finger tendon transfer	1883	2340	2908	1228	33.93
26499	Revise finger	1447	1798	2234	888	24.53
26500	Hand tendon reconstruct	855	1062	1320	788	21.78
26502	Hand tendon reconstruct	1165	1447	1798	838	23.15

CPT	SHORT DESCRIPTION	50th	75th	90th	MFS	RVU
26504	Hand tendon reconstruct	1437	1785	2218	819	22.62
26508	Release thumb contracture	1023	1271	1580	756	20.88
26510	Thumb tendon transfer	1977	2457	3053	736	20.32
26516	Fuse knuckle joint	1267	1575	1956	837	23.11
26517	Fuse knuckle joints	1408	1749	2174	930	25.68
26518	Fuse knuckle joints	1958	2433	3023	943	26.06
26520	Release knuckle contracture	1121	1393	1731	888	24.54
26525	Release finger contracture	1128	1401	1741	893	24.66
26530	Revise knuckle joint	1248	1551	1927	974	26.90
26531	Revise knuckle with implant	1368	1700	2113	1026	28.33
26535	Revise finger joint	1126	1399	1738	615	17.00
26536	Revise/implant finger joint	1378	1713	2128	910	25.14
26540	Repair hand joint	1626	2020	2510	788	21.78
26541	Repair hand joint with graft	1431	1778	2209	945	26.10
26542	Repair hand joint with graft	1679	2086	2592	802	22.16
26545	Reconstruct finger joint	1309	1626	2020	864	23.87
26546	Repair nonunion hand	1315	1635	2031	942	26.01
26548	Reconstruct finger joint	1378	1713	2128	910	25.14
26550	Construct thumb replacement	2910	3615	4492	1933	53.40
26551	Great toe-hand transfer	5149	6398	7950	2986	82.50
26553	Single transfer toe-hand	4249	5279	6560	2805	77.49
26554	Double transfer toe-hand	6180	7678	9541	3453	95.40
26555	Positional change finger	1945	2416	3002	1548	42.76
26556	Toe joint transfer	5296	6580	8176	3024	83.55
26560	Repair web finger	1205	1497	1860	671	18.53
26561	Repair web finger	1629	2024	2515	1094	30.22

NEW CODE CPT 2002 •

CPT	SHORT DESCRIPTION	50th	75th	90th	MFS	RVU
26562	Repair web finger	3427	4258	5291	1065	29.42
26565	Correct metacarpal flaw	1097	1364	1694	809	22.35
26567	Correct finger deformity	1073	1333	1657	824	22.76
26568	Lengthen metacarpal/finger	1626	2021	2511	1074	29.66
26580	Repair hand deformity	2230	2771	3443	1334	36.86
26587	Reconstruct extra finger	1086	1349	1676	717	19.80
26590	Repair finger deformity	2081	2586	3214	1227	33.90
26591	Repair muscles hand	937	1165	1447	646	17.84
26593	Release muscles hand	1057	1313	1632	698	19.28
26596	Excise constricting tissue	1144	1421	1766	727	20.08
26600	Treat metacarpal fracture	342	425	529	230	6.36
26605	Treat metacarpal fracture	530	659	818	336	9.28
26607	Treat metacarpal fracture	746	927	1152	521	14.39
26608	Treat metacarpal fracture	1039	1291	1605	541	14.94
26615	Treat metacarpal fracture	1159	1440	1790	523	14.46
26641	Treat thumb dislocation	600	745	926	396	10.94
26645	Treat thumb fracture	528	656	815	445	12.28
26650	Treat thumb fracture	850	1057	1313	561	15.51
26665	Treat thumb fracture	1189	1477	1835	645	17.81
26670	Treat hand dislocation	576	716	890	380	10.51
26675	Treat hand dislocation	659	819	1017	435	12.02
26676	Pin hand dislocation	669	831	1032	566	15.64
26685	Treat hand dislocation	938	1165	1448	609	16.81
26686	Treat hand dislocation	1241	1542	1916	682	18.83
26700	Treat knuckle dislocation	496	616	766	328	9.05
26705	Treat knuckle dislocation	600	746	927	396	10.95

CPT	SHORT DESCRIPTION	50th	75th	90th	MFS	RVU
26706	Pin knuckle dislocation	544	676	840	421	11.63
26715	Treat knuckle dislocation	829	1030	1279	547	15.11
26720	Treat finger fracture, each	262	325	404	178	4.92
26725	Treat finger fracture, each	431	535	665	327	9.03
26727	Treat finger fracture, each	787	978	1215	536	14.80
26735	Treat finger fracture, each	1073	1333	1657	570	15.74
26740	Treat finger fracture, each	356	443	550	219	6.04
26742	Treat finger fracture, each	496	616	766	418	11.55
26746	Treat finger fracture, each	1219	1515	1882	560	15.48
26750	Treat finger fracture, each	220	273	340	201	5.55
26755	Treat finger fracture, each	341	424	527	310	8.55
26756	Pin finger fracture, each	562	698	867	496	13.69
26765	Treat finger fracture, each	738	916	1139	460	12.70
26770	Treat finger dislocation	447	556	691	295	8.16
26775	Treat finger dislocation	560	695	864	370	10.21
26776	Pin finger dislocation	770	957	1189	508	14.04
26785	Treat finger dislocation	696	865	1075	460	12.70
26820	Thumb fuse with graft	1380	1715	2131	911	25.17
26841	Fuse thumb	1287	1599	1987	850	23.47
26842	Thumb fuse with graft	1361	1692	2102	899	24.83
26843	Fuse hand joint	1178	1464	1819	815	22.51
26844	Fuse/graft hand joint	1397	1736	2157	922	25.48
26850	Fuse knuckle	1086	1349	1676	814	22.49
26852	Fuse knuckle with graft	1237	1537	1910	894	24.70
26860	Fuse finger joint	887	1103	1370	678	18.74
26861	Fuse finger jnt, add-on	443	550	683	107	2.95

NEW CODE CPT 2002 •

CPT	SHORT DESCRIPTION	50th	75th	90th	MFS	RVU
26862	Fuse/graft finger joint	1141	1418	1762	850	23.47
26863	Fuse/graft added joint	495	615	764	241	6.66
26910	Amputate metacarpal bone	1137	1413	1756	814	22.48
26951	Amputate finger/thumb	898	1116	1386	659	18.21
26952	Amputate finger/thumb	1032	1282	1593	779	21.52
26989	Hand/finger surgery	0	0	0	0	.00

PELVIS AND HIP JOINT

CPT	SHORT DESCRIPTION	50th	75th	90th	MFS	RVU
26990	Drain pelvis lesion	942	1143	1416	880	24.32
26991	Drain pelvis bursa	778	944	1170	682	18.85
26992	Drain bone lesion	3782	4586	5684	1257	34.72
27000	Incise hip tendon	1510	1831	2269	502	13.86
27001	Incise hip tendon	712	864	1071	590	16.31
27003	Incise hip tendon	816	990	1227	626	17.28
27005	Incise hip tendon	960	1164	1443	779	21.52
27006	Incise hip tendons	974	1181	1464	782	21.60
27025	Incise hip/thigh fascia	1469	1782	2208	835	23.07
27030	Drain hip joint	1828	2217	2747	987	27.27
27033	Explore hip joint	1598	1937	2401	1009	27.88
27035	Denervation hip joint	1947	2361	2926	1378	38.06
27036	Excise hip joint/muscle	1919	2326	2884	1039	28.71
27040	Biopsy soft tissues	1014	1230	1524	337	9.31
27041	Biopsy soft tissues	2124	2576	3192	706	19.50
27047	Remove hip/pelvis lesion	721	874	1084	633	17.50
27048	Remove hip/pelvis lesion	1415	1716	2127	540	14.92
27049	Remove tumor hip/pelvis	3325	4032	4998	1051	29.03
27050	Biopsy sacroiliac joint	755	916	1135	449	12.41

CPT	SHORT DESCRIPTION	50th	75th	90th	MFS	RVU
27052	Biopsy hip joint	1669	2024	2508	555	15.32
27054	Remove hip joint lining	2378	2884	3574	738	20.38
27060	Remove ischial bursa	744	902	1118	479	13.24
27062	Remove femur lesion/bursa	721	874	1084	486	13.43
27065	Remove hip bone lesion	970	1176	1458	554	15.31
27066	Remove hip bone lesion	1545	1874	2323	879	24.28
27067	Remove/graft hip bone lesion	1991	2415	2993	1098	30.32
27070	Partial remove hip bone	3245	3935	4877	1078	29.79
27071	Partial remove hip bone	1639	1987	2463	1145	31.64
27075	Extensive hip surgery	2868	3477	4310	2279	62.97
27076	Extensive hip surgery	3566	4324	5360	1631	45.06
27077	Extensive hip surgery	5166	6265	7765	2669	73.73
27078	Extensive hip surgery	1406	1705	2113	1137	31.41
27079	Extensive hip surgery	2318	2811	3484	1051	29.04
27080	Remove tail bone	969	1175	1457	537	14.83
27086	Remove hip foreign body	859	1042	1292	286	7.89
27087	Remove hip foreign body	839	1017	1261	676	18.67
27090	Remove hip prosthesis	1354	1642	2035	871	24.07
27091	Remove hip prosthesis	4037	4895	6067	1462	40.39
27093	Inject for hip x-ray	1632	1979	2452	542	14.98
27095	Inject for hip x-ray	1131	1409	1778	456	12.60
27096	Inject sacroiliac joint	517	627	777	374	10.34
27097	Revise hip tendon	1784	2163	2681	657	18.15
27098	Transfer tendon to pelvis	1967	2385	2956	697	19.25
27100	Transfer abdominal muscle	2402	2912	3610	930	25.68
27105	Transfer spinal muscle	2433	2951	3657	926	25.57

NEW CODE CPT 2002 •

CPT	SHORT DESCRIPTION	50th	75th	90th	MFS	RVU
27110	Transfer iliopsoas muscle	3010	3649	4523	1000	27.63
27111	Transfer iliopsoas muscle	2010	2437	3020	919	25.40
27120	Reconstruct hip socket	2903	3521	4364	1258	34.74
27122	Reconstruct hip socket	2565	3111	3856	1142	31.54
27125	Partial hip replacement	3521	4269	5292	1113	30.76
27130	Total hip arthroplasty	5717	6933	8593	1452	40.12
27132	Total hip arthroplasty	5824	7062	8753	1649	45.56
27134	Revise hip joint replacement	7121	8634	10702	1966	54.31
27137	Revise hip joint replacement	4904	5946	7370	1509	41.68
27138	Revise hip joint replacement	4708	5709	7076	1565	43.22
27140	Transplant femur ridge	1260	1528	1894	937	25.89
27146	Incise hip bone	2322	2815	3489	1288	35.57
27147	Revise hip bone	3284	3982	4936	1486	41.06
27151	Incise hip bones	3042	3689	4572	1614	44.60
27156	Revise hip bones	3873	4697	5821	1736	47.95
27158	Revise pelvis	3654	4431	5493	1373	37.92
27161	Incise neck femur	2271	2754	3413	1213	33.50
27165	Incise/fixation femur	2890	3505	4344	1279	35.34
27170	Repair/graft femur head/neck	3061	3712	4600	1174	32.43
27175	Treat slipped epiphysis	1724	2091	2591	612	16.91
27176	Treat slipped epiphysis	2436	2954	3662	867	23.96
27177	Treat slipped epiphysis	2962	3592	4452	1065	29.41
27178	Treat slipped epiphysis	2592	3143	3896	862	23.80
27179	Revise head/neck femur	2031	2462	3052	931	25.72
27181	Treat slipped epiphysis	2841	3445	4270	1026	28.34
27185	Revise femur epiphysis	1263	1532	1899	742	20.51

CPT	SHORT DESCRIPTION	50th	75th	90th	MFS	RVU
27187	Reinforce hip bones	2714	3291	4079	1048	28.96
27193	Treat pelvic ring fracture	845	992	1203	488	13.47
27194	Treat pelvic ring fracture	1095	1286	1559	730	20.17
27200	Treat tail bone fracture	313	367	445	188	5.19
27202	Treat tail bone fracture	2915	3424	4149	1062	29.35
27215	Treat pelvic fracture(s)	2187	2569	3113	797	22.02
27216	Treat pelvic ring fracture	3262	3832	4644	1189	32.85
27217	Treat pelvic ring fracture	2344	2754	3337	1046	28.89
27218	Treat pelvic ring fracture	2630	3089	3744	1436	39.68
27220	Treat hip socket fracture	672	790	957	525	14.51
27222	Treat hip socket fracture	1369	1608	1948	899	24.84
27226	Treat hip wall fracture	2090	2455	2976	990	27.34
27227	Treat hip fracture(s)	2591	3044	3689	1590	43.91
27228	Treat hip fracture(s)	5025	5902	7154	1832	50.60
27230	Treat thigh fracture	730	858	1040	501	13.85
27232	Treat thigh fracture	1437	1688	2046	776	21.44
27235	Treat thigh fracture	3037	3567	4323	909	25.11
27236	Treat thigh fracture	3431	4031	4885	1114	30.77
27238	Treat thigh fracture	699	821	995	458	12.64
27240	Treat thigh fracture	1191	1399	1696	889	24.57
27244	Treat thigh fracture	3240	3806	4612	1137	31.42
27245	Treat thigh fracture	3122	3667	4444	1403	38.77
27246	Treat thigh fracture	1259	1479	1793	459	12.68
27248	Treat thigh fracture	846	994	1204	800	22.10
27250	Treat hip dislocation	640	752	911	513	14.18
27252	Treat hip dislocation	928	1090	1321	727	20.07

  NEW CODE CPT 2002 •

CPT	SHORT DESCRIPTION	50th	75th	90th	MFS	RVU
27253	Treat hip dislocation	1776	2086	2528	935	25.83
27254	Treat hip dislocation	2355	2766	3352	1270	35.07
27256	Treat hip dislocation	983	1154	1399	323	8.92
27257	Treat hip dislocation	1134	1332	1615	375	10.37
27258	Treat hip dislocation	2489	2923	3543	1137	31.42
27259	Treat hip dislocation	2844	3340	4048	1541	42.56
27265	Treat hip dislocation	629	739	896	427	11.79
27266	Treat hip dislocation	1133	1330	1612	580	16.03
27275	Manipulate hip joint	564	663	803	224	6.20
27280	Fuse sacroiliac joint	2267	2663	3228	1061	29.32
27282	Fuse pubic bones	2438	2863	3470	898	24.81
27284	Fuse hip joint	3148	3698	4482	1617	44.67
27286	Fuse hip joint	3463	4068	4930	1627	44.95
27290	Amputate leg at hip	4329	5085	6163	1578	43.59
27295	Amputate leg at hip	3589	4215	5109	1291	35.65
27299	Pelvis/hip joint surgery	0	0	0	0	.00

FEMUR (THIGH REGION) AND KNEE JOINT

CPT	SHORT DESCRIPTION	50th	75th	90th	MFS	RVU
27301	Drain thigh/knee lesion	986	1166	1408	818	22.59
27303	Drain bone lesion	1050	1242	1500	871	24.05
27305	Incise thigh tendon & fascia	832	984	1189	564	15.57
27306	Incise thigh tendon	644	762	920	463	12.78
27307	Incise thigh tendons	896	1060	1280	533	14.73
27310	Explore knee joint	1955	2313	2793	749	20.70
27315	Partial remove thigh nerve	1476	1745	2108	427	11.80
27320	Partial remove thigh nerve	1520	1797	2171	440	12.15
27323	Biopsy thigh soft tissues	1003	1186	1433	290	8.02

CPT	SHORT DESCRIPTION	50th	75th	90th	MFS	RVU
27324	Biopsy thigh soft tissues	754	892	1077	445	12.28
27327	Remove thigh lesion	616	728	880	487	13.44
27328	Remove thigh lesion	1086	1285	1552	486	13.42
27329	Remove tumor thigh/knee	4084	4830	5834	1116	30.84
27330	Biopsy knee joint lining	1507	1782	2153	436	12.05
27331	Explore/treat knee joint	1782	2108	2546	516	14.25
27332	Remove knee cartilage	2239	2648	3198	661	18.26
27333	Remove knee cartilage	3044	3600	4348	609	16.82
27334	Remove knee joint lining	2389	2826	3413	713	19.71
27335	Remove knee joint lining	2693	3185	3847	796	21.99
27340	Remove kneecap bursa	1028	1216	1469	391	10.79
27345	Remove knee cyst	1394	1648	1991	515	14.22
27347	Remove knee cyst	1839	2175	2627	332	9.18
27350	Remove kneecap	2042	2415	2917	661	18.27
27355	Remove femur lesion	1674	1980	2391	691	19.08
27356	Remove femur lesion/graft	1950	2306	2785	800	22.09
27357	Remove femur lesion/graft	2316	2739	3308	860	23.76
27358	Remove femur lesion/fixation	1036	1225	1479	293	8.10
27360	Partial remove leg bone(s)	1575	1863	2250	1099	30.35
27365	Extensive leg surgery	4155	4914	5935	1203	33.22
27370	Inject for knee x-ray	1516	1792	2165	439	12.12
27372	Remove foreign body	747	883	1067	519	14.35
27380	Repair kneecap tendon	1712	2024	2445	606	16.73
27381	Repair/graft kneecap tendon	1782	2107	2545	801	22.12
27385	Repair thigh muscle	2004	2370	2862	644	17.78
27386	Repair/graft thigh muscle	2137	2528	3053	839	23.17

  NEW CODE CPT 2002 •

CPT	SHORT DESCRIPTION	50th	75th	90th	MFS	RVU
27390	Incise thigh tendon	621	735	887	515	14.24
27391	Incise thigh tendons	927	1096	1324	625	17.27
27392	Incise thigh tendons	1378	1630	1969	781	21.58
27393	Lengthen thigh tendon	725	858	1036	570	15.74
27394	Lengthen thigh tendons	1277	1511	1825	730	20.18
27395	Lengthen thigh tendons	1757	2078	2510	961	26.55
27396	Transplant thigh tendon	1468	1736	2097	674	18.62
27397	Transplants thigh tendons	1610	1904	2300	889	24.57
27400	Revise thigh muscles/tendons	1384	1636	1977	755	20.87
27403	Repair knee cartilage	2060	2436	2943	665	18.37
27405	Repair knee ligament	1961	2319	2801	712	19.67
27407	Repair knee ligament	2184	2583	3119	808	22.33
27409	Repair knee ligaments	2744	3245	3920	969	26.76
27418	Repair degenerated kneecap	2650	3134	3786	845	23.35
27420	Revise unstable kneecap	2148	2540	3069	763	21.08
27422	Revise unstable kneecap	2566	3034	3665	759	20.98
27424	Revise/remove kneecap	2144	2536	3063	758	20.94
27425	Lateral retinacular release	2209	2613	3156	479	13.24
27427	Reconstruct knee	2536	2999	3622	732	20.22
27428	Reconstruct knee	3527	4171	5038	1043	28.80
27429	Reconstruct knee	3448	4078	4925	1136	31.39
27430	Revise thigh muscles	1658	1961	2368	757	20.92
27435	Incise knee joint	1584	1874	2263	742	20.50
27437	Revise kneecap	1788	2114	2554	713	19.70
27438	Revise kneecap with implant	1942	2297	2774	873	24.13
27440	Revise knee joint	2105	2489	3006	824	22.77

CPT	SHORT DESCRIPTION	50th	75th	90th	MFS	RVU
27441	Revise knee joint	2579	3050	3684	852	23.55
27442	Revise knee joint	2375	2809	3393	917	25.34
27443	Revise knee joint	2697	3189	3852	869	24.01
27445	Revise knee joint	3691	4365	5272	1272	35.15
27446	Revise knee joint	3727	4407	5324	1170	32.32
27447	Total knee arthroplasty	5559	6574	7941	1514	41.83
27448	Incise thigh	1975	2336	2822	889	24.55
27450	Incise thigh	2406	2845	3437	1078	29.77
27454	Realignment thigh bone	2428	2871	3468	1298	35.85
27455	Realignment knee	1825	2158	2606	984	27.17
27457	Realignment knee	2204	2606	3148	980	27.06
27465	Shortening thigh bone	2717	3213	3881	1079	29.82
27466	Lengthen thigh bone	3354	3966	4791	1247	34.44
27468	Shorten/lengthen thighs	4384	5185	6262	1311	36.22
27470	Repair thigh	2328	2753	3325	1245	34.38
27472	Repair/graft thigh	3029	3582	4326	1346	37.19
27475	Surgery to stop leg growth	2304	2725	3291	698	19.28
27477	Surgery to stop leg growth	2589	3062	3699	770	21.26
27479	Surgery to stop leg growth	3139	3713	4484	967	26.70
27485	Surgery to stop leg growth	1911	2260	2730	705	19.48
27486	Revise/replace knee joint	3658	4326	5225	1379	38.10
27487	Revise/replace knee joint	6693	7916	9561	1740	48.07
27488	Remove knee prosthesis	3025	3577	4321	1164	32.16
27495	Reinforce thigh	1953	2310	2790	1213	33.51
27496	Decompression thigh/knee	787	931	1124	537	14.84
27497	Decompression thigh/knee	1022	1208	1460	585	16.17

NEW CODE CPT 2002 •

CPT	SHORT DESCRIPTION	50th	75th	90th	MFS	RVU
27498	Decompression thigh/knee	1023	1210	1461	627	17.33
27499	Decompression thigh/knee	1292	1528	1845	710	19.60
27500	Treat thigh fracture	869	1052	1310	599	16.56
27501	Treat thigh fracture	1070	1295	1613	640	17.67
27502	Treat thigh fracture	1785	2161	2691	845	23.34
27503	Treat thigh fracture	1500	1815	2261	845	23.33
27506	Treat thigh fracture	3583	4336	5402	1243	34.35
27507	Treat thigh fracture	2336	2827	3522	1032	28.52
27508	Treat thigh fracture	756	915	1140	500	13.80
27509	Treat thigh fracture	1521	1840	2293	660	18.23
27510	Treat thigh fracture	1023	1238	1542	643	17.76
27511	Treat thigh fracture	2484	3006	3745	1047	28.93
27513	Treat thigh fracture	2886	3492	4350	1311	36.23
27514	Treat thigh fracture	2355	2850	3550	1240	34.26
27516	Treat thigh fracture growth plate	757	916	1141	510	14.09
27517	Treat thigh fracture growth plate	953	1154	1437	722	19.94
27519	Treat thigh fracture growth plate	2039	2468	3074	1094	30.22
27520	Treat kneecap fracture	577	699	870	316	8.72
27524	Treat kneecap fracture	2091	2530	3152	738	20.38
27530	Treat knee fracture	694	840	1047	372	10.29
27532	Treat knee fracture	762	922	1148	578	15.97
27535	Treat knee fracture	2357	2852	3553	914	25.26
27536	Treat knee fracture	2016	2440	3039	1086	30.00
27538	Treat knee fracture(s)	592	716	892	477	13.18
27540	Treat knee fracture	1722	2084	2596	929	25.65
27550	Treat knee dislocation	1205	1459	1817	508	14.04

CPT	SHORT DESCRIPTION	50th	75th	90th	MFS	RVU
27552	Treat knee dislocation	1463	1770	2205	617	17.04
27556	Treat knee dislocation	2041	2470	3076	1117	30.87
27557	Treat knee dislocation	2755	3334	4154	1264	34.92
27558	Treat knee dislocation	3103	3755	4677	1308	36.14
27560	Treat kneecap dislocation	396	479	596	366	10.11
27562	Treat kneecap dislocation	455	551	687	440	12.15
27566	Treat kneecap dislocation	1404	1699	2117	871	24.05
27570	Fixation knee joint	502	608	757	189	5.22
27580	Fuse knee	2214	2679	3337	1401	38.70
27590	Amputate leg at thigh	2093	2533	3155	943	26.05
27591	Amputate leg at thigh	1876	2270	2828	1025	28.32
27592	Amputate leg at thigh	2038	2467	3073	859	23.74
27594	Amputate follow-up surgery	760	920	1146	608	16.79
27596	Amputate follow-up surgery	1563	1892	2357	886	24.48
27598	Amputate lower leg at knee	1832	2217	2762	849	23.46
27599	Leg surgery procedure	0	0	0	0	.00

LEG (TIBIA AND FIBULA) AND ANKLE JOINT

CPT	SHORT DESCRIPTION	50th	75th	90th	MFS	RVU
27600	Decompress lower leg	661	798	989	507	14.00
27601	Decompress lower leg	733	886	1097	507	14.01
27602	Decompress lower leg	1053	1272	1576	589	16.28
27603	Drain lower leg lesion	798	964	1193	779	21.53
27604	Drain lower leg bursa	1230	1486	1840	580	16.02
27605	Incise achilles tendon	1003	1212	1500	473	13.06
27606	Incise achilles tendon	1375	1661	2057	648	17.90
27607	Treat lower leg bone lesion	993	1199	1485	790	21.83
27610	Explore/treat ankle joint	1090	1317	1631	721	19.92

NEW CODE CPT 2002 •

CPT	SHORT DESCRIPTION	50th	75th	90th	MFS	RVU
27612	Explore ankle joint	1093	1321	1635	603	16.66
27613	Biopsy lower leg soft tissue	592	715	886	279	7.71
27614	Biopsy lower leg soft tissue	1318	1592	1971	621	17.16
27615	Remove tumor lower leg	2382	2878	3564	1123	31.02
27618	Remove lower leg lesion	659	796	986	628	17.35
27619	Remove lower leg lesion	1136	1372	1699	798	22.04
27620	Explore/treat ankle joint	1153	1393	1724	543	15.01
27625	Remove ankle joint lining	1529	1847	2287	689	19.03
27626	Remove ankle joint lining	1576	1905	2358	743	20.53
27630	Remove tendon lesion	855	1033	1279	583	16.10
27635	Remove lower leg bone lesion	1267	1531	1896	723	19.97
27637	Remove/graft leg bone lesion	1778	2149	2661	854	23.59
27638	Remove/graft leg bone lesion	1593	1925	2383	890	24.59
27640	Partial remove tibia	1632	1971	2441	1136	31.37
27641	Partial remove fibula	1361	1644	2036	977	26.98
27645	Extensive lower leg surgery	1846	2231	2762	1264	34.93
27646	Extensive lower leg surgery	1659	2004	2482	1184	32.71
27647	Extensive ankle/heel surgery	1665	2011	2490	912	25.19
27648	Inject for ankle x-ray	806	974	1206	380	10.50
27650	Repair achilles tendon	1984	2396	2967	747	20.64
27652	Repair/graft achilles tendon	1665	2011	2490	785	21.68
27654	Repair achilles tendon	1727	2086	2583	788	21.77
27656	Repair leg fascia defect	743	897	1111	595	16.43
27658	Repair leg tendon, each	851	1028	1273	590	16.29
27659	Repair leg tendon, each	1074	1297	1606	744	20.54
27664	Repair leg tendon, each	1772	2140	2650	835	23.07

CPT	SHORT DESCRIPTION	50th	75th	90th	MFS	RVU
27665	Repair leg tendon, each	858	1037	1284	547	15.10
27675	Repair lower leg tendons	760	918	1137	603	16.67
27676	Repair lower leg tendons	890	1075	1332	698	19.29
27680	Release lower leg tendon	765	925	1145	536	14.81
27681	Release lower leg tendons	866	1046	1295	602	16.62
27685	Revise lower leg tendon	1212	1465	1814	644	17.78
27686	Revise lower leg tendons	1829	2209	2736	862	23.81
27687	Revise calf tendon	832	1005	1245	573	15.82
27690	Revise lower leg tendon	1236	1493	1849	707	19.54
27691	Revise lower leg tendon	1433	1731	2144	813	22.46
27692	Revise additional leg tendon	231	279	346	113	3.12
27695	Repair ankle ligament	1451	1753	2171	601	16.61
27696	Repair ankle ligaments	1797	2172	2689	687	18.97
27698	Repair ankle ligament	2342	2829	3503	738	20.39
27700	Revise ankle joint	2038	2462	3049	669	18.48
27702	Reconstruct ankle joint	3436	4151	5140	1036	28.61
27703	Reconstruct ankle joint	2871	3468	4295	1137	31.42
27704	Remove ankle implant	1224	1478	1831	638	17.63
27705	Incise tibia	1547	1869	2315	846	23.37
27707	Incise fibula	814	983	1218	487	13.45
27709	Incise tibia & fibula	1752	2117	2622	826	22.82
27712	Realignment lower leg	1955	2362	2924	1092	30.17
27715	Revise lower leg	2491	3010	3727	1144	31.61
27720	Repair tibia	2083	2516	3116	982	27.12
27722	Repair/graft tibia	2094	2530	3133	975	26.93
27724	Repair/graft tibia	2577	3113	3855	1360	37.58

    NEW CODE CPT 2002 •

CPT	SHORT DESCRIPTION	50th	75th	90th	MFS	RVU
27725	Repair lower leg	2845	3438	4257	1209	33.41
27727	Repair lower leg	2325	2809	3479	1096	30.28
27730	Repair tibia epiphysis	1156	1396	1729	1075	29.70
27732	Repair fibula epiphysis	935	1129	1399	738	20.40
27734	Repair lower leg epiphyses	1549	1871	2317	730	20.17
27740	Repair leg epiphyses	2047	2473	3062	965	26.65
27742	Repair leg epiphyses	2173	2625	3250	1024	28.29
27745	Reinforce tibia	1803	2178	2697	834	23.05
27750	Treat tibia fracture	746	901	1115	336	9.27
27752	Treat tibia fracture	1157	1398	1731	538	14.86
27756	Treat tibia fracture	1381	1668	2065	672	18.56
27758	Treat tibia fracture	2705	3268	4046	920	25.41
27759	Treat tibia fracture	2887	3488	4320	1055	29.15
27760	Treat ankle fracture	530	641	793	319	8.82
27762	Treat ankle fracture	613	741	917	490	13.53
27766	Treat ankle fracture	1598	1930	2390	644	17.79
27780	Treat fibula fracture	429	518	641	302	8.35
27781	Treat fibula fracture	871	1053	1304	411	11.35
27784	Treat fibula fracture	1055	1274	1578	605	16.72
27786	Treat ankle fracture	524	633	784	311	8.59
27788	Treat ankle fracture	805	972	1204	424	11.71
27792	Treat ankle fracture	1571	1898	2350	612	16.91
27808	Treat ankle fracture	624	754	933	349	9.65
27810	Treat ankle fracture	1085	1310	1623	493	13.61
27814	Treat ankle fracture	2097	2534	3138	837	23.11
27816	Treat ankle fracture	496	599	742	334	9.23

CPT	SHORT DESCRIPTION	50th	75th	90th	MFS	RVU
27818	Treat ankle fracture	923	1115	1380	511	14.13
27822	Treat ankle fracture	2309	2790	3454	922	25.47
27823	Treat ankle fracture	2113	2553	3161	1051	29.04
27824	Treat lower leg fracture	655	791	979	351	9.71
27825	Treat lower leg fracture	859	1037	1285	555	15.34
27826	Treat lower leg fracture	1674	2022	2504	782	21.61
27827	Treat lower leg fracture	2803	3387	4194	1123	31.02
27828	Treat lower leg fracture	2251	2720	3368	1214	33.53
27829	Treat lower leg joint	1458	1761	2181	540	14.93
27830	Treat lower leg dislocation	772	932	1154	364	10.05
27831	Treat lower leg dislocation	489	591	731	366	10.11
27832	Treat lower leg dislocation	998	1205	1493	560	15.46
27840	Treat ankle dislocation	865	1045	1293	408	11.26
27842	Treat ankle dislocation	551	666	824	442	12.22
27846	Treat ankle dislocation	1406	1699	2104	782	21.61
27848	Treat ankle dislocation	1568	1894	2345	885	24.45
27860	Fixation ankle joint	326	394	488	233	6.43
27870	Fuse ankle joint	2950	3565	4414	1072	29.62
27871	Fuse tibiofibular joint	1622	1959	2426	778	21.49
27880	Amputate lower leg	2068	2498	3093	911	25.18
27881	Amputate lower leg	1789	2162	2677	991	27.37
27882	Amputate lower leg	1251	1512	1872	836	23.10
27884	Amputate follow-up surgery	1531	1850	2291	722	19.94
27886	Amputate follow-up surgery	1653	1997	2472	786	21.71
27888	Amputate foot at ankle	1693	2045	2532	798	22.04
27889	Amputate foot at ankle	1660	2006	2484	783	21.62

NEW CODE CPT 2002 •

CPT	SHORT DESCRIPTION	50th	75th	90th	MFS	RVU
27892	Decompress leg	1029	1244	1540	603	16.66
27893	Decompress leg	1044	1262	1562	609	16.83
27894	Decompress leg	1346	1626	2014	790	21.83
27899	Leg/ankle surgery procedure	0	0	0	0	.00

FOOT AND TOES

CPT	SHORT DESCRIPTION	50th	75th	90th	MFS	RVU
28001	Drain bursa foot	561	711	1024	313	8.66
28002	Treat foot infection	603	764	1101	433	11.96
28003	Treat foot infection	876	1111	1600	754	20.84
28005	Treat foot bone lesion	1109	1406	2026	727	20.08
28008	Incise foot fascia	812	1029	1483	477	13.18
28010	Incise toe tendon	704	893	1286	393	10.87
28011	Incise toe tendons	912	1156	1666	510	14.08
28020	Explore foot joint	883	1119	1613	498	13.77
28022	Explore foot joint	787	998	1438	477	13.19
28024	Explore toe joint	632	801	1155	486	13.43
28030	Remove foot nerve	951	1206	1738	380	10.50
28035	Decompress tibia nerve	1566	1985	2860	529	14.60
28043	Excise foot lesion	544	689	993	415	11.46
28045	Excise foot lesion	847	1074	1547	489	13.52
28046	Resect tumor foot	3575	4533	6530	901	24.89
28050	Biopsy foot joint lining	927	1176	1694	518	14.32
28052	Biopsy foot joint lining	747	947	1364	451	12.46
28054	Biopsy toe joint lining	564	716	1031	420	11.60
28060	Partial remove foot fascia	988	1253	1805	530	14.64
28062	Remove foot fascia	1561	1980	2852	602	16.64
28070	Remove foot joint lining	740	939	1352	498	13.76

CPT	SHORT DESCRIPTION	50th	75th	90th	MFS	RVU
28072	Remove foot joint lining	566	717	1033	509	14.06
28080	Remove foot lesion	850	1077	1552	431	11.90
28086	Excise foot tendon sheath	971	1231	1773	627	17.31
28088	Excise foot tendon sheath	929	1178	1698	519	14.35
28090	Remove foot lesion	778	987	1422	474	13.10
28092	Remove toe lesions	501	635	915	444	12.27
28100	Remove ankle/heel lesion	1257	1594	2297	706	19.49
28102	Remove/graft foot lesion	1641	2081	2998	641	17.70
28103	Remove/graft foot lesion	1386	1758	2532	585	16.15
28104	Remove foot lesion	996	1263	1819	518	14.30
28106	Remove/graft foot lesion	1279	1622	2336	548	15.14
28107	Remove/graft foot lesion	1255	1591	2292	589	16.26
28108	Remove toe lesions	725	920	1325	441	12.17
28110	Part remove metatarsal	905	1148	1654	484	13.37
28111	Part remove metatarsal	1046	1326	1911	533	14.73
28112	Part remove metatarsal	873	1107	1595	506	13.98
28113	Part remove metatarsal	865	1096	1579	519	14.34
28114	Remove metatarsal heads	1735	2200	3170	851	23.51
28116	Revise foot	1333	1690	2435	653	18.05
28118	Remove heel bone	1244	1577	2272	584	16.12
28119	Remove heel spur	1198	1520	2189	532	14.71
28120	Part remove ankle/heel	1250	1585	2284	629	17.37
28122	Partial remove foot bone	1094	1388	1999	695	19.19
28124	Partial remove toe	758	961	1384	546	15.07
28126	Partial remove toe	700	887	1278	448	12.38
28130	Remove ankle bone	1522	1930	2781	651	17.99

NEW CODE CPT 2002 •

CPT	SHORT DESCRIPTION	50th	75th	90th	MFS	RVU
28140	Remove metatarsal	1157	1467	2114	657	18.15
28150	Remove toe	765	969	1397	484	13.36
28153	Partial remove toe	716	908	1309	454	12.54
28160	Partial remove toe	787	998	1438	463	12.80
28171	Extensive foot surgery	1371	1738	2505	688	19.00
28173	Extensive foot surgery	1132	1436	2069	748	20.67
28175	Extensive foot surgery	823	1043	1503	591	16.34
28190	Remove foot foreign body	631	821	1177	313	8.66
28192	Remove foot foreign body	566	738	1057	484	13.36
28193	Remove foot foreign body	995	1296	1856	554	15.30
28200	Repair foot tendon	995	1295	1856	494	13.66
28202	Repair/graft foot tendon	1385	1803	2583	736	20.33
28208	Repair foot tendon	543	707	1013	475	13.13
28210	Repair/graft foot tendon	734	955	1369	614	16.95
28220	Release foot tendon	886	1154	1653	481	13.28
28222	Release foot tendons	1069	1392	1994	535	14.79
28225	Release foot tendon	469	611	875	431	11.92
28226	Release foot tendons	628	818	1172	487	13.45
28230	Incise foot tendon(s)	515	670	960	474	13.09
28232	Incise toe tendon	471	613	879	434	11.99
28234	Incise foot tendon	439	572	820	428	11.81
28238	Revise foot tendon	1508	1964	2813	673	18.58
28240	Release big toe	608	792	1135	476	13.14
28250	Revise foot fascia	1074	1398	2003	571	15.78
28260	Release midfoot joint	1463	1904	2728	727	20.08
28261	Revise foot tendon	1776	2312	3313	889	24.55

CPT	SHORT DESCRIPTION	50th	75th	90th	MFS	RVU
28262	Revise foot and ankle	2720	3541	5074	1220	33.71
28264	Release midfoot joint	1660	2161	3096	825	22.79
28270	Release foot contracture	567	738	1057	513	14.18
28272	Release toe joint, each	465	605	867	435	12.02
28280	Fuse toes	752	979	1402	518	14.30
28285	Repair hammertoe	922	1201	1720	508	14.02
28286	Repair hammertoe	916	1193	1709	506	13.98
28288	Partial remove foot bone	962	1252	1794	521	14.39
28289	Repair hallux rigidus	1132	1474	2111	671	18.54
28290	Correct bunion	1321	1721	2465	579	16.00
28292	Correct bunion	1520	1980	2836	646	17.84
28293	Correct bunion	1742	2268	3249	764	21.10
28294	Correct bunion	1474	1919	2749	733	20.24
28296	Correct bunion	1922	2503	3586	771	21.30
28297	Correct bunion	1696	2208	3164	843	23.29
28298	Correct bunion	1436	1870	2679	694	19.16
28299	Correct bunion	2031	2645	3789	846	23.37
28300	Incise heel bone	1586	2065	2959	905	25.00
28302	Incise ankle bone	1475	1920	2751	733	20.25
28304	Incise midfoot bones	1267	1650	2363	713	19.69
28305	Incise/graft midfoot bones	1419	1847	2646	926	25.57
28306	Incise metatarsal	1276	1661	2380	561	15.51
28307	Incise metatarsal	1360	1771	2537	751	20.74
28308	Incise metatarsal	1052	1370	1963	507	14.00
28309	Incise metatarsals	1178	1533	2197	923	25.50
28310	Revise big toe	898	1170	1676	550	15.19

NEW CODE CPT 2002 •

CPT	SHORT DESCRIPTION	50th	75th	90th	MFS	RVU
28312	Revise toe	698	909	1302	501	13.83
28313	Repair deformity toe	605	788	1129	534	14.75
28315	Remove sesamoid bone	921	1199	1718	488	13.47
28320	Repair foot bones	1088	1417	2030	705	19.47
28322	Repair metatarsals	1119	1457	2088	768	21.22
28340	Resect enlarged toe tissue	1112	1448	2075	612	16.92
28341	Resect enlarged toe	1212	1578	2260	693	19.14
28344	Repair extra toe(s)	917	1194	1711	443	12.24
28345	Repair webbed toe(s)	1010	1315	1884	588	16.24
28360	Reconstruct cleft foot	1890	2462	3526	993	27.44
28400	Treat heel fracture	515	643	819	297	8.21
28405	Treat heel fracture	644	804	1025	429	11.86
28406	Treat heel fracture	857	1070	1363	574	15.87
28415	Treat heel fracture	2281	2848	3627	1228	33.93
28420	Treat/graft heel fracture	1889	2359	3004	1263	34.88
28430	Treat ankle fracture	497	620	790	275	7.61
28435	Treat ankle fracture	546	682	869	336	9.28
28436	Treat ankle fracture	779	973	1239	479	13.23
28445	Treat ankle fracture	1614	2016	2567	1117	30.85
28450	Treat midfoot fracture, each	434	542	691	269	7.43
28455	Treat midfoot fracture, each	532	664	846	327	9.03
28456	Treat midfoot fracture	701	876	1115	337	9.31
28465	Treat midfoot fracture, each	1051	1312	1671	584	16.13
28470	Treat metatarsal fracture	381	476	607	245	6.77
28475	Treat metatarsal fracture	551	688	877	310	8.56
28476	Treat metatarsal fracture	750	936	1193	382	10.55

CPT	SHORT DESCRIPTION	50th	75th	90th	MFS	RVU
28485	Treat metatarsal fracture	1163	1453	1850	531	14.67
28490	Treat big toe fracture	208	260	331	144	3.98
28495	Treat big toe fracture	270	337	429	166	4.59
28496	Treat big toe fracture	810	1011	1287	498	13.75
28505	Treat big toe fracture	743	927	1181	571	15.77
28510	Treat toe fracture	182	228	290	135	3.73
28515	Treat toe fracture	241	301	384	161	4.46
28525	Treat toe fracture	576	719	916	528	14.58
28530	Treat sesamoid bone fracture	246	308	392	148	4.10
28531	Treat sesamoid bone fracture	566	707	900	528	14.59
28540	Treat foot dislocation	284	355	452	218	6.03
28545	Treat foot dislocation	392	490	624	273	7.54
28546	Treat foot dislocation	955	1192	1518	587	16.21
28555	Repair foot dislocation	1086	1356	1727	748	20.67
28570	Treat foot dislocation	327	408	520	201	5.55
28575	Treat foot dislocation	519	648	825	324	8.95
28576	Treat foot dislocation	988	1234	1572	608	16.79
28585	Repair foot dislocation	1190	1486	1893	647	17.87
28600	Treat foot dislocation	264	329	419	233	6.45
28605	Treat foot dislocation	405	506	644	270	7.46
28606	Treat foot dislocation	1279	1597	2034	786	21.72
28615	Repair foot dislocation	1189	1485	1891	663	18.31
28630	Treat toe dislocation	212	265	337	153	4.22
28635	Treat toe dislocation	273	341	435	168	4.64
28636	Treat toe dislocation	428	534	680	289	7.97
28645	Repair toe dislocation	676	845	1076	416	11.49

   CPT codes and descriptions only copyright AMA   NEW CODE CPT 2002 •

CPT	SHORT DESCRIPTION	50th	75th	90th	MFS	RVU
28660	Treat toe dislocation	262	327	417	161	4.45
28665	Treat toe dislocation	211	264	336	168	4.63
28666	Treat toe dislocation	962	1201	1530	591	16.34
28675	Repair toe dislocation	522	652	831	464	12.81
28705	Fuse foot bones	2524	3152	4014	1325	36.60
28715	Fuse foot bones	2498	3119	3973	996	27.51
28725	Fuse foot bones	2223	2776	3536	895	24.72
28730	Fuse foot bones	1568	1958	2494	834	23.03
28735	Fuse foot bones	1605	2004	2553	826	22.81
28737	Revise foot bones	1379	1722	2193	725	20.04
28740	Fuse foot bones	1181	1475	1879	803	22.18
28750	Fuse big toe joint	1460	1823	2321	753	20.81
28755	Fuse big toe joint	861	1075	1369	504	13.92
28760	Fuse big toe joint	1007	1258	1602	695	19.21
28800	Amputate midfoot	1238	1545	1968	655	18.09
28805	Amputate thru metatarsal	1416	1769	2252	665	18.36
28810	Amputate toe & metatarsal	1070	1336	1701	539	14.88
28820	Amputate toe	742	926	1180	537	14.83
28825	Partial amputate toe	595	743	947	512	14.14
28899	Foot/toes surgery procedure	0	0	0	0	.00

APPLICATION OF CASTS AND STRAPPING

CPT	SHORT DESCRIPTION	50th	75th	90th	MFS	RVU
29000	Apply body cast	503	624	806	190	5.26
29010	Apply body cast	398	493	637	192	5.31
29015	Apply body cast	513	635	821	210	5.79
29020	Apply body cast	377	468	604	203	5.60
29025	Apply body cast	496	614	794	216	5.98

CPT	SHORT DESCRIPTION	50th	75th	90th	MFS	RVU
29035	Apply body cast	216	268	346	183	5.06
29040	Apply body cast	320	397	512	185	5.11
29044	Apply body cast	245	304	392	203	5.61
29046	Apply body cast	317	393	507	219	6.06
29049	Apply figure eight	111	138	179	75	2.08
29055	Apply shoulder cast	229	284	367	160	4.42
29058	Apply shoulder cast	146	181	234	101	2.78
29065	Apply long arm cast	168	208	268	76	2.09
29075	Apply forearm cast	137	169	219	70	1.93
29085	Apply hand/wrist cast	129	160	207	75	2.08
• 29086	Apply finger cast	94	116	150	54	1.50
29105	Apply long arm splint	114	142	183	73	2.03
29125	Apply forearm splint	83	103	134	55	1.53
29126	Apply forearm splint	128	158	205	74	2.04
29130	Apply finger splint	54	67	87	36	.99
29131	Apply finger splint	54	67	86	47	1.29
29200	Strap chest	97	120	155	56	1.54
29220	Strap low back	104	129	167	60	1.67
29240	Strap shoulder	106	131	170	61	1.68
29260	Strap elbow or wrist	90	112	145	52	1.44
29280	Strap hand or finger	92	114	148	53	1.46
29305	Apply hip cast	314	383	488	183	5.06
29325	Apply hip casts	344	419	534	206	5.68
29345	Apply long leg cast	237	289	369	112	3.10
29355	Apply long leg cast	241	294	375	116	3.20
29358	Apply long leg cast brace	281	343	437	121	3.34

    CPT codes and descriptions only copyright AMA   NEW CODE CPT 2002 •

CPT	SHORT DESCRIPTION	50th	75th	90th	MFS	RVU
29365	Apply long leg cast	210	255	326	99	2.73
29405	Apply short leg cast	171	208	265	73	2.01
29425	Apply short leg cast	204	248	317	80	2.20
29435	Apply short leg cast	263	320	408	98	2.70
29440	Addition walker to cast	84	102	130	45	1.25
29445	Apply rigid leg cast	342	416	531	130	3.60
29450	Apply leg cast	145	176	225	131	3.61
29505	Apply long leg splint	109	133	170	67	1.85
29515	Apply lower leg splint	96	117	150	57	1.58
29520	Strap hip	69	84	107	54	1.49
29530	Strap knee	64	77	99	52	1.44
29540	Strap ankle	50	61	78	34	.95
29550	Strap toes	47	57	73	33	.92
29580	Apply paste boot	86	105	133	45	1.23
29590	Apply foot splint	61	74	95	48	1.32
29700	Remove/revise cast	71	86	110	52	1.45
29705	Remove/revise cast	97	118	150	58	1.59
29710	Remove/revise cast	201	245	313	109	3.01
29715	Remove/revise cast	111	135	172	72	2.00
29720	Repair body cast	67	82	104	63	1.73
29730	Windowing cast	78	95	121	56	1.56
29740	Wedging cast	153	186	238	83	2.29
29750	Wedging clubfoot cast	170	207	265	92	2.55
29799	Casting/strap procedure	0	0	0	0	.00

ENDOSCOPY/ARTHROSCOPY

CPT	SHORT DESCRIPTION	50th	75th	90th	MFS	RVU
29800	Jaw arthroscopy/surgery	1366	1630	2038	594	16.42

CPT	SHORT DESCRIPTION	50th	75th	90th	MFS	RVU
29804	Jaw arthroscopy/surgery	2193	2616	3271	635	17.53
• 29805	Shoulder arthroscopy, dx	1493	1781	2227	360	9.95
• 29806	Shoulder arthroscopy/surgery	4159	4961	6204	1003	27.71
• 29807	Shoulder arthroscopy/surgery	4048	4829	6038	976	26.97
29819	Shoulder arthroscopy/surgery	1661	1981	2477	670	18.51
29820	Shoulder arthroscopy/surgery	1705	2034	2543	637	17.61
29821	Shoulder arthroscopy/surgery	2034	2427	3034	675	18.64
29822	Shoulder arthroscopy/surgery	2250	2684	3356	660	18.22
29823	Shoulder arthroscopy/surgery	2848	3398	4248	704	19.46
• 29824	Shoulder arthroscopy/surgery	2535	3024	3781	611	16.89
29825	Shoulder arthroscopy/surgery	1814	2163	2705	669	18.48
29826	Shoulder arthroscopy/surgery	2986	3562	4454	757	20.90
29830	Elbow arthroscopy	989	1180	1476	459	12.69
29834	Elbow arthroscopy/surgery	1673	1996	2495	510	14.08
29835	Elbow arthroscopy/surgery	1870	2231	2790	518	14.31
29836	Elbow arthroscopy/surgery	2256	2691	3365	588	16.23
29837	Elbow arthroscopy/surgery	1803	2151	2690	548	15.13
29838	Elbow arthroscopy/surgery	2181	2602	3253	598	16.51
29840	Wrist arthroscopy	1069	1275	1595	529	14.61
29843	Wrist arthroscopy/surgery	1153	1376	1720	562	15.53
29844	Wrist arthroscopy/surgery	1675	1998	2498	586	16.19
29845	Wrist arthroscopy/surgery	1883	2246	2808	649	17.92
29846	Wrist arthroscopy/surgery	2216	2644	3306	699	19.31
29847	Wrist arthroscopy/surgery	2180	2601	3252	718	19.84
29848	Wrist endoscopy/surgery	1599	1907	2384	529	14.62
29850	Knee arthroscopy/surgery	1683	2007	2510	594	16.42

NEW CODE CPT 2002 •

CPT	SHORT DESCRIPTION	50th	75th	90th	MFS	RVU
29851	Knee arthroscopy/surgery	1796	2142	2678	974	26.91
29855	Tibial arthroscopy/surgery	1837	2191	2740	821	22.67
29856	Tibial arthroscopy/surgery	1924	2295	2870	1036	28.63
29860	Hip arthroscopy, dx	943	1125	1406	624	17.24
29861	Hip arthroscopy/surgery	1576	1879	2350	693	19.15
29862	Hip arthroscopy/surgery	2564	3059	3825	762	21.04
29863	Hip arthroscopy/surgery	2129	2539	3175	782	21.61
29870	Knee arthroscopy, dx	1124	1341	1676	435	12.01
29871	Knee arthroscopy/drain	1403	1673	2092	572	15.81
29874	Knee arthroscopy/surgery	2147	2562	3203	582	16.07
29875	Knee arthroscopy/surgery	2207	2633	3293	539	14.88
29876	Knee arthroscopy/surgery	2718	3243	4055	660	18.22
29877	Knee arthroscopy/surgery	2387	2847	3560	603	16.67
29879	Knee arthroscopy/surgery	2637	3146	3934	646	17.85
29880	Knee arthroscopy/surgery	3260	3889	4862	675	18.64
29881	Knee arthroscopy/surgery	2680	3197	3997	629	17.38
29882	Knee arthroscopy/surgery	2898	3457	4323	679	18.75
29883	Knee arthroscopy/surgery	3183	3797	4748	825	22.79
29884	Knee arthroscopy/surgery	2268	2706	3383	624	17.23
29885	Knee arthroscopy/surgery	2632	3139	3926	732	20.21
29886	Knee arthroscopy/surgery	2058	2455	3070	637	17.59
29887	Knee arthroscopy/surgery	2450	2922	3654	729	20.14
29888	Knee arthroscopy/surgery	4785	5708	7137	1026	28.35
29889	Knee arthroscopy/surgery	3965	4729	5914	1152	31.82
29891	Ankle arthroscopy/surgery	2343	2795	3495	669	18.49
29892	Ankle arthroscopy/surgery	2705	3227	4035	699	19.30

CPT	SHORT DESCRIPTION	50th	75th	90th	MFS	RVU
29893	Scope plantar fasciotomy	1386	1654	2068	417	11.52
29894	Ankle arthroscopy/surgery	1797	2143	2680	589	16.26
29895	Ankle arthroscopy/surgery	1786	2130	2663	578	15.97
29897	Ankle arthroscopy/surgery	1682	2006	2508	612	16.92
29898	Ankle arthroscopy/surgery	2715	3239	4050	661	18.25
• **29900**	Mcp joint arthroscopy, dx	1799	2147	2684	434	11.99
• **29901**	Mcp joint arthroscopy, surgery	1984	2367	2960	479	13.22
• **29902**	Mcp joint arthroscopy, surgery	2130	2541	3177	514	14.19
• **29999**	Arthroscopy joint	0	0	0	0	.00

NEW CODE CPT 2002 •

CPT	SHORT DESCRIPTION	50th	75th	90th	MFS	RVU

RESPIRATORY SYSTEM

NOSE

CPT	SHORT DESCRIPTION	50th	75th	90th	MFS	RVU
30000	Drain nose lesion	377	462	592	147	4.06
30020	Drain nose lesion	385	472	606	150	4.15
30100	Intranasal biopsy	164	201	258	85	2.34
30110	Remove nose polyp(s)	237	290	373	165	4.55
30115	Remove nose polyp(s)	756	925	1188	333	9.20
30117	Remove intranasal lesion	590	723	928	302	8.33
30118	Remove intranasal lesion	1045	1279	1642	684	18.90
30120	Revise nose	1160	1420	1823	412	11.39
30124	Remove nose lesion	415	508	651	239	6.61
30125	Remove nose lesion	1510	1849	2372	518	14.31
30130	Remove turbinate bones	617	756	970	275	7.59
30140	Remove turbinate bones	895	1095	1406	300	8.28
30150	Partial remove nose	699	855	1098	678	18.73
30160	Remove nose	1123	1375	1764	693	19.15
30200	Inject treat nose	102	125	160	75	2.07
30210	Nasal sinus therapy	136	167	214	120	3.31
30220	Insert nasal septal button	355	435	558	151	4.17
30300	Remove nasal foreign body	347	424	545	135	3.73
30310	Remove nasal foreign body	373	457	587	146	4.02
30320	Remove nasal foreign body	926	1134	1456	367	10.14
30400	Reconstruct nose	1819	2227	2858	709	19.58
30410	Reconstruct nose	2303	2819	3618	887	24.51
30420	Reconstruct nose	3969	4859	6236	1072	29.62

CPT	SHORT DESCRIPTION	50th	75th	90th	MFS	RVU
30430	Revise nose	997	1220	1566	551	15.23
30435	Revise nose	1571	1924	2469	850	23.49
30450	Revise nose	2693	3297	4231	1251	34.55
30460	Revise nose	1358	1663	2134	723	19.97
30462	Revise nose	3325	4070	5224	1296	35.79
30465	Repair nasal stenosis	1480	1812	2325	803	22.19
30520	Repair nasal septum	1961	2400	3081	436	12.04
30540	Repair nasal defect	1392	1705	2188	543	14.99
30545	Repair nasal defect	1985	2430	3119	774	21.37
30560	Release nasal adhesions	185	226	290	135	3.72
30580	Repair upper jaw fistula	1132	1386	1779	441	12.19
30600	Repair mouth/nose fistula	1079	1321	1696	421	11.62
30620	Intranasal reconstruct	1793	2196	2818	475	13.11
30630	Repair nasal septum defect	1380	1690	2169	538	14.86
30801	Cauterize inner nose	223	274	351	135	3.74
30802	Cauterize inner nose	369	452	580	193	5.32
30901	Control nosebleed	152	186	239	99	2.73
30903	Control nosebleed	218	266	342	176	4.86
30905	Control nosebleed	370	454	582	216	5.97
30906	Repeat control nosebleed	364	445	571	249	6.89
30915	Ligate nasal sinus artery	1310	1603	2058	537	14.83
30920	Ligate upper jaw artery	1925	2357	3025	694	19.16
30930	Therapy fracture nose	285	348	447	127	3.52
30999	Nasal surgery procedure	0	0	0	0	.00

NEW CODE CPT 2002 •

CPT	SHORT DESCRIPTION	50th	75th	90th	MFS	RVU

ACCESSORY SINUSES

CPT	SHORT DESCRIPTION	50th	75th	90th	MFS	RVU
31000	Irrigate maxillary sinus	156	192	246	132	3.66
31002	Irrigate sphenoid sinus	211	258	331	149	4.12
31020	Explore maxillary sinus	650	796	1021	266	7.34
31030	Explore maxillary sinus	1429	1749	2245	405	11.19
31032	Explore sinus,remove polyps	1455	1781	2286	478	13.20
31040	Explore behind upper jaw	2868	3512	4507	632	17.47
31050	Explore sphenoid sinus	2009	2459	3156	391	10.79
31051	Sphenoid sinus surgery	2108	2580	3312	518	14.32
31070	Explore frontal sinus	1029	1260	1617	348	9.62
31075	Explore frontal sinus	1689	2067	2653	658	18.18
31080	Remove frontal sinus	1981	2426	3113	772	21.33
31081	Remove frontal sinus	2250	2755	3536	889	24.56
31084	Remove frontal sinus	2348	2875	3690	913	25.23
31085	Remove frontal sinus	2465	3018	3874	959	26.50
31086	Remove frontal sinus	2405	2944	3778	878	24.26
31087	Remove frontal sinus	2476	3032	3891	889	24.57
31090	Explore sinuses	3022	3700	4748	696	19.24
31200	Remove ethmoid sinus	1080	1323	1697	401	11.08
31201	Remove ethmoid sinus	1528	1870	2400	610	16.86
31205	Remove ethmoid sinus	1787	2187	2807	705	19.48
31225	Remove upper jaw	3347	4097	5259	1304	36.03
31230	Remove upper jaw	3783	4631	5943	1474	40.72
31231	Nasal endoscopy, dx	252	331	419	115	3.19
31233	Nasal/sinus endoscopy, dx	413	541	685	181	5.00
31235	Nasal/sinus endoscopy, dx	662	868	1100	208	5.75

CPT	SHORT DESCRIPTION	50th	75th	90th	MFS	RVU
31237	Nasal/sinus endoscopy, surgery	447	586	743	232	6.41
31238	Nasal/sinus endoscopy, surgery	515	675	855	262	7.24
31239	Nasal/sinus endoscopy, surgery	1659	2173	2755	575	15.88
31240	Nasal/sinus endoscopy, surgery	744	974	1235	160	4.41
31254	Revise ethmoid sinus	1430	1872	2374	281	7.76
31255	Remove ethmoid sinus	2021	2647	3356	420	11.59
31256	Explore maxillary sinus	1048	1373	1740	200	5.53
31267	Endoscopy maxillary sinus	1518	1988	2520	330	9.11
31276	Sinus endoscopy, surgical	1858	2434	3085	532	14.71
31287	Nasal/sinus endoscopy, surgery	1241	1625	2060	237	6.56
31288	Nasal/sinus endoscopy, surgery	1451	1900	2409	277	7.65
31290	Nasal/sinus endoscopy, surgery	2135	2797	3545	1097	30.30
31291	Nasal/sinus endoscopy, surgery	1933	2532	3209	1166	32.20
31292	Nasal/sinus endoscopy, surgery	1816	2379	3016	945	26.11
31293	Nasal/sinus endoscopy, surgery	1976	2588	3280	1026	28.34
31294	Nasal/sinus endoscopy, surgery	2291	3000	3803	1179	32.56
31299	Sinus surgery procedure	0	0	0	0	.00

LARYNX

CPT	SHORT DESCRIPTION	50th	75th	90th	MFS	RVU
31300	Remove larynx lesion	2864	3444	4273	1185	32.74
31320	Diagnostic incise larynx	1318	1585	1967	659	18.20
31360	Remove larynx	3555	4275	5304	1358	37.52
31365	Remove larynx	4962	5966	7404	1777	49.08
31367	Partial remove larynx	3629	4363	5415	1714	47.35
31368	Partial remove larynx	5461	6566	8148	2086	57.63
31370	Partial remove larynx	3580	4304	5341	1678	46.35
31375	Partial remove larynx	2785	3348	4155	1549	42.80

NEW CODE CPT 2002 •

CPT	SHORT DESCRIPTION	50th	75th	90th	MFS	RVU
31380	Partial remove larynx	2806	3373	4186	1557	43.02
31382	Partial remove larynx	2917	3507	4352	1630	45.02
31390	Remove larynx & pharynx	4643	5583	6928	2113	58.38
31395	Reconstruct larynx & pharynx	6232	7493	9298	2475	68.38
31400	Revise larynx	2475	2976	3693	969	26.78
31420	Remove epiglottis	1957	2353	2919	960	26.53
31500	Insert emergency airway	309	372	461	115	3.17
31502	Change windpipe airway	140	168	209	96	2.66
31505	Diagnostic laryngoscopy	92	111	137	90	2.50
31510	Laryngoscopy with biopsy	467	562	697	178	4.93
31511	Remove foreign body larynx	520	626	776	198	5.47
31512	Remove larynx lesion	610	733	910	189	5.23
31513	Inject into vocal cord	974	1172	1454	129	3.57
31515	Laryngoscopy for aspiration	360	433	537	153	4.22
31520	Diagnostic laryngoscopy	500	602	747	150	4.14
31525	Diagnostic laryngoscopy	464	558	692	208	5.75
31526	Diagnostic laryngoscopy	829	996	1236	157	4.34
31527	Laryngoscopy for treat	1025	1232	1529	190	5.25
31528	Laryngoscopy and dilation	613	737	915	136	3.77
31529	Laryngoscopy and dilation	513	617	765	162	4.48
31530	Operative laryngoscopy	650	781	969	200	5.52
31531	Operative laryngoscopy	777	935	1160	218	6.02
31535	Operative laryngoscopy	902	1084	1345	190	5.26
31536	Operative laryngoscopy	1152	1385	1719	216	5.97
31540	Operative laryngoscopy	841	1011	1255	250	6.90
31541	Operative laryngoscopy	1349	1622	2013	274	7.57

CPT	SHORT DESCRIPTION	50th	75th	90th	MFS	RVU
31560	Operative laryngoscopy	850	1022	1268	324	8.95
31561	Operative laryngoscopy	1073	1290	1601	340	9.38
31570	Laryngoscopy with inject	699	840	1042	292	8.08
31571	Laryngoscopy with inject	835	1004	1246	254	7.03
31575	Diagnostic laryngoscopy	293	352	436	118	3.26
31576	Laryngoscopy with biopsy	446	536	665	158	4.36
31577	Remove foreign body larynx	685	824	1022	201	5.54
31578	Remove larynx lesion	771	926	1150	223	6.17
31579	Diagnostic laryngoscopy	615	739	917	195	5.39
31580	Revise larynx	2315	2783	3453	1090	30.10
31582	Revise larynx	2154	2589	3213	1636	45.20
31584	Treat larynx fracture	2220	2670	3313	1452	40.11
31585	Treat larynx fracture	1313	1579	1959	502	13.86
31586	Treat larynx fracture	2018	2427	3012	771	21.30
31587	Revise larynx	1995	2399	2977	1001	27.64
31588	Revise larynx	2019	2427	3012	1131	31.24
31590	Reinnervate larynx	2231	2683	3329	728	20.10
31595	Larynx nerve surgery	1084	1303	1617	755	20.86
31599	Larynx surgery procedure	0	0	0	0	.00

TRACHEA AND BRONCHI

CPT	SHORT DESCRIPTION	50th	75th	90th	MFS	RVU
31600	Incise windpipe	914	1114	1339	386	10.67
31601	Incise windpipe	778	948	1140	255	7.04
31603	Incise windpipe	937	1143	1373	231	6.38
31605	Incise windpipe	712	868	1043	186	5.15
31610	Incise windpipe	1301	1586	1906	740	20.43
31611	Surgery/speech prosthesis	1533	1869	2246	591	16.32

NEW CODE CPT 2002 •

CPT	SHORT DESCRIPTION	50th	75th	90th	MFS	RVU
31612	Puncture/clear windpipe	192	234	281	90	2.50
31613	Repair windpipe opening	703	857	1030	503	13.90
31614	Repair windpipe opening	1469	1792	2153	728	20.10
31615	Visualization windpipe	469	572	687	217	5.99
31622	Dx bronchoscope/wash	663	808	971	239	6.61
31623	Dx bronchoscope/brush	656	800	962	217	5.99
31624	Dx bronchoscope/lavage	688	839	1008	209	5.76
31625	Bronchoscopy with biopsy	707	862	1036	235	6.49
31628	Bronchoscopy with biopsy	809	986	1185	265	7.33
31629	Bronchoscopy with biopsy	822	1002	1204	174	4.82
31630	Bronchoscopy with repair	673	821	986	221	6.11
31631	Bronchoscopy with dilation	801	977	1174	243	6.72
31635	Remove foreign body airway	980	1194	1435	202	5.59
31640	Bronchoscopy & remove lesion	1020	1243	1494	278	7.67
31641	Bronchoscopy, treat blockage	1381	1684	2024	273	7.53
31643	Diag bronchoscope/catheter	536	653	785	174	4.82
31645	Bronchoscopy, clear airways	671	818	983	165	4.56
31646	Bronchoscopy, reclear airway	533	649	780	143	3.96
31656	Bronchoscopy, inj for xray	452	552	663	120	3.32
31700	Insertion airway catheter	334	407	489	176	4.85
31708	Instill airway contrast dye	106	129	155	76	2.11
31710	Insertion airway catheter	145	177	213	76	2.11
31715	Inject for bronchus x-ray	142	173	208	69	1.90
31717	Bronchial brush biopsy	594	724	870	198	5.46
31720	Clearance airways	328	400	481	109	3.02
31725	Clearance airways	233	284	342	97	2.67

CPT	SHORT DESCRIPTION	50th	75th	90th	MFS	RVU
31730	Intro windpipe wire/tube	207	253	304	201	5.54
31750	Repair windpipe	2276	2775	3335	1095	30.26
31755	Repair windpipe	2773	3382	4064	1316	36.35
31760	Repair windpipe	2918	3558	4276	1326	36.62
31766	Reconstruct windpipe	3120	3805	4572	1760	48.62
31770	Repair/graft bronchus	2871	3501	4207	1464	40.45
31775	Reconstruct bronchus	2948	3595	4320	1506	41.59
31780	Reconstruct windpipe	2779	3388	4072	1167	32.24
31781	Reconstruct windpipe	3355	4090	4916	1486	41.06
31785	Remove windpipe lesion	2490	3036	3648	1145	31.64
31786	Remove windpipe lesion	2849	3474	4175	1469	40.59
31800	Repair windpipe injury	1550	1890	2271	540	14.91
31805	Repair windpipe injury	2110	2572	3091	916	25.30
31820	Close windpipe lesion	670	817	982	473	13.08
31825	Repair windpipe defect	990	1207	1451	658	18.17
31830	Revise windpipe scar	680	829	996	459	12.68
31899	Airways surgical procedure	0	0	0	0	.00

LUNGS AND PLEURA

CPT	SHORT DESCRIPTION	50th	75th	90th	MFS	RVU
32000	Drain chest	250	310	379	170	4.71
32002	Treat collapsed lung	435	539	659	115	3.17
32005	Treat lung lining chemically	292	362	443	117	3.24
32020	Insertion chest tube	613	760	930	211	5.82
32035	Explore chest	1573	1951	2386	634	17.52
32036	Explore chest	1753	2175	2660	698	19.27
32095	Biopsy through chest wall	1863	2311	2827	630	17.40
32100	Explore/biopsy chest	2480	3076	3763	977	26.99

NEW CODE CPT 2002 •

CPT	SHORT DESCRIPTION	50th	75th	90th	MFS	RVU
32110	Explore/repair chest	2241	2779	3400	1352	37.35
32120	Re-explore chest	2223	2757	3373	807	22.30
32124	Explore chest free adhesions	2086	2587	3165	860	23.76
32140	Remove lung lesion(s)	2332	2892	3538	919	25.40
32141	Remove/treat lung lesions	2387	2961	3622	930	25.70
32150	Remove lung lesion(s)	2285	2834	3467	921	25.45
32151	Remove lung foreign body	2325	2884	3528	938	25.90
32160	Open chest heart massage	2297	2849	3485	603	16.65
32200	Drain open lung lesion	1606	1992	2438	971	26.83
32201	Drain percut lung lesion	378	469	574	357	9.85
32215	Treat chest lining	1982	2458	3007	790	21.83
32220	Release lung	2542	3153	3857	1446	39.95
32225	Partial release lung	1932	2397	2932	927	25.61
32310	Remove chest lining	2260	2804	3430	903	24.95
32320	Free/remove chest lining	3145	3901	4772	1437	39.71
32400	Needle biopsy chest lining	289	359	439	135	3.72
32402	Open biopsy chest lining	1252	1553	1900	588	16.23
32405	Biopsy lung or mediastinum	460	571	699	157	4.35
32420	Puncture/clear lung	268	333	407	115	3.17
32440	Remove lung	3236	4013	4910	1489	41.13
32442	Sleeve pneumonectomy	3984	4941	6045	1582	43.71
32445	Remove lung	3719	4612	5642	1521	42.03
32480	Partial remove lung	3913	4853	5938	1403	38.77
32482	Bilobectomy	3492	4331	5299	1475	40.74
32484	Segmentectomy	3135	3889	4758	1274	35.20
32486	Sleeve lobectomy	3612	4480	5481	1457	40.24

CPT	SHORT DESCRIPTION	50th	75th	90th	MFS	RVU
32488	Completion pneumonectomy	3863	4792	5862	1549	42.78
32491	Lung volume reduce	2825	3504	4286	1324	36.58
32500	Partial remove lung	3333	4134	5058	1320	36.47
32501	Repair bronchus add-on	703	873	1067	248	6.84
32520	Remove lung & revise chest	3462	4294	5254	1338	36.95
32522	Remove lung & revise chest	4069	5047	6175	1472	40.67
32525	Remove lung & revise chest	4045	5017	6138	1592	43.97
32540	Remove lung lesion	2438	3024	3699	958	26.47
32601	Thoracoscopy, diagnostic	709	879	1076	351	9.69
32602	Thoracoscopy, diagnostic	1095	1359	1662	376	10.38
32603	Thoracoscopy, diagnostic	1070	1327	1623	467	12.90
32604	Thoracoscopy, diagnostic	1228	1523	1863	526	14.54
32605	Thoracoscopy, diagnostic	875	1085	1327	434	11.98
32606	Thoracoscopy, diagnostic	995	1235	1510	505	13.94
32650	Thoracoscopy, surgical	2130	2642	3232	741	20.47
32651	Thoracoscopy, surgical	2066	2562	3134	842	23.25
32652	Thoracoscopy, surgical	2094	2597	3177	1163	32.12
32653	Thoracoscopy, surgical	2082	2582	3159	853	23.57
32654	Thoracoscopy, surgical	2148	2664	3259	778	21.48
32655	Thoracoscopy, surgical	2178	2702	3305	850	23.49
32656	Thoracoscopy, surgical	2159	2678	3276	871	24.05
32657	Thoracoscopy, surgical	3187	3953	4836	892	24.65
32658	Thoracoscopy, surgical	2374	2944	3602	802	22.15
32659	Thoracoscopy, surgical	2484	3081	3769	799	22.08
32660	Thoracoscopy, surgical	3117	3866	4730	1088	30.05
32661	Thoracoscopy, surgical	2684	3329	4072	871	24.06

     NEW CODE CPT 2002 •

CPT	SHORT DESCRIPTION	50th	75th	90th	MFS	RVU
32662	Thoracoscopy, surgical	2674	3316	4057	1051	29.04
32663	Thoracoscopy, surgical	2974	3689	4513	1157	31.97
32664	Thoracoscopy, surgical	2696	3344	4091	917	25.33
32665	Thoracoscopy, surgical	2431	3015	3688	960	26.51
32800	Repair lung hernia	2110	2618	3202	914	25.25
32810	Close chest after drain	967	1199	1467	892	24.65
32815	Close bronchial fistula	3445	4273	5227	1423	39.31
32820	Reconstruct injured chest	3251	4033	4933	1368	37.78
32850	Donor pneumonectomy	1539	1909	2336	0	.00
32851	Lung transplant, single	4754	5896	7214	2298	63.47
32852	Lung transplant with bypass	5188	6435	7872	2475	68.37
32853	Lung transplant, double	5827	7227	8841	2803	77.43
32854	Lung transplant with bypass	6097	7563	9252	2959	81.74
32900	Remove rib(s)	1764	2188	2677	1266	34.96
32905	Revise & repair chest wall	2210	2741	3353	1305	36.06
32906	Revise & repair chest wall	3288	4078	4989	1600	44.19
32940	Revise lung	1391	1725	2110	1226	33.86
32960	Therapeutic pneumothorax	193	239	292	149	4.12
32997	Total lung lavage	611	757	927	310	8.55
32999	Chest surgery procedure	0	0	0	0	.00

CPT	SHORT DESCRIPTION	50th	75th	90th	MFS	RVU

CPT	SHORT DESCRIPTION	50th	75th	90th	MFS	RVU

NEW CODE CPT 2002 •

CPT	SHORT DESCRIPTION	50th	75th	90th	MFS	RVU

CARDIOVASCULAR SYSTEM

HEART AND PERICARDIUM

CPT	SHORT DESCRIPTION	50th	75th	90th	MFS	RVU
33010	Drain heart sac	422	524	636	122	3.38
33011	Repeat drain heart sac	203	252	306	124	3.42
33015	Incise heart sac	480	596	724	429	11.85
33020	Incise heart sac	2024	2515	3055	797	22.02
33025	Incise heart sac	2713	3371	4094	773	21.36
33030	Partial remove heart sac	2263	2812	3414	1203	33.23
33031	Partial remove heart sac	4209	5229	6350	1367	37.77
33050	Remove heart sac lesion	2276	2828	3434	953	26.33
33120	Remove heart lesion	5140	6386	7755	1567	43.30
33130	Remove heart lesion	3714	4614	5603	1314	36.30
33140	Heart revascularize (tmr)	2421	3008	3653	1189	32.84
33141	Heart tmr w/other procedure	512	636	772	254	7.02
33200	Insert heart pacemaker	3257	4047	4914	841	23.24
33201	Insert heart pacemaker	3309	4112	4993	752	20.78
33206	Insert heart pacemaker	1755	2180	2648	453	12.52
33207	Insert heart pacemaker	1961	2437	2959	529	14.61
33208	Insert heart pacemaker	2350	2920	3546	536	14.81
33210	Insert heart electrode	703	874	1061	174	4.81
33211	Insert heart electrode	869	1080	1312	180	4.98
33212	Insert pulse generator	1076	1337	1624	376	10.40
33213	Insert pulse generator	1289	1602	1946	423	11.68
33214	Upgrade pacemaker system	2030	2522	3062	515	14.22
33216	Revise eltrd pacing-defib	1037	1289	1565	387	10.70

CPT	SHORT DESCRIPTION	50th	75th	90th	MFS	RVU
33217	Revise eltrd pacing-defib	1094	1359	1650	412	11.37
33218	Revise eltrd pacing-defib	536	665	808	375	10.35
33220	Revise eltrd pacing-defib	638	792	962	375	10.36
33222	Revise pocket pacemaker	946	1176	1428	336	9.28
33223	Revise pocket pacing-defib	742	923	1120	433	11.96
33233	Remove pacemaker system	648	806	978	265	7.31
33234	Remove pacemaker system	687	853	1036	485	13.41
33235	Remove pacemaker electrode	804	999	1213	591	16.34
33236	Remove electrode/thoracotomy	2427	3016	3662	849	23.44
33237	Remove electrode/thoracotomy	2539	3155	3831	897	24.79
33238	Remove electrode/thoracotomy	2321	2884	3502	942	26.02
33240	Insert pulse generator	1437	1786	2169	493	13.62
33241	Remove pulse generator	562	699	848	248	6.84
33243	Remove eltrd/thoracotomy	2185	2715	3297	1305	36.05
33244	Remove eltrd, transven	931	1156	1404	834	23.03
33245	Insert epic eltrd pace-defib	3719	4622	5612	955	26.37
33246	Insert epic eltrd/generator	4746	5897	7161	1343	37.09
33249	Eltrd/insert pace-defib	3666	4556	5532	869	24.01
33250	Ablate heart dysrhythm focus	2517	3128	3799	1322	36.51
33251	Ablate heart dysrhythm focus	3649	4534	5506	1497	41.35
33253	Reconstruct atria	3944	4900	5951	1858	51.32
33261	Ablate heart dysrhythm focus	3103	3856	4682	1527	42.17
33282	Implant pat-active ht record	697	866	1051	325	8.98
33284	Remove pat-active ht record	538	668	812	241	6.67
33300	Repair heart wound	2384	2962	3597	1136	31.39
33305	Repair heart wound	3907	4855	5895	1352	37.36

NEW CODE CPT 2002 •

CPT	SHORT DESCRIPTION	50th	75th	90th	MFS	RVU
33310	Exploratory heart surgery	2894	3596	4367	1181	32.62
33315	Exploratory heart surgery	4830	6001	7287	1401	38.70
33320	Repair major blood vessel(s)	2630	3268	3968	1068	29.51
33321	Repair major vessel	3389	4211	5113	1305	36.05
33322	Repair major blood vessel(s)	3372	4190	5088	1309	36.15
33330	Insert major vessel graft	3699	4596	5581	1313	36.27
33332	Insert major vessel graft	4362	5420	6582	1424	39.35
33335	Insert major vessel graft	4978	6185	7511	1808	49.95
33400	Repair aortic valve	4873	5756	6662	1760	48.63
33401	Valvuloplasty, open	4575	5404	6256	1501	41.47
33403	Valvuloplasty, w/cp bypass	4682	5531	6402	1570	43.36
33404	Prepare heart-aorta conduit	5989	7074	8189	1776	49.07
33405	Replace aortic valve	6735	7956	9208	2047	56.55
33406	Replace aortic valve	5804	6856	7936	2176	60.10
33410	Replace aortic valve	6085	7188	8320	1937	53.50
33411	Replace aortic valve	6545	7730	8948	2117	58.48
33412	Replace aortic valve	6070	7170	8299	2482	68.56
33413	Replace aortic valve	7856	9279	10741	2563	70.81
33414	Repair aortic valve	5796	6846	7924	1875	51.81
33415	Revise subvalvular tissue	5243	6193	7168	1699	46.93
33416	Revise ventricle muscle	5406	6385	7391	1819	50.26
33417	Repair aortic valve	5538	6542	7572	1781	49.20
33420	Revise mitral valve	4003	4728	5472	1301	35.95
33422	Revise mitral valve	5338	6306	7299	1592	43.98
33425	Repair mitral valve	5373	6346	7346	1628	44.98
33426	Repair mitral valve	6271	7407	8574	1955	54.01

CPT	SHORT DESCRIPTION	50th	75th	90th	MFS	RVU
33427	Repair mitral valve	4575	5404	6256	2307	63.72
33430	Replace mitral valve	6957	8218	9512	1980	54.71
33460	Revise tricuspid valve	4938	5833	6751	1464	40.45
33463	Valvuloplasty, tricuspid	5746	6788	7856	1571	43.39
33464	Valvuloplasty, tricuspid	5607	6623	7667	1666	46.02
33465	Replace tricuspid valve	5241	6191	7166	1740	48.07
33468	Revise tricuspid valve	6782	8011	9272	1925	53.18
33470	Revise pulmonary valve	3911	4620	5347	1369	37.82
33471	Valvotomy pulmonary valve	3952	4669	5404	1389	38.38
33472	Revise pulmonary valve	3982	4703	5444	1386	38.30
33474	Revise pulmonary valve	5626	6646	7693	1424	39.33
33475	Replace pulmonary valve	5946	7023	8129	1952	53.92
33476	Revise heart chamber	5644	6666	7716	1535	42.40
33478	Revise heart chamber	6047	7143	8267	1619	44.73
33496	Repair prosth valve clot	5300	6260	7246	1721	47.53
33500	Repair heart vessel fistula	5848	7191	8691	1533	42.34
33501	Repair heart vessel fistula	4013	4934	5963	1089	30.07
33502	Coronary artery correct	3180	3910	4725	1455	40.19
33503	Coronary artery graft	4283	5267	6365	1343	37.10
33504	Coronary artery graft	6180	7599	9184	1602	44.25
33505	Repair artery w/tunnel	6684	8220	9934	1684	46.52
33506	Repair artery, translocation	7052	8672	10480	2098	57.96
33510	Cabg vein, single	5262	6470	7820	1725	47.66
33511	Cabg vein, two	6600	8115	9808	1788	49.39
33512	Cabg vein, three	7419	9123	11025	1888	52.15
33513	Cabg vein, four	7848	9650	11663	1910	52.76

  NEW CODE CPT 2002 •

CPT	SHORT DESCRIPTION	50th	75th	90th	MFS	RVU
33514	Cabg vein, five	7869	9676	11694	1959	54.12
33516	Cabg vein, six or more	5103	6275	7583	2076	57.36
33517	Cabg artery-vein, single	704	865	1045	136	3.75
33518	Cabg artery-vein, two	1274	1567	1894	256	7.08
33519	Cabg artery-vein, three	1686	2073	2506	376	10.39
33521	Cabg artery-vein, four	2132	2622	3169	497	13.73
33522	Cabg artery-vein, five	3681	4527	5471	618	17.06
33523	Cabg art-vein, six or more	1730	2128	2571	737	20.36
33530	Coronary artery, bypass/reop	1656	2037	2462	310	8.55
33533	Cabg arterial, single	6449	7930	9583	1827	50.48
33534	Cabg arterial, two	7153	8796	10631	1929	53.28
33535	Cabg arterial, three	7717	9490	11469	2036	56.24
33536	Cabg arterial, four or more	4435	5454	6592	2174	60.06
33542	Remove heart lesion	5572	6852	8281	1792	49.51
33545	Repair heart damage	7340	9026	10909	2207	60.97
33572	Open coronary endarterectomy	1907	2345	2835	235	6.48
33600	Close valve	6520	8017	9690	1795	49.60
33602	Close valve	6597	8112	9803	1741	48.09
33606	Anastomosis/artery-aorta	4050	4980	6019	1877	51.86
33608	Repair anomaly w/conduit	7554	9289	11227	1869	51.64
33610	Repair by enlargement	7398	9097	10994	1937	53.52
33611	Repair double ventricle	8088	9945	12020	2040	56.36
33612	Repair double ventricle	7969	9799	11843	2158	59.61
33615	Repair modified fontan	7705	9475	11451	2045	56.48
33617	Repair single ventricle	7960	9788	11830	2257	62.34
33619	Repair single ventricle	9115	11208	13546	2758	76.20

CPT	SHORT DESCRIPTION	50th	75th	90th	MFS	RVU
33641	Repair heart septum defect	5740	7058	8530	1299	35.88
33645	Revise heart veins	5290	6505	7862	1521	42.01
33647	Repair heart septum defects	6867	8444	10206	1780	49.18
33660	Repair heart defects	6146	7557	9134	1807	49.91
33665	Repair heart defects	6239	7671	9271	1784	49.28
33670	Repair heart chambers	7330	9013	10893	1950	53.86
33681	Repair heart septum defect	6739	8286	10014	1881	51.97
33684	Repair heart septum defect	6235	7666	9265	1855	51.24
33688	Repair heart septum defect	6612	8131	9827	1854	51.21
33690	Reinforce pulmonary artery	2554	3141	3796	1291	35.66
33692	Repair heart defects	6002	7381	8920	1884	52.04
33694	Repair heart defects	7232	8893	10747	2030	56.09
33697	Repair heart defects	7080	8706	10522	2142	59.16
33702	Repair heart defects	5738	7055	8527	1684	46.52
33710	Repair heart defects	7009	8618	10416	1824	50.38
33720	Repair heart defect	6799	8360	10104	1675	46.28
33722	Repair heart defect	6768	8322	10058	1783	49.26
33730	Repair heart-vein defect(s)	6889	8471	10238	2007	55.45
33732	Repair heart-vein defect	6425	7901	9549	1770	48.89
33735	Revise heart chamber	4215	5183	6264	1285	35.51
33736	Revise heart chamber	5226	6426	7767	1458	40.28
33737	Revise heart chamber	4679	5754	6954	1445	39.91
33750	Major vessel shunt	3536	4348	5255	1302	35.98
33755	Major vessel shunt	4239	5213	6300	1363	37.66
33762	Major vessel shunt	3742	4602	5562	1329	36.70
33764	Major vessel shunt & graft	4298	5285	6387	1373	37.94

NEW CODE CPT 2002 •

CPT	SHORT DESCRIPTION	50th	75th	90th	MFS	RVU
33766	Major vessel shunt	3394	4173	5044	1483	40.96
33767	Major vessel shunt	4171	5129	6199	1541	42.56
33770	Repair great vessels defect	8219	10107	12215	2190	60.50
33771	Repair great vessels defect	8117	9981	12063	2078	57.40
33774	Repair great vessels defect	7211	8867	10717	1874	51.77
33775	Repair great vessels defect	8071	9925	11995	1942	53.64
33776	Repair great vessels defect	8494	10444	12623	2043	56.45
33777	Repair great vessels defect	8361	10282	12426	2012	55.57
33778	Repair great vessels defect	8376	10299	12447	2354	65.04
33779	Repair great vessels defect	8507	10461	12643	2047	56.54
33780	Repair great vessels defect	10223	12570	15192	2459	67.94
33781	Repair great vessels defect	9052	11131	13452	2178	60.16
33786	Repair arterial trunk	7863	9669	11685	2299	63.50
33788	Revise pulmonary artery	5020	6173	7461	1622	44.81
33800	Aortic suspend	3247	3992	4825	1103	30.47
33802	Repair vessel defect	3135	3854	4658	1138	31.44
33803	Repair vessel defect	4050	4980	6019	1294	35.76
33813	Repair septal defect	4459	5482	6626	1359	37.55
33814	Repair septal defect	6372	7835	9469	1589	43.90
33820	Revise major vessel	2988	3674	4440	1062	29.34
33822	Revise major vessel	3541	4355	5263	1115	30.81
33824	Revise major vessel	3851	4735	5723	1234	34.10
33840	Remove aorta constriction	4061	4994	6036	1343	37.10
33845	Remove aorta constriction	5515	6781	8195	1443	39.87
33851	Remove aorta constriction	5584	6866	8298	1343	37.11
33852	Repair septal defect	5143	6325	7644	1486	41.04

CPT	SHORT DESCRIPTION	50th	75th	90th	MFS	RVU
33853	Repair septal defect	6737	8284	10011	1962	54.20
33860	Ascending aortic graft	6224	7653	9250	2210	61.04
33861	Ascending aortic graft	6854	8428	10186	2403	66.39
33863	Ascending aortic graft	7979	9811	11857	2559	70.70
33870	Transverse aortic arch graft	10499	12911	15603	2526	69.78
33875	Thoracic aortic graft	5954	7321	8848	1960	54.15
33877	Thoracoabdominal graft	5683	6988	8445	2448	67.63
33910	Remove lung artery emboli	5320	6541	7906	1513	41.81
33915	Remove lung artery emboli	3725	4581	5536	1250	34.53
33916	Surgery great vessel	4844	5956	7199	1606	44.36
33917	Repair pulmonary artery	6474	7961	9622	1558	43.03
33918	Repair pulmonary atresia	6291	7736	9350	1617	44.67
33919	Repair pulmonary atresia	8117	9981	12063	2335	64.50
33920	Repair pulmonary atresia	7546	9279	11214	1913	52.84
33922	Transect pulmonary artery	4856	5972	7217	1434	39.61
33924	Remove pulmonary shunt	1051	1292	1561	300	8.29
33930	Remove donor heart/lung	2254	2772	3350	0	.00
33935	Transplant heart/lung	8099	9959	12037	3513	97.04
33940	Remove donor heart	1973	2426	2932	0	.00
33945	Transplant heart	5752	7072	8548	2505	69.19
33960	External circulation assist	2418	2973	3593	998	27.56
33961	External circulation assist	2290	2816	3403	586	16.19
• 33967	Insert ia percut device	1073	1319	1594	258	7.13
33968	Remove aortic assist device	68	84	102	34	.95
33970	Aortic circulation assist	1663	2045	2471	355	9.82
33971	Aortic circulation assist	2045	2514	3039	669	18.48

NEW CODE CPT 2002 •

CPT	SHORT DESCRIPTION	50th	75th	90th	MFS	RVU
33973	Insert balloon device	1849	2274	2748	514	14.21
33974	Remove intra-aortic balloon	1928	2370	2865	962	26.58
33975	Implant ventricular device	3668	4510	5451	1077	29.76
33976	Implant ventricular device	4452	5475	6617	1216	33.60
33977	Remove ventricular device	3381	4157	5024	1165	32.19
33978	Remove ventricular device	3789	4660	5632	1291	35.66
• 33979	Insert intracorporeal device	0	0	0	0	.00
• 33980	Remove intracorporeal device	0	0	0	0	.00
33999	Cardiac surgery procedure	0	0	0	0	.00

ARTERIES AND VEINS

CPT	SHORT DESCRIPTION	50th	75th	90th	MFS	RVU
34001	Remove artery clot	1757	2075	2492	736	20.34
34051	Remove artery clot	2078	2455	2948	875	24.18
34101	Remove artery clot	1610	1901	2283	577	15.95
34111	Remove arm artery clot	2646	3125	3753	569	15.73
34151	Remove artery clot	2845	3360	4035	1353	37.38
34201	Remove artery clot	2074	2450	2942	585	16.17
34203	Remove leg artery clot	2359	2787	3346	924	25.52
34401	Remove vein clot	2154	2545	3056	1327	36.67
34421	Remove vein clot	1741	2056	2469	686	18.96
34451	Remove vein clot	2781	3285	3944	1436	39.67
34471	Remove vein clot	1814	2142	2572	589	16.26
34490	Remove vein clot	1801	2128	2555	610	16.85
34501	Repair valve, femoral vein	1696	2003	2405	954	26.35
34502	Reconstruct vena cava	4522	5341	6414	1494	41.28
34510	Transpose vein valve	1973	2331	2799	1114	30.78
34520	Cross-over vein graft	2219	2621	3148	1048	28.95

CPT	SHORT DESCRIPTION	50th	75th	90th	MFS	RVU
34530	Leg vein fuse	2087	2465	2960	984	27.18
34800	Endovasc abd repair w/tube	2220	2622	3149	1159	32.03
34802	Endovasc abd repair w/device	2450	2894	3475	1279	35.34
34804	Endovasc abd repair w/device	2450	2894	3475	1279	35.34
34808	Endovasc abd occlud device	422	498	598	220	6.07
34812	Expose for endoprosth, aortic	691	816	979	359	9.93
34813	Expose for endoprosth, femoral	490	579	696	256	7.06
34820	Expose for endoprosth, iliac	997	1177	1414	519	14.34
34825	Endovasc extend prosth, init	1326	1566	1881	694	19.16
34826	Endovasc extend prosth, addl	422	498	598	220	6.07
34830	Open aortic tube prosth repair	3455	4081	4900	1803	49.82
34831	Open aortoiliac prosth repair	3735	4411	5297	1950	53.86
34832	Open aortofemor prosth repair	3735	4411	5297	1950	53.86
35001	Repair defect artery	3407	4024	4832	1104	30.49
35002	Repair artery rupture neck	3442	4066	4882	1156	31.94
35005	Repair defect artery	3218	3800	4564	996	27.51
35011	Repair defect artery	2560	3023	3631	973	26.89
35013	Repair artery rupture arm	2732	3226	3874	1191	32.89
35021	Repair defect artery	3489	4121	4949	1094	30.22
35022	Repair artery rupture chest	2966	3503	4206	1258	34.74
35045	Repair defect arm artery	2158	2549	3060	971	26.81
35081	Repair defect artery	4692	5542	6655	1553	42.90
35082	Repair artery rupture aorta	3981	4702	5646	2087	57.65
35091	Repair defect artery	4639	5479	6579	1944	53.71
35092	Repair artery rupture aorta	5022	5932	7123	2413	66.66
35102	Repair defect artery	5228	6175	7415	1697	46.87

NEW CODE CPT 2002 •

CPT	SHORT DESCRIPTION	50th	75th	90th	MFS	RVU
35103	Repair artery rupture groin	3773	4456	5351	2176	60.10
35111	Repair defect artery	2699	3188	3828	1348	37.24
35112	Repair artery rupture,spleen	2785	3289	3950	1593	44.01
35121	Repair defect artery	3470	4098	4921	1641	45.32
35122	Repair artery rupture belly	3063	3618	4345	1892	52.27
35131	Repair defect artery	3243	3831	4600	1367	37.75
35132	Repair artery rupture groin	3444	4068	4885	1615	44.62
35141	Repair defect artery	2910	3437	4128	1097	30.31
35142	Repair artery rupture thigh	2828	3340	4010	1260	34.81
35151	Repair defect artery	2992	3534	4244	1241	34.29
35152	Repair artery rupture knee	2791	3296	3958	1377	38.05
35161	Repair defect artery	2271	2682	3220	1083	29.93
35162	Repair artery rupture	2368	2796	3358	1124	31.04
35180	Repair blood vessel lesion	2615	3089	3709	780	21.55
35182	Repair blood vessel lesion	2736	3232	3881	1603	44.27
35184	Repair blood vessel lesion	2979	3518	4225	987	27.26
35188	Repair blood vessel lesion	2633	3110	3734	815	22.51
35189	Repair blood vessel lesion	2854	3371	4048	1514	41.83
35190	Repair blood vessel lesion	2589	3057	3671	728	20.11
35201	Repair blood vessel lesion	2865	3383	4063	887	24.49
35206	Repair blood vessel lesion	2437	2879	3457	792	21.89
35207	Repair blood vessel lesion	2481	2930	3518	768	21.21
35211	Repair blood vessel lesion	4315	5097	6120	1394	38.50
35216	Repair blood vessel lesion	3530	4169	5007	1186	32.75
35221	Repair blood vessel lesion	3351	3958	4753	1321	36.49
35226	Repair blood vessel lesion	1728	2041	2451	864	23.88

CPT	SHORT DESCRIPTION	50th	75th	90th	MFS	RVU
35231	Repair blood vessel lesion	3103	3665	4401	1114	30.77
35236	Repair blood vessel lesion	3175	3750	4504	987	27.27
35241	Repair blood vessel lesion	4506	5322	6391	1452	40.11
35246	Repair blood vessel lesion	3532	4171	5009	1556	42.99
35251	Repair blood vessel lesion	3465	4093	4915	1609	44.46
35256	Repair blood vessel lesion	3100	3661	4397	1061	29.31
35261	Repair blood vessel lesion	3123	3689	4429	967	26.70
35266	Repair blood vessel lesion	2915	3443	4134	876	24.19
35271	Repair blood vessel lesion	4482	5294	6357	1387	38.32
35276	Repair blood vessel lesion	3334	3938	4729	1454	40.18
35281	Repair blood vessel lesion	3286	3881	4660	1502	41.48
35286	Repair blood vessel lesion	3088	3647	4380	956	26.40
35301	Rechannel artery	3551	4194	5037	1061	29.32
35311	Rechannel artery	3375	3986	4787	1479	40.85
35321	Rechannel artery	2976	3516	4222	877	24.23
35331	Rechannel artery	3557	4201	5045	1449	40.02
35341	Rechannel artery	2813	3323	3990	1400	38.68
35351	Rechannel artery	3134	3701	4444	1272	35.13
35355	Rechannel artery	3180	3755	4510	1036	28.63
35361	Rechannel artery	3694	4362	5239	1537	42.46
35363	Rechannel artery	3925	4636	5568	1647	45.51
35371	Rechannel artery	2581	3048	3660	825	22.79
35372	Rechannel artery	2634	3111	3736	993	27.44
35381	Rechannel artery	2546	3007	3610	904	24.96
35390	Reoperate carotid add-on	343	405	487	169	4.68
35400	Angioscopy	332	392	471	159	4.39

     NEW CODE CPT 2002 •

CPT	SHORT DESCRIPTION	50th	75th	90th	MFS	RVU
35450	Repair arterial blockage	2062	2465	2897	548	15.13
35452	Repair arterial blockage	2240	2679	3148	390	10.78
35454	Repair arterial blockage	1793	2143	2519	345	9.54
35456	Repair arterial blockage	1806	2159	2538	414	11.44
35458	Repair arterial blockage	1991	2380	2797	529	14.61
35459	Repair arterial blockage	1809	2163	2543	481	13.28
35460	Repair venous blockage	670	801	942	340	9.40
35470	Repair arterial blockage	1664	1989	2338	475	13.11
35471	Repair arterial blockage	2151	2572	3023	552	15.24
35472	Repair arterial blockage	2004	2396	2816	384	10.62
35473	Repair arterial blockage	1564	1870	2198	340	9.39
35474	Repair arterial blockage	1798	2150	2526	408	11.28
35475	Repair arterial blockage	2048	2448	2878	514	14.19
35476	Repair venous blockage	1111	1328	1561	335	9.25
35480	Atherectomy, open	2288	2735	3215	608	16.79
35481	Atherectomy, open	2436	2912	3422	434	11.99
35482	Atherectomy, open	1967	2352	2764	382	10.56
35483	Atherectomy, open	1974	2360	2773	450	12.43
35484	Atherectomy, open	2150	2571	3021	571	15.78
35485	Atherectomy, open	1989	2379	2796	529	14.60
35490	Atherectomy, percutaneous	2109	2521	2963	596	16.46
35491	Atherectomy, percutaneous	2221	2656	3121	423	11.69
35492	Atherectomy, percutaneous	1687	2017	2370	373	10.30
35493	Atherectomy, percutaneous	1756	2099	2467	451	12.47
35494	Atherectomy, percutaneous	1935	2314	2719	561	15.49
35495	Atherectomy, percutaneous	1817	2173	2554	526	14.52

CPT	SHORT DESCRIPTION	50th	75th	90th	MFS	RVU
35500	Harvest vein for bypass	633	757	890	338	9.33
35501	Artery bypass graft	3116	3726	4379	1074	29.66
35506	Artery bypass graft	3158	3775	4437	1098	30.32
35507	Artery bypass graft	3114	3723	4376	1094	30.23
35508	Artery bypass graft	3671	4389	5158	1046	28.90
35509	Artery bypass graft	3197	3822	4492	1010	27.89
35511	Artery bypass graft	3059	3658	4299	1149	31.74
35515	Artery bypass graft	3456	4132	4856	1039	28.71
35516	Artery bypass graft	3153	3770	4431	838	23.14
35518	Artery bypass graft	3648	4362	5126	1150	31.78
35521	Artery bypass graft	3237	3870	4549	1214	33.55
35526	Artery bypass graft	3356	4013	4716	1604	44.32
35531	Artery bypass graft	3947	4719	5546	1942	53.64
35533	Artery bypass graft	4828	5772	6784	1524	42.09
35536	Artery bypass graft	3639	4351	5114	1708	47.17
35541	Artery bypass graft	3436	4109	4829	1431	39.52
35546	Artery bypass graft	3967	4744	5575	1416	39.13
35548	Artery bypass graft	3710	4436	5214	1212	33.47
35549	Artery bypass graft	4905	5865	6893	1303	36.00
35551	Artery bypass graft	4137	4946	5813	1486	41.06
35556	Artery bypass graft	4092	4893	5750	1220	33.69
35558	Artery bypass graft	3090	3695	4342	1154	31.89
35560	Artery bypass graft	4046	4838	5686	1732	47.85
35563	Artery bypass graft	3304	3950	4642	1314	36.30
35565	Artery bypass graft	3310	3957	4650	1263	34.90
35566	Artery bypass graft	4608	5509	6475	1510	41.71

NEW CODE CPT 2002 •

CPT	SHORT DESCRIPTION	50th	75th	90th	MFS	RVU
35571	Artery bypass graft	3852	4605	5412	1388	38.33
35582	Vein bypass graft	3118	3728	4381	1506	41.59
35583	Vein bypass graft	3594	4297	5050	1286	35.52
35585	Vein bypass graft	3956	4730	5559	1670	46.13
35587	Vein bypass graft	3283	3925	4613	1437	39.71
35600	Harvest artery for cabg	514	615	723	273	7.53
35601	Artery bypass graft	3131	3794	4565	980	27.07
35606	Artery bypass graft	3001	3636	4375	1043	28.81
35612	Artery bypass graft	2797	3389	4078	875	24.18
35616	Artery bypass graft	2844	3447	4147	890	24.59
35621	Artery bypass graft	3236	3921	4718	1103	30.47
35623	Bypass graft, not vein	4179	5064	6093	1308	36.13
35626	Artery bypass graft	3294	3992	4803	1510	41.72
35631	Artery bypass graft	3290	3987	4797	1831	50.57
35636	Artery bypass graft	3380	4096	4928	1597	44.13
35641	Artery bypass graft	3887	4710	5668	1371	37.87
35642	Artery bypass graft	3209	3888	4678	1004	27.74
35645	Artery bypass graft	3209	3888	4678	1004	27.74
35646	Artery bypass graft	4792	5807	6987	1710	47.24
• 35647	Artery bypass graft	4968	6020	7243	1555	42.95
35650	Artery bypass graft	3304	4004	4818	1034	28.57
35651	Artery bypass graft	3985	4829	5811	1385	38.27
35654	Artery bypass graft	4360	5284	6358	1365	37.70
35656	Artery bypass graft	3781	4581	5512	1092	30.18
35661	Artery bypass graft	3288	3984	4794	1041	28.76
35663	Artery bypass graft	3451	4181	5031	1202	33.20

CPT	SHORT DESCRIPTION	50th	75th	90th	MFS	RVU
35665	Artery bypass graft	3396	4116	4952	1156	31.94
35666	Artery bypass graft	3315	4018	4834	1314	36.31
35671	Artery bypass graft	3648	4421	5319	1142	31.54
35681	Composite bypass graft	371	449	540	85	2.34
35682	Composite bypass graft	863	1046	1259	382	10.54
35683	Composite bypass graft	990	1200	1444	451	12.47
• 35685	Bypass graft patency/patch	689	835	1005	216	5.96
• 35686	Bypass graft/av fist patency	570	691	831	178	4.93
35691	Arterial transposition	3208	3888	4678	1005	27.76
35693	Arterial transposition	2790	3381	4069	862	23.82
35694	Arterial transposition	3079	3731	4489	1061	29.31
35695	Arterial transposition	3083	3736	4495	1060	29.27
35700	Reoperate bypass graft	432	524	630	163	4.51
35701	Explore carotid artery	1495	1812	2180	501	13.84
35721	Explore femoral artery	1254	1519	1828	466	12.87
35741	Explore popliteal artery	1257	1523	1833	509	14.07
35761	Explore artery/vein	1210	1466	1764	378	10.44
35800	Explore neck vessels	1360	1648	1984	426	11.76
35820	Explore chest vessels	1926	2334	2808	681	18.81
35840	Explore abdominal vessels	1724	2089	2514	581	16.04
35860	Explore limb vessels	1276	1546	1860	355	9.80
35870	Repair vessel graft defect	4284	5191	6246	1262	34.85
35875	Remove clot in graft	1725	2090	2515	642	17.73
35876	Remove clot in graft	1930	2339	2814	1015	28.04
35879	Revise graft w/vein	3620	4387	5278	909	25.12
35881	Revise graft w/vein	3647	4419	5318	1017	28.09

   NEW CODE CPT 2002 •

CPT	SHORT DESCRIPTION	50th	75th	90th	MFS	RVU
35901	Excise graft, neck	1571	1904	2291	541	14.94
35903	Excise graft, extremity	1513	1834	2206	674	18.62
35905	Excise graft, thorax	1866	2262	2721	1766	48.79
35907	Excise graft, abdomen	6031	7308	8793	1887	52.14

VASCULAR INJECTION PROCEDURES

CPT	SHORT DESCRIPTION	50th	75th	90th	MFS	RVU
36000	Place needle in vein	61	84	103	30	.84
• 36002	Pseudoaneurysm inject trt	229	319	389	181	4.99
36005	Inject ext venography	381	530	646	300	8.28
36010	Place catheter in vein	487	678	827	124	3.43
36011	Place catheter in vein	525	730	891	160	4.41
36012	Place catheter in vein	727	1012	1235	178	4.92
36013	Place catheter in artery	484	673	822	119	3.30
36014	Place catheter in artery	594	827	1009	153	4.22
36015	Place catheter in artery	682	948	1157	178	4.92
36100	Establish access to artery	527	733	894	158	4.36
36120	Establish access to artery	508	706	862	102	2.81
36140	Establish access to artery	389	541	660	102	2.82
36145	Artery to vein shunt	523	727	887	102	2.81
36160	Establish access to aorta	635	883	1078	131	3.62
36200	Place catheter in aorta	601	837	1021	154	4.26
36215	Place catheter in artery	678	944	1151	238	6.58
36216	Place catheter in artery	860	1197	1461	268	7.41
36217	Place catheter in artery	1065	1481	1807	323	8.91
36218	Place catheter in artery	216	300	367	52	1.43
36245	Place catheter in artery	740	1030	1257	242	6.69
36246	Place catheter in artery	855	1189	1451	270	7.45

CPT	SHORT DESCRIPTION	50th	75th	90th	MFS	RVU
36247	Place catheter in artery	1052	1464	1786	321	8.87
36248	Place catheter in artery	226	314	383	52	1.44
36260	Insert infuse pump	1508	2099	2561	591	16.34
36261	Revise infuse pump	760	1058	1291	341	9.42
36262	Remove infuse pump	620	862	1052	255	7.04
36299	Vessel inject procedure	0	0	0	0	.00
36400	Drawing blood	51	71	87	40	1.11
36405	Drawing blood	54	75	92	33	.90
36406	Drawing blood	52	72	88	41	1.13
36410	Drawing blood	28	38	47	25	.69
36415	Drawing blood	11	16	19	0	.00
36420	Establish access to vein	122	169	206	52	1.43
36425	Establish access to vein	196	272	332	154	4.25
36430	Blood transfuse service	129	180	220	36	1.00
36440	Blood transfuse service	172	239	291	51	1.42
36450	Exchange transfuse service	635	883	1078	112	3.10
36455	Exchange transfuse service	642	893	1090	127	3.50
36460	Transfuse service, fetal	1281	1783	2176	351	9.70
36468	Inject(s) spider veins	163	227	277	0	.00
36469	Inject(s) spider veins	88	122	149	0	.00
36470	Inject therapy vein	174	243	296	137	3.79
36471	Inject therapy veins	248	345	421	158	4.37
36481	Insert catheter vein	1237	1721	2099	371	10.25
36488	Insert catheter vein	325	452	551	80	2.20
36489	Insert catheter vein	284	395	482	264	7.28
36490	Insert catheter vein	729	1015	1238	98	2.70

NEW CODE CPT 2002 •

CPT	SHORT DESCRIPTION	50th	75th	90th	MFS	RVU
36491	Insert catheter vein	424	590	719	84	2.31
36493	Repositioning cvc	221	308	376	78	2.15
36500	Insert catheter vein	274	382	466	180	4.97
36510	Insert catheter vein	224	312	381	68	1.88
36520	Plasma and/or cell exchange	401	558	680	104	2.87
36521	Apheresis w/ adsorp/reinfuse	432	601	733	104	2.87
36522	Photopheresis	664	924	1127	281	7.77
36530	Insert infuse pump	1086	1511	1844	396	10.93
36531	Revise infuse pump	894	1244	1518	312	8.63
36532	Remove infuse pump	582	810	989	189	5.21
36533	Insert access device	1102	1533	1870	379	10.48
36534	Revise access device	734	1021	1246	164	4.54
36535	Remove access device	518	720	879	197	5.43
36540	Collect blood venous device	31	43	53	0	.00
36550	Declot vascular device	172	240	293	25	.69
36600	Withdraw arterial blood	72	101	123	28	.77
36620	Insert catheter artery	207	288	352	53	1.46
36625	Insert catheter artery	387	539	658	104	2.88
36640	Insert catheter artery	348	485	591	110	3.03
36660	Insert catheter artery	278	387	472	67	1.86
36680	Insert needle bone cavity	126	176	214	70	1.94
36800	Insert cannula	443	567	714	152	4.19
36810	Insert cannula	887	1135	1428	239	6.59
36815	Insert cannula	630	806	1013	151	4.16
36819	Av fuse/upper arm vein	1805	2310	2905	800	22.09
• 36820	Av fuse/forearm vein	2483	3177	3997	800	22.09

CPT	SHORT DESCRIPTION	50th	75th	90th	MFS	RVU
36821	Av fuse direct any site	1838	2352	2958	540	14.93
36822	Insert cannula(s)	1214	1554	1954	466	12.86
36823	Insert cannula(s)	2413	3088	3884	1224	33.81
36825	Artery-vein graft	2257	2888	3633	598	16.51
36830	Artery-vein graft	2324	2974	3741	704	19.46
36831	Open thrombect av fistula	1371	1754	2206	463	12.78
36832	Av fistula revise, open	1869	2391	3008	623	17.22
36833	Av fistula revise	1973	2525	3176	700	19.35
36834	Repair a-v aneurysm	1763	2256	2838	540	14.92
36835	Artery to vein shunt	2202	2817	3544	451	12.45
36860	External cannula declotting	370	473	595	168	4.63
36861	Cannula declotting	678	867	1091	151	4.16
36870	Percut thrombect av fistula	2499	3198	4022	1702	47.02
37140	Revise circulation	3769	4823	6067	1280	35.37
37145	Revise circulation	4055	5189	6527	1450	40.06
37160	Revise circulation	3731	4774	6006	1201	33.19
37180	Revise circulation	3987	5102	6418	1372	37.90
37181	Splice spleen/kidney veins	3956	5062	6367	1461	40.37
37195	Thrombolytic therapy, stroke	681	871	1096	291	8.03
37200	Transcatheter biopsy	805	1030	1296	230	6.35
37201	Transcatheter therapy infuse	1258	1610	2025	283	7.83
37202	Transcatheter therapy infuse	743	951	1196	340	9.39
37203	Transcatheter retrieval	942	1206	1517	285	7.88
37204	Transcatheter occlusion	3140	4018	5054	918	25.35
37205	Transcatheter stent	1565	2002	2519	456	12.61
37206	Transcatheter stent add-on	760	973	1224	213	5.89

NEW CODE CPT 2002 •

CPT	SHORT DESCRIPTION	50th	75th	90th	MFS	RVU
37207	Transcatheter stent	1468	1878	2362	463	12.78
37208	Transcatheter stent add-on	702	898	1129	218	6.02
37209	Exchange arterial catheter	330	423	532	115	3.18
37250	Iv us first vessel add-on	223	285	359	111	3.06
37251	Iv us each add vessel add-on	169	216	272	84	2.32
37565	Ligate neck vein	1233	1578	1985	603	16.67
37600	Ligate neck artery	1085	1388	1746	657	18.16
37605	Ligate neck artery	1155	1478	1859	742	20.51
37606	Ligate neck artery	1228	1571	1976	395	10.92
37607	Ligate a-v fistula	519	664	836	382	10.54
37609	Temporal artery procedure	547	700	881	379	10.46
37615	Ligate neck artery	1156	1479	1861	359	9.91
37616	Ligate chest artery	1716	2196	2763	1048	28.96
37617	Ligate abdomen artery	1732	2216	2788	1215	33.56
37618	Ligate extremity artery	959	1227	1544	324	8.94
37620	Revise major vein	2171	2778	3495	610	16.84
37650	Revise major vein	785	1004	1263	471	13.00
37660	Revise major vein	3554	4547	5720	1144	31.61
37700	Revise leg vein	922	1180	1485	265	7.33
37720	Remove leg vein	1406	1800	2264	362	9.99
37730	Remove leg veins	1692	2165	2724	459	12.69
37735	Remove leg veins/lesion	2011	2573	3237	639	17.64
37760	Revise leg veins	1986	2540	3196	628	17.36
37780	Revise leg vein	267	342	430	258	7.14
37785	Revise secondary varicosity	554	709	892	414	11.43
37788	Revascularize penis	3428	4387	5518	1355	37.44

CPT	SHORT DESCRIPTION	50th	75th	90th	MFS	RVU
37790	Penile venous occlusion	1283	1641	2064	570	15.75
37799	Vascular surgery procedure	0	0	0	0	.00

  NEW CODE CPT 2002 •

CPT	SHORT DESCRIPTION	50th	75th	90th	MFS	RVU

HEMIC AND LYMPHATIC SYSTEMS

SPLEEN

CPT	SHORT DESCRIPTION	50th	75th	90th	MFS	RVU
38100	Remove spleen, total	2498	3364	4808	816	22.53
38101	Remove spleen, partial	2273	3061	4375	867	23.96
38102	Remove spleen, total	1168	1573	2248	254	7.02
38115	Repair ruptured spleen	2150	2896	4138	885	24.45
38120	Laparoscopy, splenectomy	2170	2923	4177	952	26.31
38129	Laparoscope proc, spleen	0	0	0	0	.00
38200	Inject for spleen x-ray	408	550	786	134	3.69
• 38220	Bone marrow aspiration	997	1343	1919	208	5.75
• 38221	Bone marrow biopsy	1067	1437	2053	223	6.15
38230	Bone marrow collection	912	1228	1755	262	7.24
38231	Stem cell collection	539	726	1037	78	2.16
38240	Bone marrow/stem transplant	671	904	1292	116	3.20
38241	Bone marrow/stem transplant	1322	1781	2545	115	3.18

LYMPH NODES AND LYMPHATIC CHANNELS

CPT	SHORT DESCRIPTION	50th	75th	90th	MFS	RVU
38300	Drain lymph node lesion	1217	1640	2343	254	7.02
38305	Drain lymph node lesion	2488	3352	4790	519	14.35
38308	Incise lymph channels	511	688	984	447	12.36
38380	Thoracic duct procedure	1222	1646	2352	570	15.75
38381	Thoracic duct procedure	2648	3567	5098	875	24.18
38382	Thoracic duct procedure	2135	2875	4109	723	19.97
38500	Biopsy/remove lymph nodes	500	673	962	260	7.18
38505	Needle biopsy lymph nodes	280	378	540	161	4.44

CPT	SHORT DESCRIPTION	50th	75th	90th	MFS	RVU
38510	Biopsy/remove lymph nodes	749	1009	1442	447	12.36
38520	Biopsy/remove lymph nodes	614	826	1181	466	12.86
38525	Biopsy/remove lymph nodes	871	1173	1677	400	11.06
38530	Biopsy/remove lymph nodes	804	1083	1548	521	14.39
38542	Explore deep node(s) neck	987	1329	1899	452	12.50
38550	Remove neck/armpit lesion	720	970	1386	457	12.62
38555	Remove neck/armpit lesion	2162	2912	4162	908	25.07
38562	Remove pelvic lymph nodes	1878	2529	3614	661	18.25
38564	Remove abdomen lymph nodes	2155	2903	4149	667	18.43
38570	Laparoscopy, lymph node biopsy	2101	2830	4044	535	14.77
38571	Laparoscopy, lymphadenectomy	2251	3031	4332	796	21.98
38572	Laparoscopy, lymphadenectomy	2390	3220	4601	927	25.62
38589	Laparoscope proc, lymphatic	0	0	0	0	.00
38700	Remove lymph nodes neck	1466	1975	2822	813	22.45
38720	Remove lymph nodes neck	2875	3873	5535	1118	30.89
38724	Remove lymph nodes neck	3834	5165	7381	1175	32.46
38740	Remove armpit lymph nodes	1325	1785	2551	601	16.61
38745	Remove armpit lymph nodes	2214	2983	4263	813	22.47
38746	Remove thoracic lymph nodes	924	1245	1779	257	7.09
38747	Remove abdominal lymph nodes	706	951	1359	258	7.14
38760	Remove groin lymph nodes	1654	2228	3184	767	21.19
38765	Remove groin lymph nodes	2696	3632	5190	1196	33.05
38770	Remove pelvis lymph nodes	2400	3232	4619	773	21.35
38780	Remove abdomen lymph nodes	3682	4959	7087	1009	27.86
38790	Inject for lymphatic x-ray	2801	3772	5391	585	16.15

NEW CODE CPT 2002 •

CPT	SHORT DESCRIPTION	50th	75th	90th	MFS	RVU
38792	Identify sentinel node	347	467	668	27	.75
38794	Access thoracic lymph duct	393	530	757	224	6.19
38999	Blood/lymph system procedure	0	0	0	0	.00

CPT	SHORT DESCRIPTION	50th	75th	90th	MFS	RVU

NEW CODE CPT 2002 •

CPT	SHORT DESCRIPTION	50th	75th	90th	MFS	RVU

MEDIASTINUM AND DIAPHRAGM

MEDIASTINUM

CPT	SHORT DESCRIPTION	50th	75th	90th	MFS	RVU
39000	Explore chest	1067	1435	1786	515	14.24
39010	Explore chest	2396	3224	4012	817	22.56
39200	Remove chest lesion	2312	3111	3871	918	25.37
39220	Remove chest lesion	2452	3300	4106	1115	30.81
39400	Visualization chest	1205	1621	2017	482	13.31
39499	Chest procedure	0	0	0	0	.00

DIAPHRAGM

CPT	SHORT DESCRIPTION	50th	75th	90th	MFS	RVU
39501	Repair diaphragm laceration	1955	2630	3273	811	22.39
39502	Repair paraesophageal hernia	2050	2759	3433	956	26.42
39503	Repair diaphragm hernia	10535	14176	17639	4914	135.76
39520	Repair diaphragm hernia	2025	2724	3390	996	27.52
39530	Repair diaphragm hernia	1999	2690	3347	932	25.76
39531	Repair diaphragm hernia	2380	3203	3986	967	26.70
39540	Repair diaphragm hernia	2433	3274	4074	814	22.49
39541	Repair diaphragm hernia	1855	2496	3105	865	23.90
39545	Revise diaphragm	2320	3122	3884	877	24.24
39560	Resect diaphragm, simple	1537	2068	2573	759	20.97
39561	Resect diaphragm, complex	2103	2830	3522	1061	29.31
39599	Diaphragm surgery procedure	0	0	0	0	.00

CPT	SHORT DESCRIPTION	50th	75th	90th	MFS	RVU

NEW CODE CPT 2002 •

CPT	SHORT DESCRIPTION	50th	75th	90th	MFS	RVU

DIGESTIVE SYSTEM

LIPS

CPT	SHORT DESCRIPTION	50th	75th	90th	MFS	RVU
40490	Biopsy lip	142	182	237	105	2.91
40500	Partial excise lip	1003	1280	1667	373	10.31
40510	Partial excise lip	1022	1304	1698	428	11.83
40520	Partial excise lip	851	1086	1415	473	13.06
40525	Reconstruct lip with flap	1656	2113	2752	618	17.07
40527	Reconstruct lip with flap	1937	2472	3220	708	19.55
40530	Partial remove lip	854	1090	1420	479	13.22
40650	Repair lip	524	668	870	352	9.73
40652	Repair lip	672	857	1116	425	11.73
40654	Repair lip	928	1184	1542	497	13.74
40700	Repair cleft lip/nasal	2127	2714	3534	891	24.60
40701	Repair cleft lip/nasal	2684	3425	4460	1154	31.87
40702	Repair cleft lip/nasal	2345	2992	3897	834	23.04
40720	Repair cleft lip/nasal	1898	2423	3155	1005	27.75
40761	Repair cleft lip/nasal	2762	3524	4590	1046	28.89
40799	Lip surgery procedure	0	0	0	0	.00

VESTIBULE OF MOUTH

CPT	SHORT DESCRIPTION	50th	75th	90th	MFS	RVU
40800	Drain mouth lesion	187	239	311	118	3.27
40801	Drain mouth lesion	540	690	898	189	5.23
40804	Remove foreign body, mouth	197	251	327	142	3.92
40805	Remove foreign body, mouth	477	609	793	222	6.13
40806	Incise lip fold	270	345	449	44	1.22
40808	Biopsy mouth lesion	167	213	277	114	3.14

CPT	SHORT DESCRIPTION	50th	75th	90th	MFS	RVU
40810	Excise mouth lesion	215	275	358	148	4.10
40812	Excise/repair mouth lesion	321	410	534	197	5.43
40814	Excise/repair mouth lesion	621	793	1033	281	7.76
40816	Excise mouth lesion	804	1026	1336	299	8.26
40818	Excise oral mucosa for graft	357	455	593	239	6.60
40819	Excise lip or cheek fold	308	393	511	226	6.25
40820	Treat mouth lesion	231	294	383	135	3.74
40830	Repair mouth laceration	192	246	320	159	4.38
40831	Repair mouth laceration	432	552	718	195	5.39
40840	Reconstruct mouth	885	1129	1470	559	15.45
40842	Reconstruct mouth	762	973	1267	553	15.28
40843	Reconstruct mouth	1062	1355	1765	734	20.29
40844	Reconstruct mouth	1526	1947	2535	965	26.65
40845	Reconstruct mouth	1849	2360	3073	1169	32.30
40899	Mouth surgery procedure	0	0	0	0	.00

TONGUE AND FLOOR OF MOUTH

CPT	SHORT DESCRIPTION	50th	75th	90th	MFS	RVU
41000	Drain mouth lesion	194	248	323	137	3.79
41005	Drain mouth lesion	209	266	347	133	3.68
41006	Drain mouth lesion	572	730	951	256	7.07
41007	Drain mouth lesion	540	690	898	257	7.10
41008	Drain mouth lesion	539	687	895	264	7.30
41009	Drain mouth lesion	527	672	876	271	7.49
41010	Incise tongue fold	206	263	343	170	4.69
41015	Drain mouth lesion	550	702	914	300	8.30
41016	Drain mouth lesion	488	623	812	313	8.66
41017	Drain mouth lesion	553	705	919	313	8.65

NEW CODE CPT 2002 •

CPT	SHORT DESCRIPTION	50th	75th	90th	MFS	RVU
41018	Drain mouth lesion	594	758	988	356	9.84
41100	Biopsy tongue	210	268	349	160	4.42
41105	Biopsy tongue	225	288	375	143	3.94
41108	Biopsy floor mouth	178	227	295	127	3.51
41110	Excise tongue lesion	248	316	412	174	4.81
41112	Excise tongue lesion	510	651	848	235	6.49
41113	Excise tongue lesion	568	725	944	250	6.92
41114	Excise tongue lesion	593	757	986	568	15.70
41115	Excise tongue fold	360	460	599	165	4.56
41116	Excise mouth lesion	690	881	1147	216	5.98
41120	Partial remove tongue	1280	1634	2128	709	19.59
41130	Partial remove tongue	1927	2460	3203	786	21.72
41135	Tongue and neck surgery	3405	4345	5658	1498	41.38
41140	Remove tongue	2253	2875	3744	1620	44.74
41145	Tongue remove, neck surgery	3861	4928	6417	1938	53.53
41150	Tongue, mouth, jaw surgery	3490	4454	5800	1533	42.35
41153	Tongue, mouth, neck surgery	3732	4763	6202	1575	43.52
41155	Tongue, jaw, & neck surgery	4713	6014	7833	1816	50.18
41250	Repair tongue laceration	219	279	363	182	5.04
41251	Repair tongue laceration	319	407	530	202	5.57
41252	Repair tongue laceration	775	988	1287	233	6.43
41500	Fixation tongue	466	594	774	304	8.40
41510	Tongue to lip surgery	766	978	1273	328	9.05
41520	Reconstruct tongue fold	525	670	872	216	5.98
41599	Tongue and mouth surgery	0	0	0	0	.00

DENTOALVEOLAR STRUCTURES

CPT	SHORT DESCRIPTION	50th	75th	90th	MFS	RVU
41800	Drain gum lesion	184	235	306	117	3.22
41805	Remove foreign body, gum	211	270	351	123	3.41
41806	Remove foreign body, jawbone	259	330	430	197	5.45
41820	Excise gum, each quadrant	460	587	764	0	.00
41821	Excise gum flap	97	124	162	0	.00
41822	Excise gum lesion	269	344	447	194	5.37
41823	Excise gum lesion	522	666	868	258	7.13
41825	Excise gum lesion	220	281	365	139	3.84
41826	Excise gum lesion	408	521	679	186	5.14
41827	Excise gum lesion	601	767	1000	264	7.30
41828	Excise gum lesion	663	847	1103	231	6.38
41830	Remove gum tissue	568	725	944	252	6.97
41850	Treat gum lesion	260	332	432	0	.00
41870	Gum graft	534	682	888	0	.00
41872	Repair gum	660	842	1096	206	5.70
41874	Repair tooth socket	450	575	749	224	6.18
41899	Dental surgery procedure	0	0	0	0	.00

PALATE AND UVULA

CPT	SHORT DESCRIPTION	50th	75th	90th	MFS	RVU
42000	Drain mouth roof lesion	222	270	332	139	3.85
42100	Biopsy roof mouth	209	255	313	140	3.88
42104	Excise lesion mouth roof	320	390	478	157	4.34
42106	Excise lesion mouth roof	443	540	663	178	4.92
42107	Excise lesion mouth roof	838	1022	1254	327	9.02
42120	Remove palate/lesion	1304	1589	1950	463	12.80

NEW CODE CPT 2002 •

CPT	SHORT DESCRIPTION	50th	75th	90th	MFS	RVU
42140	Excise uvula	387	472	579	205	5.65
42145	Repair palate, pharynx/uvula	2280	2778	3409	586	16.20
42160	Treat mouth roof lesion	573	698	857	188	5.18
42180	Repair palate	261	319	391	216	5.98
42182	Repair palate	639	778	955	261	7.20
42200	Reconstruct cleft palate	2651	3231	3965	824	22.75
42205	Reconstruct cleft palate	2750	3352	4113	864	23.87
42210	Reconstruct cleft palate	3455	4210	5166	985	27.21
42215	Reconstruct cleft palate	3371	4109	5042	706	19.50
42220	Reconstruct cleft palate	2553	3111	3818	517	14.28
42225	Reconstruct cleft palate	2232	2720	3337	704	19.45
42226	Lengthen palate	2718	3312	4064	749	20.70
42227	Lengthen palate	2664	3247	3984	699	19.31
42235	Repair palate	1952	2379	2920	517	14.29
42260	Repair nose to lip fistula	1161	1415	1737	618	17.08
42280	Preparation palate mold	220	268	329	112	3.10
42281	Insert palate prosthesis	403	491	602	132	3.64
42299	Palate/uvula surgery	0	0	0	0	.00

SALIVARY GLANDS AND DUCTS

CPT	SHORT DESCRIPTION	50th	75th	90th	MFS	RVU
42300	Drain salivary gland	523	637	782	171	4.73
42305	Drain salivary gland	1317	1605	1969	431	11.91
42310	Drain salivary gland	209	255	313	144	3.99
42320	Drain salivary gland	250	304	373	192	5.31
42325	Create salivary cyst drain	344	419	514	245	6.77
42326	Create salivary cyst drain	520	633	777	270	7.45
42330	Remove salivary stone	332	404	496	188	5.18

CPT	SHORT DESCRIPTION	50th	75th	90th	MFS	RVU
42335	Remove salivary stone	802	977	1199	262	7.25
42340	Remove salivary stone	1129	1376	1688	362	10.01
42400	Biopsy salivary gland	178	217	267	122	3.36
42405	Biopsy salivary gland	316	385	472	252	6.97
42408	Excise salivary cyst	621	757	929	347	9.59
42409	Drain salivary cyst	639	779	956	230	6.35
42410	Excise parotid gland/lesion	1012	1233	1513	663	18.31
42415	Excise parotid gland/lesion	3041	3706	4548	1121	30.97
42420	Excise parotid gland/lesion	3604	4392	5389	1285	35.50
42425	Excise parotid gland/lesion	1665	2030	2490	894	24.70
42426	Excise parotid gland/lesion	3709	4521	5547	1385	38.27
42440	Excise submaxillary gland	1784	2175	2668	493	13.61
42450	Excise sublingual gland	883	1076	1320	338	9.34
42500	Repair salivary duct	941	1146	1407	353	9.74
42505	Repair salivary duct	1398	1703	2090	458	12.64
42507	Parotid duct diversion	1473	1795	2202	442	12.21
42508	Parotid duct diversion	2006	2444	2999	657	18.14
42509	Parotid duct diversion	2296	2799	3434	797	22.03
42510	Parotid duct diversion	1771	2158	2648	579	15.99
42550	Inject for salivary x-ray	1522	1854	2275	498	13.76
42600	Close salivary fistula	1201	1464	1797	472	13.05
42650	Dilation salivary duct	84	103	126	71	1.96
42660	Dilation salivary duct	108	131	161	85	2.35
42665	Ligate salivary duct	633	772	947	207	5.73
42699	Salivary surgery procedure	0	0	0	0	.00

   CPT codes and descriptions only copyright AMA   NEW CODE CPT 2002 •

CPT	SHORT DESCRIPTION	50th	75th	90th	MFS	RVU

PHARYNX, ADENOIDS, AND TONSILS

CPT	SHORT DESCRIPTION	50th	75th	90th	MFS	RVU
42700	Drain tonsil abscess	272	326	439	182	5.04
42720	Drain throat abscess	486	584	786	383	10.58
42725	Drain throat abscess	2058	2470	3325	732	20.22
42800	Biopsy throat	214	256	345	166	4.58
42802	Biopsy throat	206	248	333	177	4.89
42804	Biopsy upper nose/throat	186	224	301	158	4.37
42806	Biopsy upper nose/throat	366	439	591	189	5.23
42808	Excise pharynx lesion	452	542	730	270	7.47
42809	Remove pharynx foreign body	241	289	389	196	5.42
42810	Excise neck cyst	565	678	912	332	9.16
42815	Excise neck cyst	1748	2098	2824	517	14.27
42820	Remove tonsils and adenoids	815	978	1317	297	8.21
42821	Remove tonsils and adenoids	890	1068	1438	322	8.89
42825	Remove tonsils	756	907	1221	268	7.40
42826	Remove tonsils	847	1017	1369	269	7.42
42830	Remove adenoids	577	693	932	190	5.26
42831	Remove adenoids	624	749	1008	199	5.49
42835	Remove adenoids	475	570	768	205	5.67
42836	Remove adenoids	550	661	889	257	7.09
42842	Extensive surgery throat	3131	3758	5059	627	17.33
42844	Extensive surgery throat	4169	5003	6734	974	26.92
42845	Extensive surgery throat	4484	5382	7244	1595	44.05
42860	Excise tonsil tags	478	574	772	198	5.46
42870	Excise lingual tonsil	732	879	1183	433	11.96
42890	Partial remove pharynx	1952	2343	3154	901	24.88

CPT	SHORT DESCRIPTION	50th	75th	90th	MFS	RVU
42892	Revise pharyngeal walls	2338	2806	3777	1073	29.65
42894	Revise pharyngeal walls	4208	5051	6798	1517	41.90
42900	Repair throat wound	772	926	1247	346	9.57
42950	Reconstruct throat	1666	2000	2692	589	16.28
42953	Repair throat, esophagus	2167	2601	3501	682	18.83
42955	Surgical opening throat	679	815	1097	527	14.57
42960	Control throat bleeding	287	345	464	168	4.63
42961	Control throat bleeding	511	614	826	409	11.29
42962	Control throat bleeding	534	641	862	507	14.00
42970	Control nose/throat bleeding	439	527	709	354	9.79
42971	Control nose/throat bleeding	577	693	933	458	12.65
42972	Control nose/throat bleeding	638	765	1030	488	13.47
42999	Throat surgery procedure	0	0	0	0	.00

ESOPHAGUS

CPT	SHORT DESCRIPTION	50th	75th	90th	MFS	RVU
43020	Incise esophagus	1556	1894	2378	563	15.56
43030	Throat muscle surgery	1571	1912	2401	553	15.29
43045	Incise esophagus	2373	2889	3627	1209	33.41
43100	Excise esophagus lesion	1723	2098	2634	636	17.56
43101	Excise esophagus lesion	2291	2788	3501	973	26.89
43107	Remove esophagus	4696	5716	7177	2236	61.78
43108	Remove esophagus	4752	5785	7264	1968	54.36
43112	Remove esophagus	5021	6112	7674	2434	67.23
43113	Remove esophagus	4995	6080	7634	2026	55.98
43116	Partial remove esophagus	5596	6812	8553	1894	52.33
43117	Partial remove esophagus	4938	6011	7547	2245	62.02
43118	Partial remove esophagus	5124	6238	7832	1901	52.52

     NEW CODE CPT 2002 •

CPT	SHORT DESCRIPTION	50th	75th	90th	MFS	RVU
43121	Partial remove esophagus	4216	5132	6443	1727	47.71
43122	Partial remove esophagus	5072	6174	7751	2220	61.32
43123	Partial remove esophagus	4808	5853	7349	1909	52.74
43124	Remove esophagus	4053	4933	6194	1644	45.42
43130	Remove esophagus pouch	1820	2215	2782	791	21.86
43135	Remove esophagus pouch	2375	2891	3630	1015	28.04
43200	Esophagus endoscopy	586	714	896	348	9.62
43202	Esophagus endoscopy, biopsy	617	751	943	307	8.47
43204	Esophagus endoscopy & inject	750	913	1146	205	5.66
43205	Esophagus endoscopy/ligate	739	900	1130	205	5.67
43215	Esophagus endoscopy	791	963	1209	146	4.03
43216	Esophagus endoscopy/lesion	807	982	1233	136	3.75
43217	Esophagus endoscopy	815	992	1246	160	4.42
43219	Esophagus endoscopy	669	814	1023	159	4.39
43220	Esoph endoscopy, dilation	672	818	1027	122	3.36
43226	Esoph endoscopy, dilation	653	795	998	133	3.67
43227	Esoph endoscopy, repair	754	918	1153	196	5.42
43228	Esoph endoscopy, ablation	701	853	1071	210	5.79
43231	Esoph endoscopy w/us exam	423	515	646	181	4.99
43232	Esoph endoscopy w/us fn biopsy	492	598	751	249	6.89
43234	Upper gi endoscopy, exam	515	627	787	243	6.72
43235	Upper gi endoscopy, diagnosis	575	700	878	322	8.90
43239	Upper gi endoscopy, biopsy	692	842	1057	355	9.80
43240	Esoph endoscope w/drain cyst	747	909	1141	369	10.19
43241	Upper gi endoscopy with tube	806	981	1232	145	4.00
43242	Upper gi endo w/us fn biopsy	537	654	821	371	10.24

CPT	SHORT DESCRIPTION	50th	75th	90th	MFS	RVU
43243	Upper gi endoscopy & inject	890	1083	1360	245	6.78
43244	Upper gi endoscopy/ligate	843	1026	1288	269	7.44
43245	Operative upper gi endoscopy	790	962	1207	185	5.12
43246	Place gastrostomy tube	977	1190	1494	232	6.41
43247	Operative upper gi endoscopy	791	963	1209	185	5.12
43248	Upper gi endoscopy/guide wire	735	895	1124	173	4.79
43249	Esoph endoscopy, dilation	715	870	1093	161	4.44
43250	Upper gi endoscopy/tumor	889	1082	1358	176	4.85
43251	Operative upper gi endoscopy	874	1063	1335	201	5.56
43255	Operative upper gi endoscopy	899	1095	1375	253	6.99
43256	Upper gi endoscopy w stent	423	515	647	235	6.49
43258	Operative upper gi endoscopy	1039	1265	1589	245	6.76
43259	Endoscopic ultrasound exam	919	1119	1405	265	7.33
43260	Endo cholangiopancreatograph	1023	1246	1564	316	8.73
43261	Endo cholangiopancreatograph	1132	1378	1730	332	9.18
43262	Endo cholangiopancreatograph	1477	1797	2257	390	10.76
43263	Endo cholangiopancreatograph	1181	1438	1805	383	10.57
43264	Endo cholangiopancreatograph	1597	1944	2441	467	12.89
43265	Endo cholangiopancreatograph	1371	1669	2096	522	14.43
43267	Endo cholangiopancreatograph	1294	1576	1978	390	10.77
43268	Endo cholangiopancreatograph	1513	1842	2313	390	10.76
43269	Endo cholangiopancreatograph	1335	1625	2041	428	11.82
43271	Endo cholangiopancreatograph	1477	1798	2257	389	10.75
43272	Endo cholangiopancreatograph	938	1142	1433	390	10.77
43280	Laparoscopy, fundoplasty	3225	3926	4929	993	27.44
43289	Laparoscope proc, esoph	0	0	0	0	.00

   NEW CODE CPT 2002 •

CPT	SHORT DESCRIPTION	50th	75th	90th	MFS	RVU
43300	Repair esophagus	1643	2077	2906	626	17.30
43305	Repair esophagus and fistula	2638	3335	4664	1144	31.59
43310	Repair esophagus	3302	4174	5839	1559	43.08
43312	Repair esophagus and fistula	3709	4688	6557	1783	49.25
• **43313**	Esophagoplasty congenital	5670	7167	10025	2632	72.72
• **43314**	Tracheo-esophagoplasty cong	6228	7872	11011	2891	79.87
43320	Fuse esophagus & stomach	2510	3173	4438	1165	32.19
43324	Revise esophagus & stomach	3115	3938	5508	1161	32.08
43325	Revise esophagus & stomach	2485	3141	4394	1151	31.79
43326	Revise esophagus & stomach	2777	3511	4911	1155	31.91
43330	Repair esophagus	2162	2733	3823	1125	31.07
43331	Repair esophagus	2490	3147	4402	1212	33.47
43340	Fuse esophagus & intestine	2520	3185	4455	1138	31.45
43341	Fuse esophagus & intestine	2959	3740	5231	1237	34.16
43350	Surgical opening esophagus	1616	2042	2857	993	27.43
43351	Surgical opening esophagus	2068	2614	3656	1114	30.77
43352	Surgical opening esophagus	1557	1968	2753	946	26.13
43360	Gastrointestinal repair	3987	5039	7049	2032	56.13
43361	Gastrointestinal repair	4830	6105	8540	2243	61.95
43400	Ligate esophagus veins	2531	3199	4475	1182	32.65
43401	Esophagus surgery for veins	1408	1780	2489	1237	34.16
43405	Ligate/staple esophagus	1401	1771	2477	1125	31.09
43410	Repair esophagus wound	1431	1809	2531	868	23.97
43415	Repair esophagus wound	2461	3111	4351	1427	39.42
43420	Repair esophagus opening	1392	1760	2462	882	24.36
43425	Repair esophagus opening	2064	2609	3650	1233	34.06

CPT	SHORT DESCRIPTION	50th	75th	90th	MFS	RVU
43450	Dilate esophagus	196	247	346	106	2.92
43453	Dilate esophagus	331	418	584	82	2.27
43456	Dilate esophagus	450	569	796	137	3.78
43458	Dilate esophagus	629	795	1111	163	4.49
43460	Pressure treat esophagus	457	578	808	201	5.55
43496	Free jejunum flap, microvasc	0	0	0	0	.00
43499	Esophagus surgery procedure	0	0	0	0	.00

STOMACH

CPT	SHORT DESCRIPTION	50th	75th	90th	MFS	RVU
43500	Surgical opening stomach	1600	2012	2516	620	17.12
43501	Surgical repair stomach	2282	2870	3590	1102	30.45
43502	Surgical repair stomach	2252	2833	3543	1271	35.12
43510	Surgical opening stomach	1447	1820	2277	778	21.48
43520	Incise pyloric muscle	1602	2014	2520	599	16.56
43600	Biopsy stomach	269	338	423	111	3.07
43605	Biopsy stomach	1811	2278	2850	668	18.46
43610	Excise stomach lesion	2114	2659	3326	818	22.59
43611	Excise stomach lesion	2254	2834	3545	990	27.34
43620	Remove stomach	3750	4717	5900	1637	45.22
43621	Remove stomach	4543	5714	7147	1676	46.30
43622	Remove stomach	4788	6022	7533	1767	48.80
43631	Remove stomach, partial	2545	3201	4004	1242	34.30
43632	Remove stomach, partial	2546	3202	4005	1242	34.32
43633	Remove stomach, partial	3436	4322	5406	1268	35.02
43634	Remove stomach, partial	4023	5060	6329	1381	38.14
43635	Remove stomach, partial	797	1002	1254	109	3.01
43638	Remove stomach, partial	3528	4437	5550	1570	43.37

NEW CODE CPT 2002 •

CPT	SHORT DESCRIPTION	50th	75th	90th	MFS	RVU
43639	Remove stomach, partial	4343	5462	6832	1602	44.26
43640	Vagotomy & pylorus repair	2473	3110	3890	950	26.25
43641	Vagotomy & pylorus repair	2692	3385	4234	964	26.62
43651	Laparoscopy vagus nerve	1617	2034	2544	575	15.89
43652	Laparoscopy vagus nerve	2666	3353	4195	685	18.93
43653	Laparoscopy gastrostomy	1462	1839	2300	466	12.88
43659	Laparoscope proc, stom	0	0	0	0	.00
43750	Place gastrostomy tube	978	1230	1539	273	7.54
43752	Nasal/orogastric w/stent	0	0	0	0	.00
43760	Change gastrostomy tube	179	225	281	96	2.64
43761	Reposition gastrostomy tube	321	404	505	106	2.94
43800	Reconstruct pylorus	1780	2238	2800	773	21.36
43810	Fuse stomach and bowel	2103	2645	3309	821	22.69
43820	Fuse stomach and bowel	1986	2498	3124	858	23.70
43825	Fuse stomach and bowel	2470	3106	3885	1060	29.28
43830	Place gastrostomy tube	1617	2034	2544	553	15.28
43831	Place gastrostomy tube	1451	1825	2283	482	13.32
43832	Place gastrostomy tube	1848	2325	2908	883	24.39
43840	Repair stomach lesion	1993	2506	3135	868	23.97
43842	Gastroplasty for obesity	3692	4643	5808	1130	31.22
43843	Gastroplasty for obesity	3790	4767	5963	1138	31.43
43846	Gastric bypass for obesity	4908	6173	7722	1437	39.69
43847	Gastric bypass for obesity	4590	5773	7221	1605	44.34
43848	Revise gastroplasty	2774	3488	4363	1749	48.32
43850	Revise stomach-bowel fuse	2526	3177	3974	1343	37.11
43855	Revise stomach-bowel fuse	3039	3823	4782	1422	39.29

CPT	SHORT DESCRIPTION	50th	75th	90th	MFS	RVU
43860	Revise stomach-bowel fuse	2554	3213	4018	1361	37.61
43865	Revise stomach-bowel fuse	3151	3964	4958	1444	39.88
43870	Repair stomach opening	1308	1645	2058	565	15.62
43880	Repair stomach-bowel fistula	2089	2627	3286	1356	37.46
43999	Stomach surgery procedure	0	0	0	0	.00

INTESTINES (EXCEPT RECTUM)

CPT	SHORT DESCRIPTION	50th	75th	90th	MFS	RVU
44005	Freeing bowel adhesion	2246	2673	3296	906	25.02
44010	Incise small bowel	2079	2474	3051	726	20.05
44015	Insert needle cath bowel	957	1139	1404	138	3.80
44020	Explore small intestine	2218	2639	3255	787	21.75
44021	Decompress small bowel	1838	2187	2697	807	22.28
44025	Incise large bowel	2254	2682	3308	801	22.14
44050	Reduce bowel obstruction	1918	2283	2815	788	21.78
44055	Correct malrotation bowel	2614	3111	3836	1188	32.83
44100	Biopsy bowel	332	395	488	117	3.22
44110	Excise intestine lesion(s)	1925	2290	2825	675	18.65
44111	Excise bowel lesion(s)	2500	2975	3669	818	22.61
44120	Remove small intestine	2668	3175	3916	946	26.13
44121	Remove small intestine	1188	1414	1744	235	6.50
44125	Remove small intestine	2775	3303	4073	973	26.89
• **44126**	Enterectomy w/taper, cong	5588	6650	8201	1951	53.89
• **44127**	Enterectomy w/o taper, cong	6426	7647	9431	2243	61.97
• **44128**	Enterectomy cong, add-on	693	824	1017	242	6.68
44130	Bowel to bowel fuse	2518	2997	3696	814	22.50
44132	Enterectomy cadaver donor	0	0	0	0	.00
44133	Enterectomy live donor	0	0	0	0	.00

NEW CODE CPT 2002 •

CPT	SHORT DESCRIPTION	50th	75th	90th	MFS	RVU
44135	Intestine transplant cadaver	0	0	0	0	.00
44136	Intestine transplant live	0	0	0	0	.00
44139	Mobilization colon	401	477	588	117	3.24
44140	Partial remove colon	3001	3571	4404	1171	32.36
44141	Partial remove colon	3148	3746	4620	1209	33.39
44143	Partial remove colon	3109	3700	4563	1381	38.15
44144	Partial remove colon	3364	4003	4937	1273	35.17
44145	Partial remove colon	3620	4308	5313	1468	40.54
44146	Partial remove colon	3770	4487	5533	1634	45.15
44147	Partial remove colon	3715	4422	5453	1180	32.60
44150	Remove colon	3998	4757	5867	1451	40.08
44151	Remove colon/ileostomy	4705	5599	6906	1614	44.59
44152	Remove colon/ileostomy	4894	5824	7183	1709	47.20
44153	Remove colon/ileostomy	5616	6683	8242	1794	49.56
44155	Remove colon/ileostomy	4697	5589	6893	1643	45.40
44156	Remove colon/ileostomy	5620	6688	8248	1840	50.84
44160	Remove colon	3226	3840	4735	1043	28.82
44200	Laparoscopy, enterolysis	2163	2574	3174	821	22.69
44201	Laparoscopy, jejunostomy	1650	1963	2421	576	15.91
44202	Lap resect s/intestine single	2839	3379	4167	1231	34.02
• 44203	Lap resect s/intestine, addl	674	802	989	235	6.50
• 44204	Laparo partial colectomy	3875	4611	5687	1353	37.37
• 44205	Lap colectomy part w/ileum	3431	4083	5036	1198	33.09
44209	Laparoscope proc, intestine	0	0	0	0	.00
44300	Open bowel to skin	1751	2084	2571	716	19.78
44310	Ileostomy/jejunostomy	2196	2614	3223	998	27.58

CPT	SHORT DESCRIPTION	50th	75th	90th	MFS	RVU
44312	Revise ileostomy	838	997	1229	500	13.81
44314	Revise ileostomy	2496	2971	3664	956	26.41
44316	Devise bowel pouch	3761	4476	5520	1313	36.27
44320	Colostomy	2011	2393	2951	1124	31.05
44322	Colostomy with biopsies	2127	2531	3122	853	23.57
44340	Revise colostomy	775	922	1138	476	13.14
44345	Revise colostomy	1743	2074	2558	901	24.88
44346	Revise colostomy	2111	2512	3099	981	27.10
44360	Small bowel endoscopy	720	857	1106	149	4.12
44361	Small bowel endoscopy/biopsy	755	899	1160	164	4.52
44363	Small bowel endoscopy	789	939	1212	195	5.40
44364	Small bowel endoscopy	901	1073	1384	208	5.75
44365	Small bowel endoscopy	899	1070	1381	187	5.17
44366	Small bowel endoscopy	1050	1251	1614	242	6.68
44369	Small bowel endoscopy	921	1097	1415	246	6.80
44370	Small bowel endoscopy/stent	423	504	650	244	6.75
44372	Small bowel endoscopy	764	910	1175	243	6.72
44373	Small bowel endoscopy	732	871	1124	199	5.49
44376	Small bowel endoscopy	879	1046	1350	286	7.91
44377	Small bowel endoscopy/biopsy	997	1187	1532	300	8.28
44378	Small bowel endoscopy	1210	1441	1860	382	10.56
44379	S bowel endoscope w/stent	691	822	1061	381	10.52
44380	Small bowel endoscopy	542	645	833	70	1.92
44382	Small bowel endoscopy	638	760	981	82	2.26
44383	Ileoscopy w/stent	236	281	363	165	4.55
44385	Endoscopy bowel pouch	715	852	1099	261	7.20

        NEW CODE CPT 2002 •

CPT	SHORT DESCRIPTION	50th	75th	90th	MFS	RVU
44386	Endoscopy bowel pouch/biopsy	921	1096	1415	335	9.25
44388	Colon endoscopy	764	910	1174	359	9.91
44389	Colonoscopy with biopsy	1039	1237	1597	396	10.93
44390	Colonoscopy for foreign body	1040	1238	1598	388	10.73
44391	Colonoscopy for bleeding	1339	1595	2058	383	10.59
44392	Colonoscopy & polypectomy	1290	1536	1982	444	12.26
44393	Colonoscopy lesion remove	1250	1489	1921	491	13.56
44394	Colonoscopy w/snare	1285	1530	1975	449	12.40
44397	Colonoscopy w stent	442	527	680	257	7.09
44500	Intro gastrointestinal tube	96	115	148	32	.88
44602	Suture small intestine	1998	2379	3070	885	24.44
44603	Suture small intestine	2578	3070	3962	1024	28.30
44604	Suture large intestine	2324	2768	3572	898	24.80
44605	Repair bowel lesion	2549	3036	3917	1086	30.01
44615	Intestinal stricturoplasty	2738	3260	4207	892	24.64
44620	Repair bowel opening	1870	2226	2873	690	19.06
44625	Repair bowel opening	2656	3162	4081	840	23.21
44626	Repair bowel opening	3247	3866	4989	1381	38.15
44640	Repair bowel-skin fistula	1599	1904	2458	1188	32.81
44650	Repair bowel fistula	2258	2689	3470	1233	34.07
44660	Repair bowel-bladder fistula	2168	2582	3332	1159	32.01
44661	Repair bowel-bladder fistula	3470	4133	5333	1342	37.07
44680	Surgical revise intestine	2693	3207	4139	877	24.24
44700	Suspend bowel w/prosthesis	1918	2284	2947	901	24.89
44799	Intestine surgery procedure	0	0	0	0	.00

CPT	SHORT DESCRIPTION	50th	75th	90th	MFS	RVU

MECKEL'S DIVERTICULUM AND THE MESENTERY

CPT	SHORT DESCRIPTION	50th	75th	90th	MFS	RVU
44800	Excise bowel pouch	1824	2172	2803	650	17.95
44820	Excise mesentery lesion	1571	1871	2414	691	19.10
44850	Repair mesentery	1823	2171	2802	620	17.14
44899	Bowel surgery procedure	0	0	0	0	.00
44900	Drain app abscess, open	1196	1424	1837	613	16.94
44901	Drain app abscess, percut	951	1133	1462	310	8.56
44950	Appendectomy	1431	1704	2198	586	16.19
44955	Appendectomy add-on	611	728	940	82	2.26
44960	Appendectomy	1737	2068	2669	721	19.93
44970	Laparoscopy, appendectomy	1566	1865	2407	499	13.79
44979	Laparoscope proc, app	0	0	0	0	.00

RECTUM

CPT	SHORT DESCRIPTION	50th	75th	90th	MFS	RVU
45000	Drain pelvic abscess	470	562	679	315	8.69
45005	Drain rectal abscess	383	458	554	244	6.75
45020	Drain rectal abscess	587	702	848	338	9.34
45100	Biopsy rectum	582	695	841	321	8.87
45108	Remove anorectal lesion	1207	1442	1743	421	11.62
45110	Remove rectum	4175	4988	6031	1575	43.52
45111	Partial remove rectum	2492	2977	3599	972	26.86
45112	Remove rectum	3278	3916	4735	1687	46.59
45113	Partial proctectomy	3680	4397	5316	1669	46.10
45114	Partial remove rectum	3794	4533	5480	1528	42.21
45116	Partial remove rectum	2733	3265	3948	1381	38.16
45119	Remove rectum w/reservoir	3419	4085	4939	1673	46.22

NEW CODE CPT 2002 •

CPT	SHORT DESCRIPTION	50th	75th	90th	MFS	RVU
45120	Remove rectum	3631	4339	5245	1394	38.51
45121	Remove rectum and colon	3032	3623	4380	1529	42.23
45123	Partial proctectomy	2105	2516	3041	940	25.96
45126	Pelvic exenteration	5849	6989	8449	2444	67.51
45130	Excise rectal prolapse	2035	2431	2940	918	25.36
45135	Excise rectal prolapse	3393	4053	4901	1082	29.90
• 45136	Excise ileoanal reservoir	2965	3543	4284	1526	42.15
45150	Excise rectal stricture	883	1055	1275	435	12.02
45160	Excise rectal lesion	2261	2702	3267	852	23.53
45170	Excise rectal lesion	1311	1566	1894	661	18.27
45190	Destroy rectal tumor	1114	1331	1609	573	15.83
45300	Proctosigmoidoscopy dx	126	151	183	64	1.77
45303	Proctosigmoidoscopy dilate	138	165	200	74	2.05
45305	Proctosigmoidoscopy w/biopsy	215	256	310	99	2.74
45307	Proctosigmoidoscopy fb	250	298	361	136	3.77
45308	Proctosigmoidoscopy remove	237	284	343	92	2.55
45309	Proctosigmoidoscopy remove	251	300	362	167	4.61
45315	Proctosigmoidoscopy remove	364	434	525	161	4.44
45317	Proctosigmoidoscopy bleed	334	398	482	132	3.64
45320	Proctosigmoidoscopy ablate	354	423	512	132	3.66
45321	Proctosigmoidoscopy volvul	295	352	426	67	1.86
45327	Proctosigmoidoscopy w/stent	165	197	238	96	2.64
45330	Diagnostic sigmoidoscopy	218	261	316	106	2.93
45331	Sigmoidoscopy and biopsy	296	354	428	130	3.60
45332	Sigmoidoscopy w/fb remove	339	405	490	227	6.26
45333	Sigmoidoscopy & polypectomy	440	525	635	211	5.84

CPT	SHORT DESCRIPTION	50th	75th	90th	MFS	RVU
45334	Sigmoidoscopy for bleeding	487	582	703	145	4.01
45337	Sigmoidoscopy & decompress	397	474	573	126	3.48
45338	Sigmoidoscopy w/tumor remove	461	550	665	262	7.24
45339	Sigmoidoscopy w/ablate tumor	557	666	805	251	6.93
45341	Sigmoidoscopy w/ultrasound	325	389	470	152	4.20
45342	Sigmoidoscopy w/us guide biopsy	423	505	611	222	6.14
45345	Sigmoidoscopy w/stent	283	339	409	163	4.51
45355	Surgical colonoscopy	359	429	519	183	5.06
45378	Diagnostic colonoscopy	834	997	1205	459	12.69
45379	Colonoscopy w/fb remove	801	957	1157	477	13.19
45380	Colonoscopy and biopsy	923	1102	1333	504	13.93
45382	Colonoscopy/control bleeding	1045	1248	1509	589	16.28
45383	Lesion remove colonoscopy	1113	1330	1608	586	16.20
45384	Lesion remove colonoscopy	1100	1314	1589	531	14.68
45385	Lesion remove colonoscopy	1155	1380	1668	571	15.78
45387	Colonoscopy w/stent	574	686	829	319	8.81
45500	Repair rectum	1129	1349	1630	438	12.09
45505	Repair rectum	1154	1379	1668	432	11.94
45520	Treat rectal prolapse	88	105	127	49	1.36
45540	Correct rectal prolapse	1966	2349	2840	927	25.62
45541	Correct rectal prolapse	1868	2232	2698	771	21.31
45550	Repair rectum/remove sigmoid	2461	2941	3555	1266	34.98
45560	Repair rectocele	819	978	1183	631	17.43
45562	Explore/repair rectum	2015	2408	2911	871	24.05
45563	Explore/repair rectum	2484	2967	3588	1327	36.65
45800	Repair rect/bladder fistula	2061	2462	2977	982	27.14

  NEW CODE CPT 2002 •

CPT	SHORT DESCRIPTION	50th	75th	90th	MFS	RVU
45805	Repair fistula w/colostomy	2320	2772	3351	1193	32.97
45820	Repair rectourethral fistula	2115	2527	3056	1021	28.20
45825	Repair fistula w/colostomy	2307	2756	3332	1187	32.79
45900	Reduce rectal prolapse	269	321	388	138	3.82
45905	Dilation anal sphincter	1029	1230	1487	530	14.63
45910	Dilation rectal narrowing	1447	1728	2090	744	20.56
45915	Remove rectal obstruction	338	404	489	297	8.20
45999	Rectum surgery procedure	0	0	0	0	.00

ANUS

CPT	SHORT DESCRIPTION	50th	75th	90th	MFS	RVU
• 46020	Placement seton	401	492	628	225	6.21
46030	Remove rectal marker	274	336	429	153	4.24
46040	Incise rectal abscess	573	704	899	399	11.01
46045	Incise rectal abscess	519	637	814	275	7.60
46050	Incise anal abscess	204	250	319	180	4.98
46060	Incise rectal abscess	1314	1612	2059	363	10.04
46070	Incise anal septum	254	312	398	200	5.52
46080	Incise anal sphincter	560	687	877	236	6.53
46083	Incise external hemorrhoid	407	499	637	228	6.30
46200	Remove anal fissure	809	993	1268	280	7.73
46210	Remove anal crypt	519	637	814	291	8.05
46211	Remove anal crypts	816	1002	1279	347	9.59
46220	Remove anal tab	204	250	319	109	3.02
46221	Ligate hemorrhoid(s)	232	285	364	143	3.96
46230	Remove anal tabs	270	331	422	260	7.17
46250	Hemorrhoidectomy	762	935	1194	359	9.91
46255	Hemorrhoidectomy	1101	1352	1726	418	11.56

CPT	SHORT DESCRIPTION	50th	75th	90th	MFS	RVU
46257	Remove hemorrhoids & fissure	973	1195	1526	330	9.11
46258	Remove hemorrhoids & fistula	1042	1279	1634	350	9.67
46260	Hemorrhoidectomy	1468	1801	2300	401	11.09
46261	Remove hemorrhoids & fissure	1630	2001	2555	433	11.97
46262	Remove hemorrhoids & fistula	1336	1640	2095	456	12.61
46270	Remove anal fistula	725	890	1136	337	9.31
46275	Remove anal fistula	1232	1512	1931	348	9.61
46280	Remove anal fistula	1444	1772	2262	373	10.31
46285	Remove anal fistula	458	562	717	315	8.71
46288	Repair anal fistula	1181	1449	1851	434	11.98
46320	Remove hemorrhoid clot	209	257	328	208	5.75
46500	Inject into hemorrhoid(s)	298	366	467	167	4.62
46600	Diagnostic anoscopy	71	87	112	49	1.36
46604	Anoscopy and dilation	121	148	189	87	2.39
46606	Anoscopy and biopsy	111	136	174	63	1.75
46608	Anoscopy/ remove for body	223	273	349	125	3.45
46610	Anoscopy/remove lesion	194	238	304	105	2.90
46611	Anoscopy	211	259	331	146	4.03
46612	Anoscopy/ remove lesions	267	327	418	187	5.17
46614	Anoscopy/control bleeding	219	269	343	147	4.05
46615	Anoscopy	268	329	420	169	4.67
46700	Repair anal stricture	849	1042	1330	524	14.47
46705	Repair anal stricture	887	1088	1390	440	12.16
46715	Repair anovaginal fistula	802	984	1256	450	12.42
46716	Repair anovaginal fistula	1032	1267	1617	884	24.42
46730	Construction absent anus	2051	2517	3214	1485	41.03

NEW CODE CPT 2002 •

CPT	SHORT DESCRIPTION	50th	75th	90th	MFS	RVU
46735	Construction absent anus	2487	3053	3898	1821	50.30
46740	Construction absent anus	2537	3114	3976	1687	46.60
46742	Repair imperforate anus	2852	3500	4469	2054	56.74
46744	Repair cloacal anomaly	3539	4344	5547	2812	77.68
46746	Repair cloacal anomaly	4031	4947	6317	3183	87.92
46748	Repair cloacal anomaly	4431	5439	6945	3495	96.56
46750	Repair anal sphincter	1080	1325	1692	606	16.73
46751	Repair anal sphincter	1013	1243	1587	568	15.69
46753	Reconstruct anus	752	923	1179	471	13.00
46754	Remove suture from anus	496	608	777	278	7.68
46760	Repair anal sphincter	1443	1771	2261	809	22.36
46761	Repair anal sphincter	1943	2385	3045	780	21.55
46762	Implant artificial sphincter	2328	2857	3649	706	19.50
46900	Destroy anal lesion(s)	359	440	562	201	5.56
46910	Destroy anal lesion(s)	232	285	364	210	5.81
46916	Cryosurgery anal lesion(s)	208	255	326	188	5.19
46917	Laser surgery anal lesions	387	475	607	266	7.34
46922	Excise anal lesion(s)	360	441	564	217	5.99
46924	Destroy anal lesion(s)	682	837	1069	281	7.77
46934	Destroy hemorrhoids	405	497	635	376	10.39
46935	Destroy hemorrhoids	292	359	458	261	7.20
46936	Destroy hemorrhoids	801	983	1255	386	10.66
46937	Cryotherapy rectal lesion	318	390	498	265	7.32
46938	Cryotherapy rectal lesion	504	619	790	408	11.28
46940	Treat anal fissure	228	280	357	216	5.96
46942	Treat anal fissure	324	398	508	182	5.02

CPT	SHORT DESCRIPTION	50th	75th	90th	MFS	RVU
46945	Ligate hemorrhoids	270	331	423	219	6.05
46946	Ligate hemorrhoids	529	650	829	297	8.20
46999	Anus surgery procedure	0	0	0	0	.00

LIVER

CPT	SHORT DESCRIPTION	50th	75th	90th	MFS	RVU
47000	Needle biopsy liver	400	501	616	375	10.35
47001	Needle biopsy liver add-on	315	393	484	100	2.76
47010	Open drain liver lesion	1503	1879	2313	951	26.26
47011	Percut drain liver lesion	447	559	688	307	8.48
47015	Inject/aspirate liver cyst	1517	1896	2334	876	24.20
47100	Wedge biopsy liver	1369	1712	2107	685	18.92
47120	Partial remove liver	3018	3774	4644	1984	54.81
47122	Extensive remove liver	4018	5025	6184	2999	82.84
47125	Partial remove liver	3642	4554	5605	2696	74.49
47130	Partial remove liver	3947	4936	6075	2907	80.31
47133	Remove donor liver	3233	4043	4975	0	.00
47134	Partial remove donor liver	3641	4553	5604	2065	57.04
47135	Transplantation liver	8323	10408	12808	4812	132.93
47136	Transplantation liver	7227	9038	11123	4435	122.53
47300	Surgery for liver lesion	1847	2310	2843	862	23.80
47350	Repair liver wound	1883	2355	2898	1095	30.26
47360	Repair liver wound	2593	3243	3991	1506	41.59
47361	Repair liver wound	3247	4060	4997	2540	70.17
47362	Repair liver wound	1444	1806	2223	1068	29.50
• **47370**	Laparo ablate liver tumor rf	1205	1507	1854	943	26.04
• **47371**	Laparo ablate liver cryosug	1136	1421	1748	889	24.55
47379	Laparoscope procedure liver	0	0	0	0	.00

NEW CODE CPT 2002 •

CPT	SHORT DESCRIPTION	50th	75th	90th	MFS	RVU
• 47380	Open ablate liver tumor rf	1415	1769	2178	1107	30.58
• 47381	Open ablate liver tumor cryo	1399	1749	2153	1094	30.23
• 47382	Percut ablate liver rf	843	1054	1297	660	18.22
47399	Liver surgery procedure	0	0	0	0	.00

BILIARY TRACT

CPT	SHORT DESCRIPTION	50th	75th	90th	MFS	RVU
47400	Incise liver duct	2659	3138	3820	1785	49.30
47420	Incise bile duct	2189	2583	3145	1124	31.04
47425	Incise bile duct	2820	3328	4052	1115	30.81
47460	Incise bile duct sphincter	2130	2513	3060	1033	28.54
47480	Incise gallbladder	1855	2189	2665	669	18.47
47490	Incise gallbladder	815	962	1171	551	15.23
47500	Inject for liver x-rays	406	479	584	99	2.73
47505	Inject for liver x-rays	257	304	370	133	3.67
47510	Insert catheter bile duct	1000	1180	1437	639	17.65
47511	Insert bile duct drain	1286	1518	1848	780	21.54
47525	Change bile duct catheter	580	684	833	330	9.13
47530	Revise/reinsert bile tube	502	593	722	406	11.21
47550	Bile duct endoscopy add-on	370	436	531	159	4.40
47552	Biliary endoscopy thru skin	506	597	727	325	8.98
47553	Biliary endoscopy thru skin	563	664	808	338	9.35
47554	Biliary endoscopy thru skin	668	788	959	483	13.35
47555	Biliary endoscopy thru skin	636	751	914	400	11.06
47556	Biliary endoscopy thru skin	603	712	866	450	12.43
47560	Laparoscopy w/cholangio	1181	1394	1697	263	7.27
47561	Lap w/cholangio/biopsy	1307	1542	1878	285	7.86
47562	Lap cholecystectomy	2520	2974	3621	629	17.37

CPT	SHORT DESCRIPTION	50th	75th	90th	MFS	RVU
47563	Lap cholecystectomy/graph	2569	3031	3691	673	18.58
47564	Lap cholecystectomy/explore	2383	2812	3424	794	21.93
47570	Lap cholecystoenterostomy	1936	2285	2782	707	19.53
47579	Lap procedure biliary	0	0	0	0	.00
47600	Remove gallbladder	2190	2585	3147	782	21.60
47605	Remove gallbladder	2276	2685	3270	839	23.17
47610	Remove gallbladder	2399	2831	3446	1058	29.23
47612	Remove gallbladder	3635	4290	5223	1053	29.08
47620	Remove gallbladder	2633	3107	3783	1150	31.76
47630	Remove bile duct stone	753	889	1083	462	12.77
47700	Explore bile ducts	2066	2439	2969	934	25.81
47701	Bile duct revise	3659	4318	5257	1608	44.41
47711	Excise bile duct tumor	3259	3846	4683	1316	36.35
47712	Excise bile duct tumor	3290	3883	4727	1698	46.91
47715	Excise bile duct cyst	2368	2795	3403	1062	29.34
47716	Fuse bile duct cyst	1879	2217	2700	943	26.04
47720	Fuse gallbladder & bowel	1860	2194	2672	939	25.94
47721	Fuse upper gi structures	2541	2999	3651	1110	30.65
47740	Fuse gallbladder & bowel	2123	2506	3051	1075	29.71
47741	Fuse gallbladder & bowel	2851	3364	4096	1223	33.78
47760	Fuse bile ducts and bowel	2833	3343	4070	1460	40.34
47765	Fuse liver ducts & bowel	2870	3386	4123	1440	39.79
47780	Fuse bile ducts and bowel	3379	3987	4855	1494	41.26
47785	Fuse bile ducts and bowel	3929	4637	5645	1768	48.84
47800	Reconstruct bile ducts	3030	3576	4354	1333	36.82
47801	Place bile duct support	1759	2075	2527	944	26.07

 NEW CODE CPT 2002 •

CPT	SHORT DESCRIPTION	50th	75th	90th	MFS	RVU
47802	Fuse liver duct & intestine	3093	3650	4444	1267	34.99
47900	Suture bile duct injury	1669	1969	2398	1151	31.80
47999	Bile tract surgery procedure	0	0	0	0	.00

PANCREAS

CPT	SHORT DESCRIPTION	50th	75th	90th	MFS	RVU
48000	Drain abdomen	1648	1944	2367	1520	41.98
48001	Place drain, pancreas	4220	4980	6064	1896	52.39
48005	Resect/debride pancreas	2817	3324	4047	2238	61.82
48020	Remove pancreatic stone	2309	2725	3317	887	24.50
48100	Biopsy pancreas, open	1845	2178	2652	736	20.34
48102	Needle biopsy pancreas	640	756	920	501	13.84
48120	Remove pancreas lesion	2394	2825	3440	901	24.89
48140	Partial remove pancreas	2743	3237	3941	1297	35.84
48145	Partial remove pancreas	2944	3474	4230	1367	37.75
48146	Pancreatectomy	3754	4431	5394	1549	42.79
48148	Remove pancreatic duct	3215	3794	4619	1017	28.10
48150	Partial remove pancreas	4725	5576	6789	2669	73.72
48152	Pancreatectomy	4368	5155	6277	2482	68.56
48153	Pancreatectomy	4711	5560	6769	2696	74.47
48154	Pancreatectomy	4406	5200	6331	2498	69.02
48155	Remove pancreas	4507	5318	6475	1478	40.83
48160	Pancreas remove/transplant	0	0	0	0	.00
48180	Fuse pancreas and bowel	3643	4300	5235	1380	38.12
48400	Inject, intraop add-on	359	424	516	99	2.74
48500	Surgery pancreatic cyst	1841	2173	2645	882	24.37
48510	Drain pancreatic pseudocyst	2622	3094	3767	826	22.83
48511	Drain pancreatic pseudocyst	675	796	970	294	8.12

CPT	SHORT DESCRIPTION	50th	75th	90th	MFS	RVU
48520	Fuse pancreas cyst and bowel	2204	2600	3166	887	24.49
48540	Fuse pancreas cyst and bowel	2723	3214	3913	1100	30.38
48545	Pancreatorrhaphy	2442	2882	3509	1038	28.67
48547	Duodenal exclusion	4477	5283	6432	1418	39.17
48550	Donor pancreatectomy	0	0	0	0	.00
48554	Transpl allograft pancreas	3569	4212	5129	1801	49.74
48556	Remove allograft pancreas	1770	2089	2543	939	25.94
48999	Pancreas surgery procedure	0	0	0	0	.00

ABDOMEN, PERITONEUM, AND OMENTUM

CPT	SHORT DESCRIPTION	50th	75th	90th	MFS	RVU
49000	Explore abdomen	1948	2402	3150	690	19.07
49002	Reopening abdomen	1652	2038	2672	639	17.65
49010	Explore behind abdomen	2092	2581	3384	744	20.55
49020	Drain abdominal abscess	1690	2084	2733	1287	35.56
49021	Drain abdominal abscess	939	1159	1519	340	9.38
49040	Drain, open, abdom abscess	1786	2203	2888	810	22.38
49041	Drain, percut, abdom abscess	475	586	769	371	10.25
49060	Drain, open, retrop abscess	1678	2069	2713	950	26.25
49061	Drain, percut, retroper absc	749	924	1211	357	9.86
49062	Drain to peritoneal cavity	1367	1686	2211	706	19.50
49080	Puncture peritoneal cavity	238	294	385	216	5.98
49081	Remove abdominal fluid	201	247	324	161	4.46
49085	Remove abdomen foreign body	1200	1480	1940	715	19.74
49180	Biopsy abdominal mass	432	532	698	373	10.31
49200	Remove abdominal lesion	2144	2645	3468	642	17.73
49201	Remove abdominal lesion	3175	3916	5134	911	25.18
49215	Excise sacral spine tumor	2920	3602	4722	1864	51.50

NEW CODE CPT 2002 •

CPT	SHORT DESCRIPTION	50th	75th	90th	MFS	RVU
49220	Multiple surgery abdomen	2511	3098	4061	881	24.33
49250	Excise umbilicus	967	1193	1564	523	14.45
49255	Remove omentum	1535	1894	2483	685	18.92
49320	Diag laparo separate proc	1275	1573	2062	314	8.68
49321	Laparoscopy, biopsy	1473	1818	2383	326	9.00
49322	Laparoscopy, aspiration	1513	1867	2448	355	9.80
49323	Laparo drain lymphocele	1415	1746	2289	526	14.54
49329	Laparo proc, abdm/per/oment	0	0	0	0	.00
49400	Air inject into abdomen	169	209	273	102	2.81
49420	Insert abdominal drain	388	479	628	121	3.33
49421	Insert abdominal drain	1078	1330	1743	368	10.17
49422	Remove perm cannula/catheter	1022	1260	1652	358	9.89
49423	Exchange drain catheter	294	363	476	81	2.23
49424	Assess cyst, contrast inject	158	195	255	45	1.24
49425	Insert abdomen-venous drain	1624	2003	2626	701	19.37
49426	Revise abdomen-venous shunt	1684	2078	2724	606	16.73
49427	Inject abdominal shunt	155	192	251	52	1.44
49428	Ligate shunt	528	651	854	346	9.56
49429	Remove shunt	1214	1497	1963	426	11.76
• 49491	Repairing hern premie reduc	1835	2264	2968	644	17.78
• 49492	Rpr ing hern premie, blocked	2255	2782	3647	791	21.85
49495	Rpr ing hernia baby, reduc	1431	1765	2314	368	10.16
49496	Rpr ing hernia baby, blocked	1477	1822	2389	565	15.62
49500	Rpr ing hernia, init, reduce	1322	1631	2138	341	9.42
49501	Rpr ing hernia, init blocked	1445	1782	2337	516	14.26
49505	Rpr i/hern init reduc>5 yr	1380	1703	2232	464	12.83

CPT	SHORT DESCRIPTION	50th	75th	90th	MFS	RVU
49507	Rpr i/hern init block>5 yr	1613	1989	2608	600	16.57
49520	Rerepair ing hernia, reduce	1640	2023	2652	578	15.96
49521	Rerepair ing hernia, blocked	1678	2069	2713	683	18.86
49525	Repair ing hernia, sliding	1586	1957	2565	517	14.28
49540	Repair lumbar hernia	1394	1720	2255	613	16.94
49550	Rpr fem hernia, init, reduce	1360	1678	2200	504	13.93
49553	Rpr fem hernia, init blocked	1367	1686	2211	551	15.22
49555	Rerepair fem hernia, reduce	1276	1573	2063	547	15.12
49557	Rerepair fem hernia, blocked	1474	1818	2383	641	17.71
49560	Rpr ventral hern init, reduc	1713	2113	2771	676	18.68
49561	Rpr ventral hern init, block	1960	2418	3170	803	22.19
49565	Rerepair ventral hern, reduce	1905	2349	3080	682	18.84
49566	Rerepair ventral hern, block	2126	2623	3439	812	22.43
49568	Hernia repair w/mesh	624	770	1009	259	7.15
49570	Rpr epigastric hern, reduce	1069	1319	1730	352	9.73
49572	Rpr epigastric hern, blocked	1356	1672	2193	409	11.31
49580	Rpr umbil hern, reduc <5 yr	1080	1333	1747	271	7.48
49582	Rpr umbil hern, block < 5 yr	1220	1505	1973	443	12.24
49585	Rpr umbil hern, reduc > 5 yr	1207	1489	1952	395	10.91
49587	Rpr umbil hern, block > 5 yr	1419	1750	2294	452	12.48
49590	Repair spigelian hernia	1307	1613	2114	515	14.24
49600	Repair umbilical lesion	1475	1819	2385	666	18.39
49605	Repair umbilical lesion	11288	13924	18255	3959	109.36
49606	Repair umbilical lesion	1952	2408	3157	1102	30.43
49610	Repair umbilical lesion	1421	1753	2298	657	18.14
49611	Repair umbilical lesion	1561	1925	2524	584	16.13

NEW CODE CPT 2002 •

CPT	SHORT DESCRIPTION	50th	75th	90th	MFS	RVU
49650	Laparo hernia repair initial	1522	1877	2461	371	10.24
49651	Laparo hernia repair recur	1401	1729	2266	488	13.48
49659	Laparo proc hernia repair	0	0	0	0	.00
49900	Repair abdominal wall	1334	1645	2157	735	20.31
49905	Omental flap	991	1222	1602	348	9.60
49906	Free omental flap, microvasc	0	0	0	0	.00
49999	Abdomen surgery procedure	0	0	0	0	.00

CPT	SHORT DESCRIPTION	50th	75th	90th	MFS	RVU

NEW CODE CPT 2002 •

CPT	SHORT DESCRIPTION	50th	75th	90th	MFS	RVU

URINARY SYSTEM

KIDNEY

CPT	SHORT DESCRIPTION	50th	75th	90th	MFS	RVU
50010	Explore kidney	1932	2376	3021	682	18.84
50020	Renal abscess, open drain	1809	2225	2828	1056	29.18
50021	Renal abscess, percut drain	1729	2126	2703	506	13.99
50040	Drain kidney	2369	2912	3703	989	27.32
50045	Explore kidney	2514	3091	3929	908	25.07
50060	Remove kidney stone	2435	2994	3806	1103	30.47
50065	Incise kidney	3113	3828	4867	1176	32.48
50070	Incise kidney	2986	3671	4667	1166	32.22
50075	Remove kidney stone	3201	3935	5003	1430	39.50
50080	Remove kidney stone	2649	3257	4141	963	26.60
50081	Remove kidney stone	3590	4414	5612	1317	36.37
50100	Revise kidney blood vessels	1584	1948	2477	980	27.07
50120	Explore kidney	2392	2941	3740	937	25.88
50125	Explore and drain kidney	2461	3025	3846	980	27.07
50130	Remove kidney stone	2585	3179	4041	998	27.57
50135	Explore kidney	2916	3585	4558	1096	30.29
50200	Biopsy kidney	526	647	822	134	3.71
50205	Biopsy kidney	1238	1522	1935	679	18.77
50220	Remove kidney, open	3013	3704	4709	999	27.60
50225	Remove kidney open, complex	3038	3736	4750	1151	31.79
50230	Remove kidney open, radical	4005	4924	6260	1243	34.34
50234	Remove kidney & ureter	2855	3510	4462	1260	34.82
50236	Remove kidney & ureter	3258	4006	5094	1471	40.63

CPT	SHORT DESCRIPTION	50th	75th	90th	MFS	RVU
50240	Partial remove kidney	2928	3600	4577	1328	36.68
50280	Remove kidney lesion	2039	2507	3187	918	25.35
50290	Remove kidney lesion	2220	2729	3470	881	24.33
50300	Remove donor kidney	2500	3073	3907	0	.00
50320	Remove donor kidney	4322	5314	6756	1266	34.97
50340	Remove kidney	2313	2844	3616	818	22.61
50360	Transplantation kidney	6171	7587	9646	1896	52.37
50365	Transplantation kidney	6427	7902	10047	2230	61.61
50370	Remove transplanted kidney	2296	2823	3589	900	24.86
50380	Reimplantation kidney	4302	5289	6725	1306	36.08
50390	Drain kidney lesion	433	532	677	99	2.73
50392	Insert kidney drain	659	811	1031	170	4.71
50393	Insert ureteral tube	783	962	1224	209	5.78
50394	Inject for kidney x-ray	198	244	310	123	3.40
50395	Create passage to kidney	763	938	1192	170	4.71
50396	Measure kidney pressure	144	177	226	111	3.08
50398	Change kidney tube	216	265	337	94	2.59
50400	Revise kidney/ureter	2876	3537	4496	1114	30.77
50405	Revise kidney/ureter	3121	3838	4879	1347	37.22
50500	Repair kidney wound	2180	2680	3408	1172	32.39
50520	Close kidney-skin fistula	2298	2825	3592	1096	30.29
50525	Repair renal-abdomen fistula	2887	3549	4513	1342	37.08
50526	Repair renal-abdomen fistula	3092	3802	4833	1466	40.50
50540	Revise horseshoe kidney	3729	4585	5829	1145	31.63
50541	Laparo ablate renal cyst	2148	2640	3357	861	23.78
50544	Laparoscopy, pyeloplasty	2571	3161	4019	1189	32.85

   NEW CODE CPT 2002 •

CPT	SHORT DESCRIPTION	50th	75th	90th	MFS	RVU
50545	Laparo radical nephrectomy	2381	2928	3723	1273	35.18
50546	Laparoscopic nephrectomy	2379	2925	3718	1095	30.25
50547	Laparo remove donor kidney	4262	5241	6663	1405	38.81
50548	Laparo remove k/ureter	2389	2937	3735	1288	35.59
50549	Laparoscope proc, renal	0	0	0	0	.00
50551	Kidney endoscopy	1342	1650	2098	393	10.86
50553	Kidney endoscopy	2792	3432	4364	818	22.59
50555	Kidney endoscopy & biopsy	3339	4106	5220	978	27.02
50557	Kidney endoscopy & treat	3366	4139	5262	986	27.24
50559	Renal endoscopy/radiotracer	836	1028	1307	343	9.47
50561	Kidney endoscopy & treat	3255	4002	5089	953	26.34
50570	Kidney endoscopy	1649	2027	2577	483	13.34
50572	Kidney endoscopy	582	716	910	525	14.51
50574	Kidney endoscopy & biopsy	612	753	957	563	15.54
50575	Kidney endoscopy	1015	1248	1587	708	19.55
50576	Kidney endoscopy & treat	808	994	1263	557	15.39
50578	Renal endoscopy/radiotracer	904	1111	1413	580	16.03
50580	Kidney endoscopy & treat	940	1155	1469	601	16.59
50590	Fragmenting kidney stone	2643	3249	4131	739	20.41

URETER

CPT	SHORT DESCRIPTION	50th	75th	90th	MFS	RVU
50600	Explore ureter	1974	2251	2834	938	25.90
50605	Insert ureteral support	1194	1362	1714	922	25.47
50610	Remove ureter stone	1988	2268	2855	944	26.09
50620	Remove ureter stone	1876	2140	2694	891	24.62
50630	Remove ureter stone	1853	2114	2661	880	24.32
50650	Remove ureter	2148	2450	3085	1020	28.19

CPT	SHORT DESCRIPTION	50th	75th	90th	MFS	RVU
50660	Remove ureter	2376	2709	3411	1128	31.17
50684	Inject for ureter x-ray	1206	1375	1731	573	15.82
50686	Measure ureter pressure	509	581	731	242	6.68
50688	Change ureter tube	228	260	327	108	2.99
50690	Inject for ureter x-ray	1267	1445	1818	602	16.62
50700	Revise ureter	2107	2403	3025	911	25.16
50715	Release ureter	2155	2457	3094	1193	32.95
50722	Release ureter	1826	2083	2622	1020	28.18
50725	Release/revise ureter	2708	3089	3888	1106	30.54
50727	Revise ureter	1299	1482	1866	551	15.23
50728	Revise ureter	1836	2094	2636	763	21.08
50740	Fuse ureter & kidney	2462	2808	3535	1070	29.57
50750	Fuse ureter & kidney	2594	2958	3724	1131	31.23
50760	Fuse ureters	2466	2813	3541	1078	29.78
50770	Splicing ureters	2606	2972	3741	1129	31.19
50780	Reimplant ureter in bladder	3415	3895	4903	1070	29.57
50782	Reimplant ureter in bladder	2636	3007	3785	1179	32.58
50783	Reimplant ureter in bladder	2707	3088	3887	1199	33.12
50785	Reimplant ureter in bladder	2720	3103	3906	1182	32.65
50800	Implant ureter in bowel	2324	2651	3337	922	25.46
50810	Fuse ureter & bowel	3414	3894	4902	1233	34.06
50815	Urine shunt to intestine	3441	3925	4941	1193	32.95
50820	Construct bowel bladder	3607	4114	5179	1291	35.65
50825	Construct bowel bladder	3968	4526	5697	1639	45.29
50830	Revise urine flow	2444	2787	3509	1790	49.44
50840	Replace ureter by bowel	3577	4079	5135	1198	33.09

NEW CODE CPT 2002 •

CPT	SHORT DESCRIPTION	50th	75th	90th	MFS	RVU
50845	Appendico-vesicostomy	2674	3050	3840	1171	32.35
50860	Transplant ureter to skin	1928	2199	2768	916	25.30
50900	Repair ureter	2042	2330	2933	821	22.68
50920	Close ureter/skin fistula	1959	2235	2813	852	23.54
50930	Close ureter/bowel fistula	2500	2852	3590	1125	31.09
50940	Release ureter	1961	2237	2816	868	23.99
50945	Laparoscopy ureterolithotomy	1949	2223	2798	926	25.57
50947	Laparo new ureter/bladder	2567	2928	3686	1384	38.23
50948	Laparo new ureter/bladder	2347	2677	3370	1265	34.94
50949	Laparoscope proc ureter	0	0	0	0	.00
50951	Endoscopy ureter	874	997	1255	415	11.47
50953	Endoscopy ureter	1765	2013	2534	838	23.16
50955	Ureter endoscopy & biopsy	2152	2455	3090	1022	28.24
50957	Ureter endoscopy & treat	2045	2332	2936	971	26.83
50959	Ureter endoscopy & tracer	653	745	938	223	6.16
50961	Ureter endoscopy & treat	2270	2589	3259	1078	29.78
50970	Ureter endoscopy	762	869	1094	362	10.00
50972	Ureter endoscopy & catheter	539	614	773	355	9.80
50974	Ureter endoscopy & biopsy	669	763	961	466	12.86
50976	Ureter endoscopy & treat	655	747	941	458	12.66
50978	Ureter endoscopy & tracer	688	785	988	264	7.28
50980	Ureter endoscopy & treat	732	834	1050	348	9.60

BLADDER

CPT	SHORT DESCRIPTION	50th	75th	90th	MFS	RVU
51000	Drain bladder	123	167	229	104	2.86
51005	Drain bladder	192	260	358	162	4.47
51010	Drain bladder	304	411	565	296	8.18

CPT	SHORT DESCRIPTION	50th	75th	90th	MFS	RVU
51020	Incise & treat bladder	1181	1598	2197	465	12.85
51030	Incise & treat bladder	1243	1682	2312	478	13.20
51040	Incise & drain bladder	1140	1542	2121	331	9.14
51045	Incise bladder/drain ureter	1165	1576	2167	480	13.25
51050	Remove bladder stone	1180	1597	2196	456	12.61
51060	Remove ureter stone	1656	2240	3080	576	15.92
51065	Remove ureter calculus	1433	1939	2665	559	15.44
51080	Drain bladder abscess	881	1192	1639	434	11.98
51500	Remove bladder cyst	1304	1765	2426	621	17.15
51520	Remove bladder lesion	1402	1897	2608	598	16.53
51525	Remove bladder lesion	1766	2390	3285	831	22.97
51530	Remove bladder lesion	1457	1972	2711	761	21.01
51535	Repair ureter lesion	1462	1978	2720	786	21.70
51550	Partial remove bladder	1303	1763	2424	919	25.39
51555	Partial remove bladder	1706	2309	3174	1216	33.60
51565	Revise bladder & ureter(s)	2126	2876	3954	1254	34.64
51570	Remove bladder	2343	3170	4358	1391	38.43
51575	Remove bladder & nodes	3728	5044	6935	1726	47.68
51580	Remove bladder/revise tract	3750	5075	6977	1775	49.03
51585	Remove bladder & nodes	4738	6410	8813	1982	54.75
51590	Remove bladder/revise tract	4818	6519	8962	1835	50.68
51595	Remove bladder/revise tract	5572	7540	10365	2060	56.92
51596	Remove bladder/create pouch	4883	6607	9083	2203	60.85
51597	Remove pelvic structures	5699	7711	10601	2132	58.90
51600	Inject for bladder x-ray	277	375	515	233	6.43
51605	Preparation for bladder xray	750	1014	1394	630	17.41

  NEW CODE CPT 2002 •

CPT	SHORT DESCRIPTION	50th	75th	90th	MFS	RVU
51610	Inject for bladder x-ray	745	1008	1386	626	17.30
51700	Irrigate bladder	90	122	168	81	2.25
51705	Change bladder tube	122	165	227	117	3.23
51710	Change bladder tube	252	341	469	242	6.69
51715	Endoscopic inject/implant	534	723	994	305	8.42
51720	Treat bladder lesion	155	210	289	136	3.76
51725	Simple cystometrogram	323	410	517	274	7.56
51726	Complex cystometrogram	253	321	405	236	6.51
51736	Urine flow measurement	97	122	154	63	1.73
51741	Electro-uroflowmetry, first	148	188	237	114	3.16
51772	Urethra pressure profile	278	353	445	235	6.50
51784	Anal/urinary muscle study	215	272	343	182	5.02
51785	Anal/urinary muscle study	214	271	342	185	5.11
51792	Urinary reflex study	188	239	301	168	4.63
51795	Urine voiding pressure study	281	356	448	237	6.55
51797	Intraabdominal pressure test	283	359	452	239	6.61
51800	Revise bladder/urethra	2350	2744	3254	1020	28.18
51820	Revise urinary tract	3470	4051	4805	1095	30.25
51840	Attach bladder/urethra	2071	2417	2867	668	18.46
51841	Attach bladder/urethra	2342	2733	3242	820	22.64
51845	Repair bladder neck	2265	2644	3135	624	17.25
51860	Repair bladder wound	1693	1976	2343	753	20.81
51865	Repair bladder wound	2270	2650	3143	904	24.98
51880	Repair bladder opening	1116	1302	1545	513	14.18
51900	Repair bladder/vagina lesion	2478	2893	3431	801	22.13
51920	Close bladder-uterus fistula	2203	2572	3050	736	20.32

CPT	SHORT DESCRIPTION	50th	75th	90th	MFS	RVU
51925	Hysterectomy/bladder repair	2636	3077	3650	967	26.71
51940	Correct bladder defect	1758	2052	2434	1694	46.81
51960	Revise bladder & bowel	3940	4599	5454	1369	37.81
51980	Construct bladder opening	2097	2448	2903	702	19.40
51990	Laparo urethral suspend	1972	2302	2730	735	20.31
51992	Laparo sling operation	1909	2228	2642	787	21.75
52000	Cystoscopy	331	407	529	202	5.58
• **52001**	Cystoscopy, remove clots	288	354	459	133	3.67
52005	Cystoscopy & ureter catheter	1249	1536	1993	576	15.92
52007	Cystoscopy and biopsy	470	578	750	153	4.22
52010	Cystoscopy & duct catheter	515	634	822	330	9.11
52204	Cystoscopy	530	652	846	315	8.69
52214	Cystoscopy and treat	649	798	1036	379	10.46
52224	Cystoscopy and treat	622	765	993	352	9.73
52234	Cystoscopy and treat	962	1184	1536	238	6.58
52235	Cystoscopy and treat	1530	1882	2441	280	7.74
52240	Cystoscopy and treat	2147	2641	3425	497	13.73
52250	Cystoscopy and radiotracer	494	608	788	228	6.30
52260	Cystoscopy and treat	550	677	878	199	5.49
52265	Cystoscopy and treat	492	606	786	249	6.89
52270	Cystoscopy & revise urethra	535	658	853	378	10.45
52275	Cystoscopy & revise urethra	637	783	1016	449	12.40
52276	Cystoscopy and treat	1053	1295	1680	465	12.85
52277	Cystoscopy and treat	637	784	1017	314	8.67
52281	Cystoscopy and treat	1373	1689	2191	634	17.51
52282	Cystoscopy implant stent	1737	2136	2771	801	22.14

    NEW CODE CPT 2002 •

CPT	SHORT DESCRIPTION	50th	75th	90th	MFS	RVU
52283	Cystoscopy and treat	443	545	706	382	10.54
52285	Cystoscopy and treat	622	765	992	394	10.89
52290	Cystoscopy and treat	450	553	717	232	6.42
52300	Cystoscopy and treat	583	717	930	269	7.43
52301	Cystoscopy and treat	606	745	966	279	7.72
52305	Cystoscopy and treat	582	716	929	269	7.42
52310	Cystoscopy and treat	615	757	981	247	6.83
52315	Cystoscopy and treat	942	1159	1503	795	21.95
52317	Remove bladder stone	1324	1628	2112	1202	33.21
52318	Remove bladder stone	1733	2132	2765	465	12.84
52320	Cystoscopy and treat	931	1146	1486	238	6.57
52325	Cystoscopy stone remove	1368	1683	2184	312	8.61
52327	Cystoscopy inject material	848	1043	1353	264	7.28
52330	Cystoscopy and treat	2050	2521	3270	946	26.13
52332	Cystoscopy and treat	796	979	1270	791	21.84
52334	Create passage to kidney	529	650	844	244	6.74
52341	Cysto w/ureter stricture tx	600	738	957	317	8.77
52342	Cysto w/up stricture tx	649	799	1036	344	9.49
52343	Cysto w/renal stricture tx	719	885	1148	380	10.51
52344	Cysto/uretero stone remove	769	946	1227	407	11.24
52345	Cysto/uretero w/up stricture	819	1008	1308	433	11.97
52346	Cystouretero w/renal strict	922	1134	1471	488	13.48
• 52347	Cystoscopy resect ducts	608	748	970	281	7.75
52351	Cystouretro & or pyeloscope	612	753	977	297	8.21
52352	Cystouretro w/stone remove	758	932	1209	349	9.63
52353	Cystouretero w/lithotripsy	878	1080	1401	404	11.15

CPT	SHORT DESCRIPTION	50th	75th	90th	MFS	RVU
52354	Cystouretero w/biopsy	768	945	1226	372	10.28
52355	Cystouretero w/excise tumor	902	1109	1439	447	12.36
52400	Cystouretero w/congen repair	1073	1320	1712	580	16.03
52450	Incise prostate	946	1163	1509	531	14.66
52500	Revise bladder neck	1467	1805	2341	571	15.78
52510	Dilation prostatic urethra	1013	1247	1617	468	12.92
52601	Prostatectomy (turp)	2417	2973	3856	770	21.27
52606	Control postop bleeding	1168	1437	1864	539	14.89
52612	Prostatectomy, first stage	1384	1703	2209	550	15.18
52614	Prostatectomy, second stage	913	1123	1456	490	13.55
52620	Remove residual prostate	735	905	1173	479	13.22
52630	Remove prostate regrowth	1976	2431	3153	511	14.13
52640	Relieve bladder contracture	1042	1282	1663	461	12.74
52647	Laser surgery prostate	3855	4742	6151	2545	70.30
52648	Laser surgery prostate	1410	1734	2250	706	19.50
52700	Drain prostate abscess	844	1039	1347	490	13.53

URETHRA

CPT	SHORT DESCRIPTION	50th	75th	90th	MFS	RVU
53000	Incise urethra	456	648	900	358	9.88
53010	Incise urethra	439	624	866	288	7.96
53020	Incise urethra	277	394	547	228	6.31
53025	Incise urethra	277	394	547	218	6.01
53040	Drain urethra abscess	994	1413	1963	780	21.55
53060	Drain urethra abscess	418	595	826	328	9.07
53080	Drain urinary leakage	696	989	1374	546	15.08
53085	Drain urinary leakage	979	1392	1934	769	21.23
53200	Biopsy urethra	387	550	764	304	8.39

  NEW CODE CPT 2002 •

CPT	SHORT DESCRIPTION	50th	75th	90th	MFS	RVU
53210	Remove urethra	1188	1688	2345	774	21.38
53215	Remove urethra	1449	2060	2861	917	25.32
53220	Treat urethra lesion	852	1211	1683	476	13.15
53230	Remove urethra lesion	1134	1612	2239	599	16.54
53235	Remove urethra lesion	1128	1603	2227	624	17.23
53240	Surgery for urethra pouch	543	772	1072	441	12.19
53250	Remove urethra gland	988	1405	1951	397	10.98
53260	Treat urethra lesion	430	611	849	337	9.32
53265	Treat urethra lesion	458	650	903	359	9.92
53270	Remove urethra gland	476	677	941	374	10.33
53275	Repair urethra defect	381	541	752	298	8.24
53400	Revise urethra, stage 1	994	1413	1963	794	21.93
53405	Revise urethra, stage 2	1179	1676	2327	869	24.00
53410	Reconstruct urethra	1491	2120	2945	964	26.64
53415	Reconstruct urethra	1504	2138	2970	1112	30.73
53420	Reconstruct urethra, stage 1	1625	2311	3209	862	23.80
53425	Reconstruct urethra, stage 2	1479	2102	2920	940	25.97
53430	Reconstruct urethra	1256	1786	2481	966	26.69
• 53431	Reconstruct urethra/bladder	1341	1907	2649	1053	29.08
53440	Correct bladder function	1503	2137	2969	766	21.16
53442	Remove perineal prosthesis	683	970	1348	539	14.90
• 53444	Insert tandem cuff	962	1367	1899	755	20.85
53445	Insert uro/ves neck sphincter	1434	2039	2832	855	23.62
• 53446	Remove uro sphincter	890	1266	1758	699	19.30
53447	Remove/replace ur sphincter	1253	1782	2475	803	22.18
• 53448	Rem/repl ur sphincter comp	1604	2280	3167	1259	34.77

CPT	SHORT DESCRIPTION	50th	75th	90th	MFS	RVU
53449	Repair uro sphincter	840	1194	1658	615	17.00
53450	Revise urethra	730	1038	1441	422	11.67
53460	Revise urethra	602	856	1189	472	13.05
53502	Repair urethra injury	907	1290	1792	504	13.93
53505	Repair urethra injury	906	1288	1789	496	13.71
53510	Repair urethra injury	1170	1663	2310	626	17.29
53515	Repair urethra injury	1870	2659	3694	795	21.95
53520	Repair urethra defect	703	999	1388	555	15.33
53600	Dilate urethra stricture	119	169	235	89	2.47
53601	Dilate urethra stricture	106	150	209	85	2.35
53605	Dilate urethra stricture	122	173	241	65	1.80
53620	Dilate urethra stricture	176	250	347	131	3.63
53621	Dilate urethra stricture	157	224	311	124	3.43
53660	Dilation urethra	98	139	194	71	1.97
53661	Dilation urethra	90	128	177	71	1.97
53665	Dilation urethra	104	148	205	39	1.08
53670	Insert urinary catheter	105	149	207	82	2.27
53675	Insert urinary catheter	156	222	308	152	4.19
53850	Prostatic microwave thermotx	4499	6397	8885	3531	97.55
53852	Prostatic rf thermotx	3966	5639	7832	3113	85.99
• 53853	Prostatic water thermother	2641	3756	5216	2073	57.27
53899	Urology surgery procedure	0	0	0	0	.00

NEW CODE CPT 2002 •

MALE GENITAL SYSTEM

PENIS

CPT	SHORT DESCRIPTION	50th	75th	90th	MFS	RVU
54000	Slitting prepuce	508	666	899	264	7.30
54001	Slitting prepuce	619	811	1095	322	8.89
54015	Drain penis lesion	947	1241	1675	492	13.60
54050	Destroy penis lesion(s)	290	380	512	151	4.16
54055	Destroy penis lesion(s)	552	724	977	287	7.93
54056	Cryosurgery penis lesion(s)	457	599	809	154	4.26
54057	Laser surgery penis lesion(s)	460	603	814	155	4.29
54060	Excise penis lesion(s)	322	422	569	279	7.70
54065	Destroy penis lesion(s)	523	685	924	287	7.93
54100	Biopsy penis	201	264	356	201	5.54
54105	Biopsy penis	729	954	1288	379	10.46
54110	Treat penis lesion	1040	1362	1839	685	18.93
54111	Treat penis lesion, graft	1572	2059	2779	859	23.73
54112	Treat penis lesion, graft	1900	2490	3360	973	26.88
54115	Treat penis lesion	742	972	1311	658	18.17
54120	Partial remove penis	1211	1587	2141	677	18.71
54125	Remove penis	1616	2118	2858	858	23.71
54130	Remove penis & nodes	2750	3602	4862	1207	33.33
54135	Remove penis & nodes	3489	4571	6169	1543	42.62
54150	Circumcision	559	732	988	290	8.02
54152	Circumcision	350	459	619	153	4.23
54160	Circumcision	535	701	946	278	7.68
54161	Circumcision	549	719	970	202	5.57

CPT	SHORT DESCRIPTION	50th	75th	90th	MFS	RVU
• 54162	Lysis penile circumcise lesion	424	556	750	220	6.09
• 54163	Repair circumcision	398	522	704	207	5.72
• 54164	Frenulotomy penis	350	458	618	182	5.02
54200	Treat penis lesion	278	364	491	144	3.99
54205	Treat penis lesion	867	1135	1532	576	15.90
54220	Treat penis lesion	324	425	573	168	4.65
54230	Prepare penis study	251	329	444	68	1.88
54231	Dynamic cavernosometry	372	487	657	161	4.44
54235	Penile inject	137	180	242	89	2.45
54240	Penis study	213	279	377	110	3.03
54250	Penis study	258	338	456	191	5.28
54300	Revise penis	1286	1685	2274	722	19.94
54304	Revise penis	1621	2123	2866	842	23.27
54308	Reconstruct urethra	1859	2435	3287	813	22.47
54312	Reconstruct urethra	2182	2858	3857	909	25.11
54316	Reconstruct urethra	2411	3159	4263	1068	29.49
54318	Reconstruct urethra	1224	1603	2163	813	22.46
54322	Reconstruct urethra	1779	2330	3145	845	23.34
54324	Reconstruct urethra	2297	3009	4061	1063	29.36
54326	Reconstruct urethra	2199	2881	3888	1007	27.82
54328	Revise penis/urethra	2695	3531	4765	1019	28.16
54332	Revise penis/urethra	2464	3228	4357	1085	29.96
54336	Revise penis/urethra	2763	3620	4885	1286	35.53
54340	Secondary urethral surgery	1389	1819	2455	703	19.43
54344	Secondary urethral surgery	1947	2551	3442	1012	27.95
54348	Secondary urethral surgery	2170	2843	3837	1096	30.27

NEW CODE CPT 2002 •

CPT	SHORT DESCRIPTION	50th	75th	90th	MFS	RVU
54352	Reconstruct urethra/penis	3432	4496	6067	1553	42.89
54360	Penis plastic surgery	1900	2489	3359	777	21.47
54380	Repair penis	1597	2092	2823	910	25.13
54385	Repair penis	2429	3182	4294	1024	28.30
54390	Repair penis and bladder	2981	3905	5270	1360	37.58
54400	Insert semi-rigid prosthesis	1363	1786	2410	581	16.05
54401	Insert self-contd prosthesis	1556	2039	2751	661	18.26
54405	Insert multi-comp penis pros	3715	4867	6569	821	22.68
• 54406	Remove multi-comp penis pros	1323	1733	2339	687	18.99
• 54408	Repair multi-comp penis pros	1394	1826	2465	724	20.01
• 54410	Rem/rep penis prosth	1648	2159	2914	856	23.66
• 54411	Rem/rep penis prosth, comp	1796	2353	3175	933	25.78
• 54415	Rem self-cont penis prosth	982	1287	1737	510	14.10
• 54416	Rem/rep penis contain pros	1279	1675	2261	665	18.36
• 54417	Rem/rep penis prosth, comp	1576	2065	2787	819	22.63
54420	Revise penis	1654	2167	2924	754	20.84
54430	Revise penis	1634	2140	2888	685	18.92
54435	Revise penis	968	1268	1711	463	12.78
54440	Repair penis	0	0	0	0	.00
54450	Preputial stretching	132	172	233	83	2.29

TESTIS

CPT	SHORT DESCRIPTION	50th	75th	90th	MFS	RVU
54500	Biopsy testis	432	525	645	277	7.65
54505	Biopsy testis	409	497	611	232	6.42
54512	Excise lesion testis	847	1029	1264	519	14.33
54520	Remove testis	1039	1263	1551	337	9.31
54522	Orchiectomy, partial	962	1169	1436	589	16.27

CPT	SHORT DESCRIPTION	50th	75th	90th	MFS	RVU
54530	Remove testis	1535	1865	2291	527	14.57
54535	Extensive testis surgery	1164	1414	1738	746	20.61
54550	Explore for testis	788	957	1176	479	13.24
54560	Explore for testis	1133	1376	1690	689	19.02
54600	Reduce testis torsion	838	1017	1250	429	11.84
54620	Suspend testis	479	581	714	307	8.47
54640	Suspend testis	1714	2082	2558	427	11.79
54650	Orchiopexy (fowler-stephens)	1175	1427	1754	708	19.55
54660	Revise testis	430	522	642	330	9.11
54670	Repair testis injury	783	951	1169	403	11.12
54680	Relocation testis(es)	1043	1267	1557	769	21.24
54690	Laparoscopy, orchiectomy	1120	1360	1671	689	19.03
54692	Laparoscopy, orchiopexy	1161	1411	1733	709	19.59
54699	Laparoscope proc testis	0	0	0	0	.00

EPIDIDYMIS

CPT	SHORT DESCRIPTION	50th	75th	90th	MFS	RVU
54700	Drain scrotum	704	855	1051	451	12.46
54800	Biopsy epididymis	504	612	752	323	8.92
54820	Explore epididymis	508	617	758	329	9.08
54830	Remove epididymis lesion	540	656	806	346	9.57
54840	Remove epididymis lesion	1053	1279	1572	337	9.30
54860	Remove epididymis	891	1082	1330	402	11.10
54861	Remove epididymis	1234	1499	1842	532	14.70
54900	Fuse spermatic ducts	1091	1325	1628	779	21.53
54901	Fuse spermatic ducts	1488	1808	2221	1051	29.04

CPT	SHORT DESCRIPTION	50th	75th	90th	MFS	RVU
TUNICA VAGINALIS						
55000	Drain hydrocele	150	183	224	136	3.77
55040	Remove hydrocele	1110	1349	1657	336	9.27
55041	Remove hydroceles	1210	1470	1806	466	12.87
55060	Repair hydrocele	645	783	962	345	9.53
SCROTUM						
55100	Drain scrotum abscess	697	847	1040	447	12.34
55110	Explore scrotum	650	789	970	354	9.77
55120	Remove scrotum lesion	409	497	611	324	8.94
55150	Remove scrotum	1022	1241	1525	451	12.45
55175	Revise scrotum	775	942	1157	342	9.45
55180	Revise scrotum	1076	1307	1606	645	17.82
VAS DEFERENS						
55200	Incise sperm duct	435	529	650	275	7.59
55250	Remove sperm duct(s)	553	671	825	479	13.22
55300	Prepare sperm duct x-ray	493	598	735	191	5.27
55400	Repair sperm duct	2010	2442	3000	518	14.31
55450	Ligate sperm duct	703	853	1049	450	12.44
SPERMATIC CORD						
55500	Remove hydrocele	700	851	1045	354	9.78
55520	Remove sperm cord lesion	818	994	1221	377	10.41
55530	Revise spermatic cord veins	1337	1624	1995	360	9.94
55535	Revise spermatic cord veins	1252	1521	1868	406	11.21
55540	Revise hernia & sperm veins	1054	1281	1574	463	12.78
55550	Laparo ligate spermatic vein	1163	1413	1736	388	10.71

CPT	SHORT DESCRIPTION	50th	75th	90th	MFS	RVU
55559	Laparo proc spermatic cord	0	0	0	0	.00

SEMINAL VESICLES

CPT	SHORT DESCRIPTION	50th	75th	90th	MFS	RVU
55600	Incise sperm duct pouch	900	1093	1343	404	11.17
55605	Incise sperm duct pouch	1489	1808	2222	503	13.89
55650	Remove sperm duct pouch	2260	2745	3373	686	18.96
55680	Remove sperm pouch lesion	2407	2924	3592	336	9.27

PROSTATE

CPT	SHORT DESCRIPTION	50th	75th	90th	MFS	RVU
55700	Biopsy prostate	337	409	503	230	6.35
55705	Biopsy prostate	914	1111	1365	317	8.75
55720	Drain prostate abscess	945	1148	1411	505	13.96
55725	Drain prostate abscess	1097	1333	1638	571	15.77
55801	Remove prostate	1975	2418	2942	1037	28.66
55810	Extensive prostate surgery	2974	3641	4431	1295	35.78
55812	Extensive prostate surgery	3541	4336	5276	1561	43.11
55815	Extensive prostate surgery	3983	4877	5935	1713	47.31
55821	Remove prostate	2267	2776	3378	843	23.30
55831	Remove prostate	2132	2611	3177	913	25.23
55840	Extensive prostate surgery	4288	5251	6390	1317	36.38
55842	Extensive prostate surgery	2715	3325	4046	1402	38.72
55845	Extensive prostate surgery	5105	6251	7607	1612	44.52
55859	Percut/needle insert, pros	1716	2101	2556	759	20.97
55860	Surgical exposure prostate	886	1085	1320	840	23.20
55862	Extensive prostate surgery	1455	1782	2169	1058	29.22
55865	Extensive prostate surgery	2638	3231	3931	1293	35.73
55870	Electroejaculation	314	384	467	169	4.68

     NEW CODE CPT 2002 •

CPT	SHORT DESCRIPTION	50th	75th	90th	MFS	RVU
55873	Cryoablate prostate	1984	2430	2957	1127	31.14
55899	Genital surgery procedure	0	0	0	0	.00

INTERSEX SURGERY

CPT	SHORT DESCRIPTION	50th	75th	90th	MFS	RVU
55970	Sex transformation, M to F	0	0	0	0	.00
55980	Sex transformation, F to M	0	0	0	0	.00

CPT	SHORT DESCRIPTION	50th	75th	90th	MFS	RVU

NEW CODE CPT 2002 •

CPT	SHORT DESCRIPTION	50th	75th	90th	MFS	RVU

FEMALE GENITAL SYSTEM

VULVA, PERINEUM AND INTROITUS

CPT	SHORT DESCRIPTION	50th	75th	90th	MFS	RVU
56405	I & D vulva/perineum	228	289	372	148	4.08
56420	Drain gland abscess	215	272	351	145	4.00
56440	Surgery for vulva lesion	728	923	1188	252	6.95
56441	Lysis labial lesion(s)	285	362	466	177	4.88
56501	Destroy vulva lesions, simp	166	210	270	148	4.10
56515	Destroy vulva lesion/s comp	586	742	956	222	6.14
56605	Biopsy vulva/perineum	183	232	299	113	3.11
56606	Biopsy vulva/perineum	105	133	171	83	2.30
56620	Partial remove vulva	1746	2211	2849	484	13.36
56625	Complete remove vulva	1907	2416	3112	559	15.44
56630	Extensive vulva surgery	2486	3149	4057	779	21.52
56631	Extensive vulva surgery	3019	3824	4926	1036	28.63
56632	Extensive vulva surgery	3685	4668	6014	1258	34.74
56633	Extensive vulva surgery	3186	4036	5199	1007	27.83
56634	Extensive vulva surgery	3942	4993	6432	1119	30.91
56637	Extensive vulva surgery	4271	5409	6969	1351	37.31
56640	Extensive vulva surgery	3896	4935	6357	1340	37.01
56700	Partial remove hymen	539	683	880	215	5.94
56720	Incise hymen	220	278	358	92	2.54
56740	Remove vagina gland lesion	792	1004	1293	327	9.02
56800	Repair vagina	763	966	1245	258	7.12
56805	Repair clitoris	2628	3328	4288	1099	30.37
56810	Repair perineum	871	1103	1421	270	7.45

VAGINA

CPT	SHORT DESCRIPTION	50th	75th	90th	MFS	RVU
57000	Explore vagina	655	829	1068	208	5.74
57010	Drain pelvic abscess	814	1032	1329	387	10.68
57020	Drain pelvic fluid	241	305	393	119	3.28
57022	I & D vaginal hematoma, pp	296	374	482	179	4.94
57023	I & D vaginal hematoma, non-ob	296	374	482	290	8.00
57061	Destroy vag lesions, simple	180	228	293	136	3.75
57065	Destroy vag lesions, complex	718	910	1172	216	5.96
57100	Biopsy vagina	170	215	277	106	2.94
57105	Biopsy vagina	373	472	608	152	4.21
57106	Remove vagina wall, partial	1368	1733	2233	348	9.61
57107	Remove vagina tissue, part	2053	2600	3350	1297	35.82
57109	Vaginectomy partial w/nodes	2766	3503	4513	1551	42.86
57110	Remove vagina wall, complete	1864	2362	3042	843	23.28
57111	Remove vagina tissue, compl	2422	3068	3953	1541	42.56
57112	Vaginectomy w/nodes, compl	3524	4463	5750	1650	45.57
57120	Close vagina	1602	2030	2615	471	13.01
57130	Remove vagina lesion	680	862	1110	178	4.91
57135	Remove vagina lesion	552	699	900	218	6.02
57150	Treat vagina infection	65	83	106	60	1.65
• **57155**	Insert uteri tandems/ovoids	915	1158	1492	383	10.57
57160	Insert pessary/other device	84	106	137	76	2.10
57170	Fitting diaphragm/cap	98	124	160	89	2.46
57180	Treat vaginal bleeding	284	360	464	149	4.11
57200	Repair vagina	649	823	1060	270	7.46
57210	Repair vagina/perineum	731	926	1193	339	9.36

NEW CODE CPT 2002 •

CPT	SHORT DESCRIPTION	50th	75th	90th	MFS	RVU
57220	Revise urethra	754	955	1231	299	8.25
57230	Repair urethral lesion	826	1046	1347	385	10.63
57240	Repair bladder & vagina	1340	1697	2187	406	11.22
57250	Repair rectum & vagina	1279	1620	2087	365	10.08
57260	Repair vagina	1902	2410	3104	517	14.27
57265	Extensive repair vagina	2248	2847	3668	713	19.70
57268	Repair bowel bulge	1263	1600	2062	433	11.96
57270	Repair bowel pouch	1338	1695	2183	719	19.86
57280	Suspend vagina	2317	2935	3781	877	24.22
57282	Repair vaginal prolapse	2070	2622	3378	549	15.16
57284	Repair paravaginal defect	2444	3095	3988	772	21.32
57287	Revise/remove sling repair	1262	1599	2060	685	18.92
57288	Repair bladder defect	2411	3054	3934	765	21.12
57289	Repair bladder & vagina	1581	2002	2579	711	19.65
57291	Construction vagina	1320	1673	2155	531	14.66
57292	Construct vagina with graft	2344	2969	3825	781	21.58
57300	Repair rectum-vagina fistula	1252	1586	2044	475	13.13
57305	Repair rectum-vagina fistula	1912	2422	3120	800	22.10
57307	Fistula repair & colostomy	2005	2539	3271	914	25.24
57308	Fistula repair, transperine	1533	1941	2501	609	16.81
57310	Repair urethrovaginal lesion	1484	1880	2422	441	12.18
57311	Repair urethrovaginal lesion	2303	2917	3758	505	13.94
57320	Repair bladder-vagina lesion	1490	1888	2432	517	14.29
57330	Repair bladder-vagina lesion	1745	2211	2848	730	20.17
57335	Repair vagina	1109	1405	1810	1094	30.23
57400	Dilation vagina	284	360	464	133	3.67

CPT	SHORT DESCRIPTION	50th	75th	90th	MFS	RVU
57410	Pelvic examination	275	349	449	168	4.64
57415	Remove vaginal foreign body	289	366	471	220	6.07
57452	Examination vagina	224	284	366	101	2.78
57454	Vagina examination & biopsy	318	403	520	119	3.28
57460	Cervix excise	766	970	1250	191	5.28

CERVIX UTERI

CPT	SHORT DESCRIPTION	50th	75th	90th	MFS	RVU
57500	Biopsy cervix	168	215	285	122	3.36
57505	Endocervical curettage	178	228	302	120	3.31
57510	Cauterize cervix	200	256	339	198	5.47
57511	Cryocautery cervix	236	303	401	167	4.62
57513	Laser surgery cervix	826	1060	1403	174	4.81
57520	Conization cervix	1010	1296	1715	321	8.88
57522	Conization cervix	903	1159	1533	279	7.72
57530	Remove cervix	710	910	1205	328	9.05
57531	Remove cervix, radical	3604	4624	6118	1625	44.90
57540	Remove residual cervix	1338	1717	2272	721	19.92
57545	Remove cervix/repair pelvis	1637	2100	2779	770	21.28
57550	Remove residual cervix	1047	1342	1776	364	10.06
57555	Remove cervix/repair vagina	1371	1758	2327	570	15.74
57556	Remove cervix, repair bowel	1251	1604	2123	518	14.31
57700	Revise cervix	632	810	1072	239	6.59
57720	Revise cervix	765	982	1299	288	7.95
57800	Dilation cervical canal	155	199	263	75	2.07
57820	D & C residual cervix	423	542	718	164	4.54

NEW CODE CPT 2002 •

CPT	SHORT DESCRIPTION	50th	75th	90th	MFS	RVU

CORPUS UTERI

CPT	SHORT DESCRIPTION	50th	75th	90th	MFS	RVU
58100	Biopsy uterus lining	195	250	331	114	3.16
58120	Dilation and curettage	816	1047	1386	275	7.61
58140	Remove uterus lesion	2673	3429	4537	849	23.44
58145	Remove uterus lesion	1991	2554	3379	505	13.95
58150	Total hysterectomy	2789	3578	4734	893	24.67
58152	Total hysterectomy	3340	4284	5669	1169	32.29
58180	Partial hysterectomy	3045	3905	5168	895	24.73
58200	Extensive hysterectomy	4180	5361	7094	1280	35.36
58210	Extensive hysterectomy	6211	7967	10542	1681	46.43
58240	Remove pelvis contents	5387	6911	9144	2239	61.86
58260	Vaginal hysterectomy	2552	3274	4332	764	21.11
58262	Vaginal hysterectomy	2746	3522	4660	863	23.85
58263	Vaginal hysterectomy	3209	4116	5446	935	25.83
58267	Hysterectomy & vagina repair	2955	3790	5015	990	27.36
58270	Hysterectomy & vagina repair	2960	3797	5024	835	23.06
58275	Hysterectomy/revise vagina	2457	3151	4169	913	25.21
58280	Hysterectomy/revise vagina	2719	3487	4614	978	27.01
58285	Extensive hysterectomy	3073	3942	5216	1277	35.29
58300	Insert intrauterine device	197	253	335	92	2.53
58301	Remove intrauterine device	110	141	186	109	3.02
58321	Artificial insemination	161	206	273	74	2.05
58322	Artificial insemination	183	234	310	82	2.26
58323	Sperm washing	113	146	193	28	.78
58340	Catheter for hysterography	1165	1495	1978	484	13.38
58345	Reopen fallopian tube	580	744	984	244	6.75

CPT	SHORT DESCRIPTION	50th	75th	90th	MFS	RVU
• **58346**	Insert Heyman uteri capsule	982	1259	1666	408	11.27
58350	Reopen fallopian tube	240	308	408	118	3.26
58353	Endometr ablate, thermal	405	519	687	225	6.21
58400	Suspend uterus	1360	1745	2309	404	11.15
58410	Suspend uterus	1800	2309	3056	748	20.66
58520	Repair ruptured uterus	1256	1611	2132	700	19.33
58540	Revise uterus	1825	2341	3098	828	22.88
58550	Laparo-asst vag hysterectomy	3096	3971	5255	823	22.74
58551	Laparoscopy, remove myoma	2021	2592	3430	824	22.75
58555	Hysteroscopy, dx, sep proc	831	1066	1410	240	6.62
58558	Hysteroscopy, biopsy	1164	1493	1976	318	8.79
58559	Hysteroscopy, lysis	1498	1922	2543	340	9.38
58560	Hysteroscopy, resect septum	1351	1733	2293	388	10.72
58561	Hysteroscopy, remove myoma	1827	2343	3100	536	14.80
58562	Hysteroscopy, remove fb	1223	1569	2076	292	8.07
58563	Hysteroscopy, ablation	1759	2256	2985	341	9.41
58578	Laparo proc uterus	0	0	0	0	.00
58579	Hysteroscope procedure	0	0	0	0	.00

OVIDUCT/OVARY

CPT	SHORT DESCRIPTION	50th	75th	90th	MFS	RVU
58600	Division fallopian tube	1413	1746	2267	344	9.50
58605	Division fallopian tube	1079	1334	1731	313	8.65
58611	Ligate oviduct(s) add-on	660	816	1059	77	2.13
58615	Occlude fallopian tube(s)	1179	1458	1892	277	7.65
58660	Laparoscopy, lysis	1832	2265	2940	659	18.21
58661	Laparoscopy, remove adnexa	2148	2655	3446	639	17.64
58662	Laparoscopy, excise lesions	1930	2386	3097	678	18.72

     NEW CODE CPT 2002 •

CPT	SHORT DESCRIPTION	50th	75th	90th	MFS	RVU
58670	Laparoscopy, tubal cautery	1408	1741	2260	358	9.88
58671	Laparoscopy, tubal block	1375	1699	2206	358	9.90
58672	Laparoscopy, fimbrioplasty	2977	3680	4777	757	20.91
58673	Laparoscopy, salpingostomy	3076	3803	4937	807	22.30
58679	Laparo proc, oviduct-ovary	0	0	0	0	.00
58700	Remove fallopian tube	1723	2130	2765	678	18.74
58720	Remove ovary/tube(s)	2049	2533	3288	671	18.55
58740	Revise fallopian tube(s)	1831	2263	2938	794	21.93
58750	Repair oviduct	2896	3580	4647	867	23.96
58752	Revise ovarian tube(s)	2704	3343	4340	879	24.27
58760	Remove tubal obstruction	2796	3456	4486	777	21.47
58770	Create new tubal opening	2716	3357	4358	819	22.63

OVARY

CPT	SHORT DESCRIPTION	50th	75th	90th	MFS	RVU
58800	Drain ovarian cyst(s)	870	1076	1396	323	8.93
58805	Drain ovarian cyst(s)	1100	1359	1764	366	10.10
58820	Drain ovary abscess, open	1094	1352	1755	286	7.89
58822	Drain ovary abscess, percut	1282	1585	2057	588	16.25
58823	Drain pelvic abscess, percut	327	404	524	215	5.94
58825	Transposition ovary(s)	1453	1796	2332	635	17.55
58900	Biopsy ovary(s)	1312	1622	2106	369	10.19
58920	Partial remove ovary(s)	1502	1857	2411	648	17.89
58925	Remove ovarian cyst(s)	2051	2536	3292	662	18.29
58940	Remove ovary(s)	1890	2336	3033	442	12.20
58943	Remove ovary(s)	2480	3065	3979	1094	30.21
58950	Resect ovarian malignancy	2434	3009	3906	1010	27.89
58951	Resect ovarian malignancy	3788	4682	6078	1317	36.39

CPT	SHORT DESCRIPTION	50th	75th	90th	MFS	RVU
58952	Resect ovarian malignancy	6026	7449	9670	1466	40.50
• 58953	TAH, rad dissect for debulk	7230	8938	11603	1839	50.79
• 58954	Tah rad debulk/lymph remove	7860	9716	12613	1999	55.21
58960	Explore abdomen	2620	3239	4204	892	24.64

IN VITRO FERTILIZATION

CPT	SHORT DESCRIPTION	50th	75th	90th	MFS	RVU
58970	Retrieval oocyte	1645	2034	2640	451	12.45
58974	Transfer embryo	839	1037	1346	0	.00
58976	Transfer embryo	1174	1451	1883	236	6.52
58999	Genital surgery procedure	0	0	0	0	.00

NEW CODE CPT 2002 •

CPT	SHORT DESCRIPTION	50th	75th	90th	MFS	RVU

MATERNITY CARE AND DELIVERY

CPT	SHORT DESCRIPTION	50th	75th	90th	MFS	RVU
59000	Amniocentesis, diagnostic	339	421	545	130	3.58
• 59001	Amniocentesis, therapeutic	412	511	662	167	4.60
59012	Fetal cord puncture, prenatal	518	642	832	209	5.78
59015	Chorion biopsy	448	556	720	153	4.24
59020	Fetal contract stress test	135	168	217	59	1.64
59025	Fetal non-stress test	130	161	208	39	1.09
59030	Fetal scalp blood sample	277	343	445	126	3.49
59050	Fetal monitor w/report	214	265	343	52	1.43
59051	Fetal monitor/interpret only	83	103	133	43	1.19
59100	Remove uterus lesion	1615	2004	2595	766	21.17
59120	Treat ectopic pregnancy	2087	2589	3353	720	19.90
59121	Treat ectopic pregnancy	1805	2239	2900	729	20.15
59130	Treat ectopic pregnancy	1599	1983	2569	866	23.92
59135	Treat ectopic pregnancy	1939	2406	3116	856	23.64
59136	Treat ectoplc pregnancy	1962	2433	3152	793	21.90
59140	Treat ectopic pregnancy	1196	1484	1922	367	10.14
59150	Treat ectopic pregnancy	1939	2405	3115	709	19.59
59151	Treat ectopic pregnancy	2257	2800	3627	689	19.02
59160	D & C after delivery	693	860	1114	251	6.93
59200	Insert cervical dilator	186	231	299	85	2.35
59300	Episiotomy or vaginal repair	383	475	616	176	4.85
59320	Revise cervix	979	1214	1573	153	4.24
59325	Revise cervix	1031	1279	1657	245	6.77
59350	Repair uterus	1195	1482	1920	290	8.02

CPT	SHORT DESCRIPTION	50th	75th	90th	MFS	RVU
59400	Obstetrical care	2694	3342	4329	1542	42.61
59409	Obstetrical care	1707	2118	2743	778	21.49
59410	Obstetrical care	1795	2226	2883	884	24.41
59412	Antepartum manipulate	439	545	706	123	3.40
59414	Deliver placenta	388	482	624	117	3.24
59425	Antepartum care only	462	573	742	399	11.03
59426	Antepartum care only	945	1172	1518	685	18.91
59430	Care after delivery	492	611	792	138	3.80
59510	Cesarean delivery	3247	4029	5218	1757	48.53
59514	Cesarean delivery only	2020	2506	3246	919	25.40
59515	Cesarean delivery	2206	2737	3545	1050	29.01
59525	Remove uterus after cesarean	784	973	1260	492	13.59
59610	Vbac delivery	3029	3758	4868	1641	45.32
59612	Vbac delivery only	2179	2703	3501	876	24.19
59614	Vbac care after delivery	2304	2858	3702	976	26.97
59618	Attempted vbac delivery	3394	4210	5453	1851	51.14
59620	Attempted vbac delivery only	1653	2051	2656	997	27.55
59622	Attempted vbac after care	1843	2287	2962	1131	31.23
59812	Treat miscarriage	785	973	1261	302	8.34
59820	Care miscarriage	851	1055	1367	308	8.52
59821	Treat miscarriage	954	1183	1532	328	9.06
59830	Treat uterus infection	1008	1251	1620	400	11.06
59840	Abortion	614	762	987	274	7.56
59841	Abortion	906	1123	1455	433	11.96
59850	Abortion	1262	1565	2027	352	9.72
59851	Abortion	1301	1615	2091	370	10.21

NEW CODE CPT 2002 •

CPT	SHORT DESCRIPTION	50th	75th	90th	MFS	RVU
59852	Abortion	1719	2132	2761	518	14.30
59855	Abortion	1218	1511	1957	384	10.60
59856	Abortion	1125	1395	1807	455	12.56
59857	Abortion	1729	2145	2778	558	15.41
59866	Abortion (mpr)	459	569	737	229	6.32
59870	Evacuate mole uterus	912	1132	1466	384	10.61
59871	Remove cerclage suture	255	316	410	170	4.70
59898	Laparo proc ob care/deliver	0	0	0	0	.00
59899	Maternity care procedure	0	0	0	0	.00

CPT	SHORT DESCRIPTION	50th	75th	90th	MFS	RVU

NEW CODE CPT 2002 •

CPT	SHORT DESCRIPTION	50th	75th	90th	MFS	RVU

ENDOCRINE SYSTEM

THYROID GLAND

CPT	SHORT DESCRIPTION	50th	75th	90th	MFS	RVU
60000	Drain thyroid/tongue cyst	187	228	286	156	4.30
60001	Aspirate/inject thyroid cyst	187	228	286	101	2.80
60100	Biopsy thyroid	232	283	355	156	4.31
60200	Remove thyroid lesion	1443	1758	2205	625	17.27
60210	Partial thyroid excise	2112	2573	3227	670	18.52
60212	Partial thyroid excise	2186	2664	3340	947	26.16
60220	Partial remove thyroid	2223	2709	3397	729	20.14
60225	Partial remove thyroid	2865	3491	4377	852	23.55
60240	Remove thyroid	3024	3685	4621	973	26.88
60252	Remove thyroid	3544	4318	5415	1225	33.84
60254	Extensive thyroid surgery	3789	4617	5789	1641	45.34
60260	Repeat thyroid surgery	2301	2804	3516	1069	29.52
60270	Remove thyroid	2807	3420	4289	1216	33.59
60271	Remove thyroid	2372	2890	3624	1027	28.38
60280	Remove thyroid duct lesion	1704	2077	2604	420	11.61
60281	Remove thyroid duct lesion	1531	1865	2339	560	15.47

PARATHYROID, THYMUS, ADRENAL GLANDS, AND CAROTID BODY

CPT	SHORT DESCRIPTION	50th	75th	90th	MFS	RVU
60500	Explore parathyroid glands	3006	3663	4593	935	25.83
60502	Re-explore parathyroids	2629	3204	4017	1170	32.32
60505	Explore parathyroid glands	2945	3589	4500	1273	35.16
60512	Autotransplant parathyroid	463	564	707	239	6.61
60520	Remove thymus gland	2508	3056	3832	1021	28.20

CPT	SHORT DESCRIPTION	50th	75th	90th	MFS	RVU
60521	Remove thymus gland	2739	3338	4186	1187	32.78
60522	Remove thymus gland	3394	4136	5186	1405	38.80
60540	Explore adrenal gland	2268	2764	3465	961	26.54
60545	Explore adrenal gland	2936	3578	4487	1135	31.36
60600	Remove carotid body lesion	2671	3255	4082	1203	33.23
60605	Remove carotid body lesion	3224	3928	4925	1471	40.64
60650	Laparoscopy adrenalectomy	2534	3088	3871	1098	30.32
60659	Laparo proc endocrine	0	0	0	0	.00
60699	Endocrine surgery procedure	0	0	0	0	.00

NEW CODE CPT 2002 •

CPT	SHORT DESCRIPTION	50th	75th	90th	MFS	RVU

NERVOUS SYSTEM

SKULL, MENINGES AND BRAIN

CPT	SHORT DESCRIPTION	50th	75th	90th	MFS	RVU
61000	Remove cranial cavity fluid	306	380	485	127	3.50
61001	Remove cranial cavity fluid	191	238	304	135	3.72
61020	Remove brain cavity fluid	303	376	481	155	4.29
61026	Inject into brain canal	321	400	510	151	4.18
61050	Remove brain canal fluid	291	362	462	116	3.20
61055	Inject into brain canal	446	555	709	146	4.03
61070	Brain canal shunt procedure	1238	1539	1965	301	8.31
61105	Twist drill hole	1409	1752	2237	357	9.86
61107	Drill skull for implantation	1833	2279	2911	331	9.14
61108	Drill skull for drain	2762	3434	4386	699	19.32
61120	Burr hole for puncture	1536	1910	2440	595	16.45
61140	Pierce skull for biopsy	3073	3821	4880	1052	29.05
61150	Pierce skull for drain	3066	3813	4869	1152	31.83
61151	Pierce skull for drain	3430	4265	5447	834	23.03
61154	Pierce skull & remove clot	3638	4524	5777	994	27.47
61156	Pierce skull for drain	3231	4018	5131	1087	30.04
61210	Pierce skull implant device	1908	2372	3029	381	10.53
61215	Insert brain-fluid device	1633	2031	2593	366	10.12
61250	Pierce skull & explore	1824	2269	2897	694	19.17
61253	Pierce skull & explore	2793	3473	4436	806	22.27
61304	Open skull for explore	4274	5064	5782	1417	39.14
61305	Open skull for explore	4715	5586	6378	1708	47.17
61312	Open skull for drain	5625	6665	7610	1597	44.13

CPT	SHORT DESCRIPTION	50th	75th	90th	MFS	RVU
61313	Open skull for drain	5337	6324	7220	1620	44.76
61314	Open skull for drain	4116	4877	5569	1440	39.78
61315	Open skull for drain	4805	5693	6501	1793	49.52
61320	Open skull for drain	4760	5640	6440	1666	46.02
61321	Open skull for drain	4741	5618	6414	1808	49.94
61330	Decompress eye socket	3910	4633	5290	1641	45.33
61332	Explore/biopsy eye socket	4145	4911	5607	1877	51.86
61333	Explore orbit/remove lesion	4451	5274	6022	1688	46.64
61334	Explore orbit/remove object	3839	4549	5194	1136	31.37
61340	Relieve cranial pressure	2804	3322	3794	1233	34.07
61343	Incise skull (press relief)	7011	8307	9485	1946	53.77
61345	Relieve cranial pressure	2887	3421	3906	1759	48.60
61440	Incise skull for surgery	3379	4004	4571	1605	44.34
61450	Incise skull for surgery	4403	5217	5957	1648	45.52
61458	Incise skull for brain wound	5820	6896	7874	1754	48.46
61460	Incise skull for surgery	5341	6328	7225	1820	50.29
61470	Incise skull for surgery	3614	4282	4889	1609	44.45
61480	Incise skull for surgery	3156	3740	4270	1606	44.37
61490	Incise skull for surgery	3076	3644	4161	1673	46.21
61500	Remove skull lesion	4294	5087	5809	1166	32.21
61501	Remove infected skull bone	3522	4173	4765	981	27.09
61510	Remove brain lesion	6811	8070	9214	1840	50.82
61512	Remove brain lining lesion	6570	7785	8888	2259	62.41
61514	Remove brain abscess	5424	6427	7338	1639	45.29
61516	Remove brain lesion	5374	6368	7271	1613	44.56
61518	Remove brain lesion	6430	7619	8700	2432	67.19

NEW CODE CPT 2002 •

CPT	SHORT DESCRIPTION	50th	75th	90th	MFS	RVU
61519	Remove brain lining lesion	7024	8322	9502	2677	73.96
61520	Remove brain lesion	6620	7844	8956	3507	96.87
61521	Remove brain lesion	7556	8953	10223	2880	79.55
61522	Remove brain abscess	5347	6335	7233	1881	51.95
61524	Remove brain lesion	5322	6306	7200	1799	49.70
61526	Remove brain lesion	5249	6219	7101	3274	90.44
61530	Remove brain lesion	6376	7555	8626	2804	77.46
61531	Implant brain electrodes	3480	4124	4708	978	27.03
61533	Implant brain electrodes	4761	5642	6442	1293	35.72
61534	Remove brain lesion	5121	6068	6928	1391	38.42
61535	Remove brain electrodes	3171	3757	4290	799	22.08
61536	Remove brain lesion	5871	6956	7942	2294	63.38
61538	Remove brain tissue	5860	6944	7928	1755	48.49
61539	Remove brain tissue	5976	7080	8084	2085	57.61
61541	Incise brain tissue	6830	8093	9240	1855	51.24
61542	Remove brain tissue	6980	8271	9443	2009	55.51
61543	Remove brain tissue	7031	8331	9513	1910	52.75
61544	Remove & treat brain lesion	4767	5649	6450	1651	45.62
61545	Excise brain tumor	7223	8558	9772	2815	77.77
61546	Remove pituitary gland	5894	6983	7974	2031	56.10
61548	Remove pituitary gland	6683	7919	9041	1408	38.90
61550	Release skull seams	3081	3650	4168	749	20.68
61552	Release skull seams	4040	4787	5466	1097	30.31
61556	Incise skull/sutures	3981	4716	5385	1360	37.57
61557	Incise skull/sutures	5014	5941	6783	1465	40.47
61558	Excise skull/sutures	5200	6161	7035	1479	40.86

CPT	SHORT DESCRIPTION	50th	75th	90th	MFS	RVU
61559	Excise skull/sutures	6080	7204	8225	2119	58.54
61563	Excise skull tumor	5438	6444	7357	1721	47.54
61564	Excise skull tumor	6951	8236	9404	2159	59.64
61570	Remove foreign body brain	5732	6792	7755	1557	43.00
61571	Incise skull for brain wound	6272	7431	8485	1703	47.05
61575	Skull base/brainstem surgery	4335	5137	5865	2199	60.76
61576	Skull base/brainstem surgery	5040	5972	6818	3113	86.00
61580	Craniofacial approach skull	3611	4278	4885	1921	53.06
61581	Craniofacial approach skull	4864	5763	6580	2191	60.54
61582	Craniofacial approach skull	5396	6393	7300	2082	57.52
61583	Craniofacial approach skull	5337	6324	7220	2384	65.86
61584	Orbitocranial approach/skull	3662	4340	4955	2251	62.17
61585	Orbitocranial approach/skull	4679	5544	6330	2426	67.01
61586	Resect nasopharynx skull	3722	4410	5036	1629	45.01
61590	Infratemporal approach/skull	5028	5957	6802	2613	72.18
61591	Infratemporal approach/skull	5307	6288	7180	2745	75.83
61592	Orbitocranial approach/skull	4888	5792	6613	2562	70.78
61595	Transtemporal approach/skull	4868	5768	6586	1895	52.36
61596	Transcochlear approach/skull	5066	6003	6854	2236	61.76
61597	Transcondylar approach/skull	6890	8164	9322	2426	67.02
61598	Transpetrosal approach/skull	4048	4796	5476	2133	58.93
61600	Resect/excise cranial lesion	4671	5535	6320	1592	43.98
61601	Resect/excise cranial lesion	5172	6128	6997	1829	50.52
61605	Resect/excise cranial lesion	5170	6125	6994	1839	50.81
61606	Resect/excise cranial lesion	7104	8417	9611	2491	68.81
61607	Resect/excise cranial lesion	6582	7799	8905	2321	64.13

NEW CODE CPT 2002 •

CPT	SHORT DESCRIPTION	50th	75th	90th	MFS	RVU
61608	Resect/excise cranial lesion	7750	9183	10485	2726	75.30
61609	Transect artery sinus	1953	2315	2643	618	17.07
61610	Transect artery sinus	5926	7021	8017	1722	47.57
61611	Transect artery sinus	1425	1688	1927	432	11.93
61612	Transect artery sinus	5371	6364	7266	1655	45.73
61613	Remove aneurysm sinus	7568	8967	10239	2625	72.52
61615	Resect/excise lesion skull	5859	6943	7927	2082	57.52
61616	Resect/excise lesion skull	7950	9420	10756	2799	77.32
61618	Repair dura	4178	4950	5652	1134	31.34
61619	Repair dura	5881	6968	7956	1368	37.80
61624	Occlusion/embolization cath	4347	5204	6108	1041	28.76
61626	Occlusion/embolization cath	3404	4075	4783	845	23.34
61680	Intracranial vessel surgery	6628	7934	9312	1996	55.13
61682	Intracranial vessel surgery	7388	8843	10379	3942	108.91
61684	Intracranial vessel surgery	7287	8722	10238	2544	70.28
61686	Intracranial vessel surgery	9169	10975	12882	4141	114.39
61690	Intracranial vessel surgery	5598	6701	7865	1899	52.46
61692	Intracranial vessel surgery	6202	7424	8714	3314	91.55
61697	Brain aneurysm repair, comp	6036	7226	8481	3231	89.25
61698	Brain aneurysm repair, comp	5810	6955	8163	3103	85.71
61700	Brain aneurysm repair, simp	8052	9638	11313	3226	89.12
61702	Inner skull vessel surgery	8153	9760	11455	3094	85.47
61703	Clamp neck artery	3670	4393	5157	1166	32.22
61705	Revise circulation to head	6694	8013	9405	2272	62.76
61708	Revise circulation to head	5695	6817	8001	1955	54.00
61710	Revise circulation to head	2326	2784	3268	1693	46.77

CPT	SHORT DESCRIPTION	50th	75th	90th	MFS	RVU
61711	Fuse skull arteries	6259	7493	8794	2331	64.40
61720	Incise skull/brain surgery	5062	6059	7112	1129	31.18
61735	Incise skull/brain surgery	5290	6333	7433	1352	37.36
61750	Incise skull/brain biopsy	5276	6316	7413	1194	32.99
61751	Brain biopsy w/ ct/mr guide	5571	6669	7827	1162	32.11
61760	Implant brain electrodes	4993	5977	7015	1437	39.71
61770	Incise skull for treat	4942	5915	6943	1404	38.79
61790	Treat trigeminal nerve	3182	3809	4471	710	19.60
61791	Treat trigeminal tract	3335	3992	4685	978	27.03
61793	Focus radiation beam	6519	7803	9159	1152	31.82
61795	Brain surgery using computer	891	1067	1258	253	6.99
61850	Implant neuroelectrodes	2904	3476	4080	824	22.75
61860	Implant neuroelectrodes	4122	4934	5792	1357	37.50
61862	Implant neurostimul, subcort	2425	2903	3408	1284	35.47
61870	Implant neuroelectrodes	4320	5171	6069	963	26.61
61875	Implant neuroelectrodes	4155	4974	5838	900	24.87
61880	Revise/remove neuroelectrode	3246	3886	4561	466	12.86
61885	Implant neurostim one array	1216	1456	1709	414	11.43
61886	Implant neurostim arrays	1261	1509	1771	571	15.77
61888	Revise/remove neuroreceiver	772	924	1084	362	10.01
62000	Treat skull fracture	2963	3547	4163	709	19.59
62005	Treat skull fracture	3972	4755	5581	1008	27.85
62010	Treat head injury	4623	5534	6496	1292	35.69
62100	Repair brain fluid leakage	4769	5708	6700	1451	40.07
62115	Reduce skull defect	2637	3156	3704	1347	37.22
62116	Reduce skull defect	2981	3568	4188	1538	42.48

NEW CODE CPT 2002 •

CPT	SHORT DESCRIPTION	50th	75th	90th	MFS	RVU
62117	Reduce skull defect	3350	4011	4707	1623	44.84
62120	Repair skull cavity lesion	4206	5035	5909	1504	41.56
62121	Incise skull repair	4400	5267	6182	1360	37.57
62140	Repair skull defect	3685	4411	5177	899	24.83
62141	Repair skull defect	4489	5373	6307	1001	27.65
62142	Remove skull plate/flap	2632	3151	3698	731	20.20
62143	Replace skull plate/flap	3301	3951	4638	884	24.41
62145	Repair skull & brain	4654	5571	6539	1245	34.40
62146	Repair skull with graft	4651	5568	6535	1075	29.69
62147	Repair skull with graft	5566	6663	7821	1280	35.36
62180	Establish brain cavity shunt	3595	4304	5051	1392	38.46
62190	Establish brain cavity shunt	3140	3758	4411	761	21.02
62192	Establish brain cavity shunt	3293	3942	4627	831	22.96
62194	Replace/irrigate catheter	1263	1512	1775	282	7.78
62200	Establish brain cavity shunt	4955	5932	6962	1221	33.74
62201	Establish brain cavity shunt	4365	5225	6133	982	27.14
62220	Establish brain cavity shunt	3474	4159	4881	873	24.13
62223	Establish brain cavity shunt	4266	5107	5994	868	23.99
62225	Replace/irrigate catheter	1515	1814	2129	384	10.61
62230	Replace/revise brain shunt	2978	3564	4184	690	19.06
62252	Csf shunt reprogram	150	179	211	82	2.27
62256	Remove brain cavity shunt	1674	2004	2352	483	13.34
62258	Replace brain cavity shunt	3752	4491	5272	951	26.27

SPINE AND SPINAL CORD

CPT	SHORT DESCRIPTION	50th	75th	90th	MFS	RVU
62263	Lysis epidural adhesions	1267	1550	2047	424	11.71
62268	Drain spinal cord cyst	1536	1879	2482	281	7.77

CPT	SHORT DESCRIPTION	50th	75th	90th	MFS	RVU
62269	Needle biopsy spinal cord	1318	1613	2130	279	7.71
62270	Spinal fluid tap, diagnostic	207	253	334	191	5.27
62272	Drain cerebro spinal fluid	296	362	478	176	4.86
62273	Treat epidural spine lesion	473	578	764	140	3.86
62280	Treat spinal cord lesion	377	462	610	239	6.59
62281	Treat spinal cord lesion	545	666	880	265	7.32
62282	Treat spinal canal lesion	630	771	1018	291	8.04
62284	Inject for myelogram	468	573	756	260	7.17
62287	Percutaneous diskectomy	3587	4389	5796	499	13.79
62290	Inject for spine disk x-ray	576	705	931	321	8.88
62291	Inject for spine disk x-ray	572	700	924	337	9.32
62292	Inject into disk lesion	2392	2926	3865	501	13.85
62294	Inject into spinal artery	2204	2696	3560	726	20.05
62310	Inject spine c/t	573	701	926	207	5.73
62311	Inject spine l/s (cd)	520	637	841	212	5.85
62318	Inject spine w/cath, c/t	613	750	991	217	5.99
62319	Inject spine w/cath l/s (cd)	555	679	897	205	5.65
62350	Implant spinal canal cath	1612	1973	2605	409	11.30
62351	Implant spinal canal cath	3034	3712	4903	677	18.69
62355	Remove spinal canal catheter	1240	1517	2003	324	8.94
62360	Insert spine infuse device	1212	1483	1958	191	5.29
62361	Implant spine infuse pump	1288	1576	2081	347	9.59
62362	Implant spine infuse pump	1624	1987	2624	433	11.96
62365	Remove spine infuse device	933	1142	1508	362	9.99
63001	Remove spinal lamina	3501	4284	5657	1105	30.53
63003	Remove spinal lamina	4059	4966	6558	1118	30.88

NEW CODE CPT 2002 •

CPT	SHORT DESCRIPTION	50th	75th	90th	MFS	RVU
63005	Remove spinal lamina	3618	4426	5845	1051	29.03
63011	Remove spinal lamina	3979	4868	6428	986	27.24
63012	Remove spinal lamina	4192	5129	6774	1030	28.45
63015	Remove spinal lamina	4238	5185	6847	1335	36.87
63016	Remove spinal lamina	4599	5627	7431	1321	36.48
63017	Remove spinal lamina	4479	5480	7237	1117	30.85
63020	Neck spine disk surgery	4745	5805	7667	1051	29.03
63030	Low back disk surgery	4371	5348	7063	873	24.13
63035	Spinal disk surgery add-on	1114	1363	1801	195	5.39
63040	Laminotomy, single cervical	4475	5475	7231	1287	35.56
63042	Laminotomy, single lumbar	5274	6453	8522	1214	33.53
63043	Laminotomy, addl cervical	0	0	0	0	.00
63044	Laminotomy, addl lumbar	0	0	0	0	.00
63045	Remove spinal lamina	5284	6465	8537	1155	31.91
63046	Remove spinal lamina	4673	5717	7551	1112	30.71
63047	Remove spinal lamina	5187	6346	8380	1037	28.64
63048	Remove spinal lamina add-on	1214	1485	1962	202	5.59
63055	Decompress spinal cord	5197	6359	8397	1491	41.19
63056	Decompress spinal cord	5408	6616	8738	1381	38.14
63057	Decompress spine cord add-on	1778	2175	2872	322	8.89
63064	Decompress spinal cord	4889	5982	7900	1681	46.45
63066	Decompress spine cord add-on	1488	1820	2404	205	5.65
63075	Neck spine disk surgery	4628	5662	7477	1338	36.97
63076	Neck spine disk surgery	1324	1619	2139	253	6.99
63077	Spine disk surgery thorax	4173	5105	6742	1461	40.35
63078	Spine disk surgery thorax	1460	1786	2359	199	5.50

• NEW CODE CPT 2002   CPT codes and descriptions only copyright AMA

CPT	SHORT DESCRIPTION	50th	75th	90th	MFS	RVU
63081	Remove vertebral body	6200	7585	10017	1624	44.87
63082	Rem vertebral body add-on	1440	1761	2326	273	7.53
63085	Rem vertebral body	5343	6536	8632	1792	49.51
63086	Rem vertebral body add-on	1506	1842	2433	195	5.40
63087	Remove vertebral body	5281	6461	8533	2313	63.89
63088	Rem vertebral body add-on	1580	1934	2554	268	7.40
63090	Remove vertebral body	5459	6679	8820	1830	50.55
63091	Rem vertebral body add-on	1361	1666	2200	180	4.96
63170	Incise spinal cord tract(s)	4095	5010	6616	1349	37.26
63172	Drain spinal cyst	4314	5278	6971	1249	34.49
63173	Drain spinal cyst	4940	6043	7981	1508	41.67
63180	Revise spinal cord ligaments	3862	4725	6240	1272	35.14
63182	Revise spinal cord ligaments	4543	5559	7341	1361	37.59
63185	Incise spinal column/nerves	3967	4853	6409	971	26.82
63190	Incise spinal column/nerves	4787	5856	7734	1159	32.01
63191	Incise spinal column/nerves	3483	4261	5628	1147	31.69
63194	Incise spinal column & cord	3701	4528	5980	1328	36.68
63195	Incise spinal column & cord	3557	4351	5746	1278	35.30
63196	Incise spinal column & cord	4096	5011	6618	1484	40.99
63197	Incise spinal column & cord	4019	4917	6493	1412	39.02
63198	Incise spinal column & cord	4587	5611	7411	1571	43.39
63199	Incise spinal column & cord	4537	5551	7331	1697	46.89
63200	Release spinal cord	4294	5254	6938	1311	36.21
63250	Revise spinal cord vessels	4998	6495	8557	2590	71.56
63251	Revise spinal cord vessels	4326	5622	7407	2631	72.69
63252	Revise spinal cord vessels	5767	7494	9873	2617	72.30

     NEW CODE CPT 2002 •

CPT	SHORT DESCRIPTION	50th	75th	90th	MFS	RVU
63265	Excise intraspinal lesion	4281	5563	7330	1414	39.06
63266	Excise intraspinal lesion	4018	5222	6879	1465	40.47
63267	Excise intraspinal lesion	3945	5127	6755	1192	32.93
63268	Excise intraspinal lesion	3065	3984	5248	1183	32.67
63270	Excise intraspinal lesion	4526	5881	7749	1749	48.31
63271	Excise intraspinal lesion	4367	5675	7477	1761	48.65
63272	Excise intraspinal lesion	4933	6411	8446	1654	45.70
63273	Excise intraspinal lesion	4159	5405	7121	1600	44.21
63275	Biopsy/excise spinal tumor	4725	6140	8089	1550	42.83
63276	Biopsy/excise spinal tumor	4669	6068	7994	1533	42.35
63277	Biopsy/excise spinal tumor	4548	5910	7786	1370	37.85
63278	Biopsy/excise spinal tumor	3697	4805	6330	1363	37.66
63280	Biopsy/excise spinal tumor	5569	7238	9535	1843	50.91
63281	Biopsy/excise spinal tumor	5495	7140	9407	1826	50.45
63282	Biopsy/excise spinal tumor	5584	7256	9560	1720	47.51
63283	Biopsy/excise spinal tumor	4275	5555	7319	1636	45.19
63285	Biopsy/excise spinal tumor	6010	7810	10290	2321	64.13
63286	Biopsy/excise spinal tumor	6067	7884	10387	2288	63.21
63287	Biopsy/excise spinal tumor	6154	7997	10536	2361	65.21
63290	Biopsy/excise spinal tumor	4842	6292	8289	2411	66.61
63300	Remove vertebral body	3497	4544	5987	1587	43.84
63301	Remove vertebral body	3463	4500	5928	1748	48.28
63302	Remove vertebral body	3553	4617	6082	1792	49.51
63303	Remove vertebral body	3753	4877	6426	1934	53.42
63304	Remove vertebral body	3692	4798	6321	1913	52.85
63305	Remove vertebral body	4031	5239	6902	2051	56.66

• NEW CODE CPT 2002   CPT codes and descriptions only copyright AMA

CPT	SHORT DESCRIPTION	50th	75th	90th	MFS	RVU
63306	Remove vertebral body	3711	4823	6354	1911	52.80
63307	Remove vertebral body	3923	5098	6717	1924	53.15
63308	Remove vertebral body add-on	1155	1501	1977	326	9.00
63600	Remove spinal cord lesion	2767	3596	4738	783	21.62
63610	Stimulation spinal cord	2107	2738	3607	473	13.06
63615	Remove lesion spinal cord	3362	4369	5756	1036	28.63
63650	Implant neuroelectrodes	2482	3226	4250	369	10.19
63655	Implant neuroelectrodes	5355	6959	9168	702	19.40
63660	Revise/remove neuroelectrode	2004	2604	3431	379	10.48
63685	Implant neuroreceiver	1842	2393	3153	440	12.15
63688	Revise/remove neuroreceiver	1344	1747	2302	354	9.78
63700	Repair spinal herniation	3089	4014	5289	1075	29.69
63702	Repair spinal herniation	3481	4524	5961	1077	29.74
63704	Repair spinal herniation	3905	5075	6686	1353	37.39
63706	Repair spinal herniation	4031	5239	6902	1536	42.44
63707	Repair spinal fluid leakage	4044	5255	6923	770	21.28
63709	Repair spinal fluid leakage	4232	5499	7245	963	26.60
63710	Graft repair spine defect	3748	4871	6417	949	26.22
63740	Install spinal shunt	3211	4173	5498	771	21.30
63741	Install spinal shunt	1709	2221	2925	508	14.02
63744	Revise spinal shunt	1636	2125	2800	555	15.33
63746	Remove spinal shunt	1152	1497	1973	454	12.54

EXTRACRANIAL NERVES, PERIPHERAL NERVES, AND AUTONOMIC NERVOUS SYSTEM

CPT	SHORT DESCRIPTION	50th	75th	90th	MFS	RVU
64400	Inject for nerve block	165	220	299	140	3.87
64402	Inject for nerve block	427	569	771	206	5.70

NEW CODE CPT 2002 •

CPT	SHORT DESCRIPTION	50th	75th	90th	MFS	RVU
64405	Inject for nerve block	227	303	411	99	2.74
64408	Inject for nerve block	334	444	602	161	4.45
64410	Inject for nerve block	358	477	647	173	4.78
64412	Inject for nerve block	381	507	688	136	3.75
64413	Inject for nerve block	215	287	389	156	4.30
64415	Inject for nerve block	416	555	752	152	4.21
64417	Inject for nerve block	429	572	776	172	4.74
64418	Inject for nerve block	232	309	419	140	3.88
64420	Inject for nerve block	271	362	490	131	3.62
64421	Inject for nerve block	383	510	691	170	4.69
64425	Inject for nerve block	266	354	480	152	4.19
64430	Inject for nerve block	196	261	354	161	4.46
64435	Inject for nerve block	342	455	617	165	4.56
64445	Inject for nerve block	279	372	504	114	3.16
64450	Inject for nerve block	135	180	243	114	3.14
64470	Inj paravertebral c/t	412	549	744	217	5.99
64472	Inj paravertebral c/t add-on	316	421	571	191	5.28
64475	Inj paravertebral l/s	398	531	720	193	5.32
64476	Inj paravertebral l/s add-on	305	406	551	177	4.90
64479	Inj foramen epidural c/t	529	705	955	244	6.74
64480	Inj foramen epidural add-on	416	554	751	206	5.70
64483	Inj foramen epidural l/s	515	687	931	234	6.46
64484	Inj foramen epidural add-on	373	497	673	198	5.46
64505	Inject for nerve block	232	309	418	139	3.85
64508	Inject for nerve block	262	350	474	127	3.50
64510	Inject for nerve block	422	563	763	138	3.82

• NEW CODE CPT 2002   CPT codes and descriptions only copyright AMA

CPT	SHORT DESCRIPTION	50th	75th	90th	MFS	RVU
64520	Inject for nerve block	465	619	839	178	4.92
64530	Inject for nerve block	415	553	749	172	4.74
64550	Apply neurostimulator	85	113	153	27	.75
64553	Implant neuroelectrodes	504	672	911	244	6.73
64555	Implant neuroelectrodes	356	475	644	172	4.76
64560	Implant neuroelectrodes	183	244	331	175	4.83
• 64561	Implant neuroelectrodes	1658	2210	2995	801	22.13
64565	Implant neuroelectrodes	393	524	711	190	5.25
64573	Implant neuroelectrodes	1077	1435	1946	521	14.38
64575	Implant neuroelectrodes	307	409	554	281	7.75
64577	Implant neuroelectrodes	331	441	598	310	8.56
64580	Implant neuroelectrodes	321	427	579	299	8.27
• 64581	Implant neuroelectrodes	1542	2056	2786	745	20.59
64585	Revise/remove neuroelectrode	278	371	503	187	5.17
64590	Implant neuroreceiver	299	398	540	180	4.97
64595	Revise/remove neuroreceiver	223	298	403	146	4.03
64600	Inject treat nerve	250	313	411	243	6.71
64605	Inject treat nerve	372	465	612	353	9.76
64610	Inject treat nerve	502	628	825	451	12.46
64612	Destroy nerve face muscle	319	399	524	183	5.05
64613	Destroy nerve spine muscle	417	521	685	140	3.88
64614	Destroy nerve extrem musc	397	496	652	200	5.52
64620	Inject treat nerve	615	769	1011	217	5.99
64622	Destroy paravertebral nerve l/s	659	824	1083	287	7.94
64623	Destroy paravertebral n add-on	345	431	567	177	4.90
64626	Destroy paravertebral nerve c/t	434	543	714	284	7.84

  NEW CODE CPT 2002 •

CPT	SHORT DESCRIPTION	50th	75th	90th	MFS	RVU
64627	Destroy paravertebral n add-on	392	490	644	180	4.98
64630	Inject treat nerve	367	458	602	247	6.82
64640	Inject treat nerve	313	392	515	237	6.54
64680	Inject treat nerve	317	396	521	205	5.66
64702	Revise finger/toe nerve	812	1015	1335	318	8.79
64704	Revise hand/foot nerve	1147	1433	1884	304	8.39
64708	Revise arm/leg nerve	1702	2128	2798	439	12.13
64712	Revise sciatic nerve	1567	1959	2576	503	13.90
64713	Revise arm nerve(s)	1917	2396	3151	676	18.67
64714	Revise low back nerve(s)	1451	1814	2385	551	15.22
64716	Revise cranial nerve	1438	1797	2363	437	12.08
64718	Revise ulnar nerve at elbow	1865	2330	3065	440	12.15
64719	Revise ulnar nerve at wrist	1257	1571	2067	371	10.26
64721	Carpal tunnel surgery	1409	1761	2316	415	11.47
64722	Relieve pressure on nerve(s)	1039	1299	1708	308	8.51
64726	Release foot/toe nerve	493	616	810	286	7.89
64727	Internal nerve revise	324	405	674	188	5.18
64732	Incise brow nerve	737	943	1228	321	8.87
64734	Incise cheek nerve	741	948	1235	346	9.55
64736	Incise chin nerve	786	1006	1310	300	8.29
64738	Incise jaw nerve	959	1226	1597	380	10.49
64740	Incise tongue nerve	1251	1600	2085	367	10.13
64742	Incise facial nerve	1299	1662	2165	430	11.87
64744	Incise nerve back head	788	1008	1314	368	10.16
64746	Incise diaphragm nerve	592	757	986	408	11.26
64752	Incise vagus nerve	1622	2075	2703	465	12.85

CPT	SHORT DESCRIPTION	50th	75th	90th	MFS	RVU
64755	Incise stomach nerves	2423	3099	4037	763	21.08
64760	Incise vagus nerve	1541	1971	2568	417	11.52
64761	Incise pelvis nerve	596	763	994	367	10.15
64763	Incise hip/thigh nerve	793	1014	1321	504	13.91
64766	Incise hip/thigh nerve	1090	1394	1817	521	14.39
64771	Sever cranial nerve	1198	1532	1996	511	14.11
64772	Incise spinal nerve	812	1039	1353	481	13.29
64774	Remove skin nerve lesion	537	687	895	351	9.69
64776	Remove digit nerve lesion	633	810	1055	349	9.64
64778	Digit nerve surgery add-on	263	337	439	186	5.13
64782	Remove limb nerve lesion	747	956	1245	396	10.95
64783	Limb nerve surgery add-on	382	489	637	223	6.15
64784	Remove nerve lesion	1174	1502	1957	651	17.98
64786	Remove sciatic nerve lesion	1673	2140	2788	1017	28.09
64787	Implant nerve end	811	1037	1352	258	7.14
64788	Remove skin nerve lesion	775	991	1291	313	8.65
64790	Remove nerve lesion	1376	1760	2293	743	20.52
64792	Remove nerve lesion	1512	1934	2519	939	25.93
64795	Biopsy nerve	505	646	842	189	5.22
64802	Remove sympathetic nerves	1576	2016	2627	550	15.19
64804	Remove sympathetic nerves	2375	3038	3957	842	23.26
64809	Remove sympathetic nerves	2343	2997	3905	748	20.67
64818	Remove sympathetic nerves	1653	2115	2755	620	17.14
64820	Remove sympathetic nerves	952	1218	1587	652	18.02
• 64821	Remove sympathetic nerves	1306	1670	2176	609	16.83
• 64822	Remove sympathetic nerves	1306	1670	2176	609	16.83

      NEW CODE CPT 2002 •

CPT	SHORT DESCRIPTION	50th	75th	90th	MFS	RVU
• 64823	Remove sympathetic nerves	1508	1928	2512	703	19.43
64831	Repair digit nerve	1271	1626	2118	652	18.02
64832	Repair nerve add-on	615	787	1025	342	9.45
64834	Repair hand or foot nerve	1028	1315	1713	681	18.82
64835	Repair hand or foot nerve	1145	1464	1907	737	20.36
64836	Repair hand or foot nerve	1344	1719	2240	731	20.20
64837	Repair nerve add-on	627	802	1045	381	10.53
64840	Repair leg nerve	1603	2050	2671	784	21.67
64856	Repair/transpose nerve	1953	2498	3254	911	25.17
64857	Repair arm/leg nerve	1514	1936	2523	958	26.46
64858	Repair sciatic nerve	1736	2221	2893	1097	30.31
64859	Nerve surgery	669	855	1114	253	7.00
64861	Repair arm nerves	1726	2207	2876	1256	34.71
64862	Repair low back nerves	2375	3038	3958	1238	34.20
64864	Repair facial nerve	1731	2214	2885	808	22.31
64865	Repair facial nerve	2101	2687	3500	980	27.07
64866	Fuse facial/other nerve	2716	3474	4526	964	26.64
64868	Fuse facial/other nerve	2774	3548	4622	905	25.01
64870	Fuse facial/other nerve	2685	3434	4474	967	26.72
64872	Subsequent repair nerve	237	304	396	120	3.31
64874	Repair & revise nerve add-on	351	449	585	180	4.96
64876	Repair nerve/shorten bone	375	480	625	185	5.12
64885	Nerve graft head or neck	2093	2677	3487	1111	30.70
64886	Nerve graft head or neck	2465	3153	4108	1306	36.08
64890	Nerve graft hand or foot	1611	2060	2684	983	27.16
64891	Nerve graft hand or foot	1850	2367	3083	842	23.27

CPT	SHORT DESCRIPTION	50th	75th	90th	MFS	RVU
64892	Nerve graft arm or leg	1753	2243	2922	914	25.26
64893	Nerve graft arm or leg	1957	2504	3262	1018	28.12
64895	Nerve graft hand or foot	2369	3030	3947	1083	29.91
64896	Nerve graft hand or foot	2800	3582	4666	1234	34.09
64897	Nerve graft arm or leg	2468	3156	4112	1151	31.80
64898	Nerve graft arm or leg	2901	3711	4834	1193	32.96
64901	Nerve graft add-on	885	1131	1474	614	16.96
64902	Nerve graft add-on	1197	1531	1994	697	19.25
64905	Nerve pedicle transfer	936	1198	1560	886	24.47
64907	Nerve pedicle transfer	1617	2068	2694	1183	32.69
64999	Nervous system surgery	0	0	0	0	.00

NEW CODE CPT 2002 •

CPT	SHORT DESCRIPTION	50th	75th	90th	MFS	RVU

EYE AND OCULAR ADNEXA

EYEBALL

CPT	SHORT DESCRIPTION	50th	75th	90th	MFS	RVU
65091	Revise eye	1388	1836	2451	663	18.31
65093	Revise eye with implant	1439	1903	2541	687	18.98
65101	Remove eye	1467	1940	2590	700	19.35
65103	Remove eye/insert implant	1520	2009	2683	725	20.04
65105	Remove eye/attach implant	1688	2232	2980	778	21.50
65110	Remove eye	2358	3118	4163	1105	30.53
65112	Remove eye/revise socket	2695	3564	4758	1252	34.60
65114	Remove eye/revise socket	2806	3711	4954	1340	37.01
65125	Revise ocular implant	513	679	906	344	9.50
65130	Insert ocular implant	1433	1894	2529	684	18.89
65135	Insert ocular implant	1516	2004	2676	724	19.99
65140	Attach ocular implant	1701	2249	3003	749	20.69
65150	Revise ocular implant	1323	1750	2336	632	17.45
65155	Reinsert ocular implant	1758	2324	3102	784	21.65
65175	Remove ocular implant	1011	1337	1785	648	17.89
65205	Remove foreign body from eye	96	128	170	50	1.37
65210	Remove foreign body from eye	131	173	231	60	1.65
65220	Remove foreign body from eye	682	901	1203	325	8.99
65222	Remove foreign body from eye	146	194	259	64	1.77
65235	Remove foreign body from eye	1416	1872	2500	540	14.91
65260	Remove foreign body from eye	1772	2343	3128	871	24.05
65265	Remove foreign body from eye	2028	2681	3580	994	27.47
65270	Repair eye wound	459	606	810	219	6.05

CPT	SHORT DESCRIPTION	50th	75th	90th	MFS	RVU
65272	Repair eye wound	739	977	1304	353	9.74
65273	Repair eye wound	416	550	734	350	9.68
65275	Repair eye wound	843	1114	1487	402	11.11
65280	Repair eye wound	1378	1822	2432	573	15.84
65285	Repair eye wound	2068	2734	3650	987	27.27
65286	Repair eye wound	733	969	1294	537	14.84
65290	Repair eye socket wound	930	1230	1642	444	12.27

ANTERIOR SEGMENT

CPT	SHORT DESCRIPTION	50th	75th	90th	MFS	RVU
65400	Remove eye lesion	953	1243	1755	540	14.91
65410	Biopsy cornea	160	208	294	119	3.29
65420	Remove eye lesion	868	1132	1597	460	12.70
65426	Remove eye lesion	1345	1754	2476	487	13.46
65430	Corneal smear	1120	1460	2061	370	10.21
65435	Curette/treat cornea	136	178	251	84	2.33
65436	Curette/treat cornea	1138	1485	2096	376	10.38
65450	Treat corneal lesion	1247	1626	2295	412	11.37
65600	Revise cornea	632	824	1163	329	9.08
65710	Corneal transplant	2407	3140	4431	944	26.09
65730	Corneal transplant	3896	5081	7171	976	26.97
65750	Corneal transplant	3108	4054	5722	1091	30.13
65755	Corneal transplant	3090	4030	5688	1084	29.95
65760	Revise cornea	2040	2660	3755	0	.00
65765	Revise cornea	3147	4105	5793	0	.00
65767	Corneal tissue transplant	2983	3891	5492	0	.00
65770	Revise cornea with implant	3103	4047	5711	1221	33.73
65771	Radial keratotomy	1722	2246	3170	0	.00

NEW CODE CPT 2002 •

CPT	SHORT DESCRIPTION	50th	75th	90th	MFS	RVU
65772	Correct astigmatism	750	978	1380	433	11.97
65775	Correct astigmatism	949	1238	1747	530	14.64
65800	Drain eye	204	266	375	156	4.32
65805	Drain eye	205	267	377	157	4.33
65810	Drain eye	974	1271	1794	507	14.01
65815	Drain eye	1012	1320	1863	530	14.65
65820	Relieve inner eye pressure	1454	1896	2676	704	19.44
65850	Incise eye	1451	1892	2670	770	21.28
65855	Laser surgery eye	1363	1778	2509	333	9.19
65860	Incise inner eye adhesions	860	1121	1582	284	7.84
65865	Incise inner eye adhesions	1380	1800	2541	461	12.74
65870	Incise inner eye adhesions	1054	1375	1940	498	13.76
65875	Incise inner eye adhesions	923	1203	1698	513	14.16
65880	Incise inner eye adhesions	985	1285	1814	543	15.01
65900	Remove eye lesion	1316	1716	2422	874	24.14
65920	Remove implant eye	1863	2430	3430	615	16.99
65930	Remove blood clot from eye	1081	1411	1991	599	16.56
66020	Inject treat eye	224	292	413	148	4.09
66030	Inject treat eye	150	196	277	129	3.55
66130	Remove eye lesion	1189	1575	2079	566	15.63
66150	Glaucoma surgery	1927	2552	3369	710	19.61
66155	Glaucoma surgery	1759	2329	3074	708	19.55
66160	Glaucoma surgery	1779	2356	3110	812	22.42
66165	Glaucoma surgery	1722	2281	3010	689	19.04
66170	Glaucoma surgery	2029	2688	3548	1077	29.75
66172	Incise eye	2421	3207	4232	1133	31.30

• NEW CODE CPT 2002   CPT codes and descriptions only copyright AMA

CPT	SHORT DESCRIPTION	50th	75th	90th	MFS	RVU
66180	Implant eye shunt	2335	3092	4081	998	27.56
66185	Revise eye shunt	1398	1852	2444	613	16.93
66220	Repair eye lesion	2182	2890	3814	654	18.08
66225	Repair/graft eye lesion	2669	3535	4665	765	21.14
66250	Follow-up surgery eye	1482	1963	2591	517	14.29
66500	Incise iris	551	730	964	314	8.68
66505	Incise iris	491	650	858	335	9.26
66600	Remove iris and lesion	1738	2302	3038	649	17.92
66605	Remove iris	2448	3242	4279	939	25.94
66625	Remove iris	1316	1743	2301	479	13.23
66630	Remove iris	1339	1774	2341	513	14.16
66635	Remove iris	1248	1653	2182	476	13.14
66680	Repair iris & ciliary body	1118	1481	1954	433	11.95
66682	Repair iris & ciliary body	1348	1785	2356	514	14.20
66700	Destroy ciliary body	1140	1511	1994	439	12.14
66710	Destroy ciliary body	1137	1507	1988	502	13.88
66720	Destroy ciliary body	1125	1490	1967	484	13.37
66740	Destroy ciliary body	1304	1727	2279	416	11.49
66761	Revise iris	1249	1655	2184	358	9.89
66762	Revise iris	1097	1453	1918	377	10.41
66770	Remove inner eye lesion	1147	1519	2005	410	11.32
66820	Incise secondary cataract	978	1258	1582	454	12.55
66821	After cataract laser surgery	888	1143	1437	230	6.34
66825	Reposition intraocular lens	1772	2280	2867	692	19.11
66830	Remove lens lesion	1275	1641	2062	564	15.58
66840	Remove lens material	2296	2955	3715	548	15.14

NEW CODE CPT 2002 •

CPT	SHORT DESCRIPTION	50th	75th	90th	MFS	RVU
66850	Remove lens material	2520	3243	4077	615	16.99
66852	Remove lens material	2822	3631	4565	664	18.35
66920	Extraction lens	2352	3027	3806	602	16.63
66930	Extraction lens	2721	3502	4402	707	19.53
66940	Extraction lens	2457	3162	3975	640	17.67
66982	Cataract surgery, complex	1611	2073	2606	846	23.37
66983	Cataract surgery w/iol, 1 stage	2575	3314	4166	568	15.70
66984	Cataract surgery w/iol, I stage	2857	3676	4622	669	18.49
66985	Insert lens prosthesis	2241	2884	3626	571	15.77
66986	Exchange lens prosthesis	2501	3218	4046	783	21.63
66999	Eye surgery procedure	0	0	0	0	.00

POSTERIOR SEGMENT

CPT	SHORT DESCRIPTION	50th	75th	90th	MFS	RVU
67005	Partial remove eye fluid	1785	2146	2492	314	8.67
67010	Partial remove eye fluid	1969	2367	2750	379	10.46
67015	Release eye fluid	854	1027	1193	564	15.57
67025	Replace eye fluid	1196	1438	1670	917	25.34
67027	Implant eye drug system	3601	4330	5029	957	26.43
67028	Inject eye drug	1380	1829	2413	527	14.55
67030	Incise inner eye strands	1215	1461	1697	434	11.99
67031	Laser surgery eye strands	977	1175	1364	291	8.04
67036	Remove inner eye fluid	3877	4661	5414	784	21.66
67038	Strip retinal membrane	4933	5930	6889	1379	38.09
67039	Laser treat retina	3098	3724	4326	1007	27.83
67040	Laser treat retina	4519	5432	6310	1158	31.99
67101	Repair detached retina	1825	2194	2549	692	19.11
67105	Repair detached retina	2082	2503	2907	561	15.50

CPT	SHORT DESCRIPTION	50th	75th	90th	MFS	RVU
67107	Repair detached retina	3659	4399	5110	1052	29.05
67108	Repair detached retina	5481	6589	7653	1446	39.94
67110	Repair detached retina	2607	3135	3641	1119	30.90
67112	Rerepair detached retina	2269	2728	3169	1201	33.18
67115	Release encircling material	777	934	1084	442	12.20
67120	Remove eye implant material	1073	1289	1498	861	23.78
67121	Remove eye implant material	1291	1552	1803	853	23.56
67141	Treat retina	1572	1890	2195	496	13.69
67145	Treat retina	1482	1781	2069	399	11.01
67208	Treat retinal lesion	1384	1664	1932	564	15.58
67210	Treat retinal lesion	1558	1873	2176	603	16.66
67218	Treat retinal lesion	2769	3329	3867	1282	35.42
67220	Treat choroid lesion	1670	2008	2332	898	24.82
67221	Ocular photodynamic ther	611	735	854	325	8.97
• 67225	Eye photodynamic ther add-on	121	146	169	44	1.21
67227	Treat retinal lesion	1540	1851	2150	584	16.13
67228	Treat retinal lesion	1690	2032	2360	847	23.41
67250	Reinforce eye wall	2087	2508	2914	765	21.12
67255	Reinforce/graft eye wall	2336	2808	3262	773	21.36
67299	Eye surgery procedure	0	0	0	0	.00

     NEW CODE CPT 2002 •

CPT	SHORT DESCRIPTION	50th	75th	90th	MFS	RVU

OCULAR ADNEXA

CPT	SHORT DESCRIPTION	50th	75th	90th	MFS	RVU
67311	Revise eye muscle	1669	2102	2677	481	13.28
67312	Revise two eye muscles	1982	2497	3180	592	16.35
67314	Revise eye muscle	1795	2261	2880	534	14.76
67316	Revise two eye muscles	2298	2894	3687	653	18.05
67318	Revise eye muscle(s)	2060	2594	3305	562	15.53
67320	Revise eye muscle(s) add-on	1005	1266	1612	239	6.59
67331	Eye surgery follow-up add-on	521	656	835	226	6.25
67332	Rerevise eye muscles add-on	1929	2429	3094	247	6.83
67334	Revise eye muscle w/suture	990	1247	1588	219	6.04
67335	Eye suture during surgery	642	808	1029	137	3.79
67340	Revise eye muscle add-on	1016	1279	1630	273	7.53
67343	Release eye tissue	849	1070	1363	540	14.91
67345	Destroy nerve eye muscle	550	693	883	273	7.55
67350	Biopsy eye muscle	508	640	815	181	4.99
67399	Eye muscle surgery procedure	0	0	0	0	.00
67400	Explore/biopsy eye socket	2224	2801	3569	870	24.04
67405	Explore/drain eye socket	1885	2374	3024	755	20.85
67412	Explore/treat eye socket	2278	2869	3655	939	25.93
67413	Explore/treat eye socket	2146	2703	3444	877	24.23
67414	Explore/decompress eye socket	1662	2093	2666	1032	28.51
67415	Aspiration orbital contents	340	428	545	96	2.65
67420	Explore/treat eye socket	3904	4917	6263	1509	41.69
67430	Explore/treat eye socket	3512	4423	5635	1185	32.74
67440	Explore/drain eye socket	3473	4374	5572	1162	32.10
67445	Explore/decompress eye socket	2052	2584	3292	1203	33.24

CPT	SHORT DESCRIPTION	50th	75th	90th	MFS	RVU
67450	Explore/biopsy eye socket	2661	3352	4269	1143	31.58
67500	Inject/treat eye socket	219	275	351	64	1.78
67505	Inject/treat eye socket	253	319	406	66	1.81
67515	Inject/treat eye socket	160	201	256	54	1.49
67550	Insert eye socket implant	1506	1896	2415	878	24.26
67560	Revise eye socket implant	1490	1877	2391	889	24.57
67570	Decompress optic nerve	2777	3498	4456	1156	31.93
67599	Orbit surgery procedure	0	0	0	0	.00
67700	Drain eyelid abscess	695	873	1097	333	9.21
67710	Incise eyelid	677	851	1070	325	8.98
67715	Incise eyelid fold	140	176	221	67	1.86
67800	Remove eyelid lesion	207	260	327	149	4.11
67801	Remove eyelid lesions	768	966	1214	369	10.19
67805	Remove eyelid lesions	809	1016	1278	388	10.72
67808	Remove eyelid lesion(s)	480	603	758	301	8.31
67810	Biopsy eyelid	513	645	810	246	6.80
67820	Revise eyelashes	222	280	352	107	2.95
67825	Revise eyelashes	538	677	851	258	7.14
67830	Revise eyelashes	1005	1263	1587	482	13.32
67835	Revise eyelashes	1183	1487	1869	387	10.68
67840	Remove eyelid lesion	777	977	1229	373	10.31
67850	Treat eyelid lesion	796	1000	1258	382	10.55
67875	Close eyelid by suture	983	1235	1553	472	13.03
67880	Revise eyelid	1262	1586	1994	606	16.73
67882	Revise eyelid	914	1149	1444	749	20.70
67900	Repair brow defect	1029	1294	1627	642	17.73

  NEW CODE CPT 2002 •

CPT	SHORT DESCRIPTION	50th	75th	90th	MFS	RVU
67901	Repair eyelid defect	1421	1786	2245	525	14.51
67902	Repair eyelid defect	1438	1807	2272	526	14.54
67903	Repair eyelid defect	2160	2716	3414	633	17.48
67904	Repair eyelid defect	1897	2385	2997	778	21.49
67906	Repair eyelid defect	1956	2459	3091	620	17.12
67908	Repair eyelid defect	1563	1966	2471	542	14.98
67909	Revise eyelid defect	1424	1790	2250	574	15.85
67911	Revise eyelid defect	2068	2600	3268	450	12.42
67914	Repair eyelid defect	707	889	1118	618	17.06
67915	Repair eyelid defect	1134	1426	1792	544	15.04
67916	Repair eyelid defect	974	1224	1539	825	22.79
67917	Repair eyelid defect	1209	1520	1910	612	16.90
67921	Repair eyelid defect	1429	1796	2258	597	16.48
67922	Repair eyelid defect	1125	1414	1778	540	14.92
67923	Repair eyelid defect	1017	1279	1608	813	22.45
67924	Repair eyelid defect	1322	1663	2090	579	15.99
67930	Repair eyelid wound	1228	1543	1940	589	16.28
67935	Repair eyelid wound	1707	2145	2697	819	22.63
67938	Remove eyelid foreign body	833	1047	1316	400	11.04
67950	Revise eyelid	1534	1928	2424	548	15.13
67961	Revise eyelid	1663	2090	2628	555	15.34
67966	Revise eyelid	1860	2339	2939	576	15.91
67971	Reconstruct eyelid	1558	1959	2462	654	18.06
67973	Reconstruct eyelid	1765	2219	2790	847	23.41
67974	Reconstruct eyelid	2021	2541	3194	842	23.25
67975	Reconstruct eyelid	1283	1614	2028	616	17.02

CPT	SHORT DESCRIPTION	50th	75th	90th	MFS	RVU
67999	Revise eyelid	0	0	0	0	.00

CONJUNCTIVA

CPT	SHORT DESCRIPTION	50th	75th	90th	MFS	RVU
68020	Incise/drain eyelid lining	562	753	925	334	9.22
68040	Treat eyelid lesions	522	699	858	310	8.56
68100	Biopsy eyelid lining	569	762	936	338	9.34
68110	Remove eyelid lining lesion	659	883	1085	392	10.82
68115	Remove eyelid lining lesion	666	892	1096	396	10.93
68130	Remove eyelid lining lesion	656	878	1078	271	7.50
68135	Remove eyelid lining lesion	618	828	1017	367	10.14
68200	Treat eyelid by inject	142	190	234	46	1.27
68320	Revise/graft eyelid lining	1278	1712	2103	410	11.33
68325	Revise/graft eyelid lining	1579	2115	2598	506	13.99
68326	Revise/graft eyelid lining	1417	1897	2331	496	13.71
68328	Revise/graft eyelid lining	1757	2353	2890	567	15.65
68330	Revise eyelid lining	753	1009	1239	447	12.36
68335	Revise/graft eyelid lining	958	1283	1576	476	13.16
68340	Separate eyelid adhesions	1117	1496	1838	732	20.21
68360	Revise eyelid lining	847	1134	1393	409	11.31
68362	Revise eyelid lining	1092	1463	1797	567	15.65
68399	Eyelid lining surgery	0	0	0	0	.00
68400	Incise/drain tear gland	807	1080	1327	479	13.24
68420	Incise/drain tear sac	871	1167	1433	517	14.29
68440	Incise tear duct opening	539	721	886	320	8.84
68500	Remove tear gland	1499	2007	2465	751	20.75
68505	Partial remove tear gland	1241	1662	2041	790	21.82
68510	Biopsy tear gland	1090	1460	1794	648	17.89

  NEW CODE CPT 2002 •

CPT	SHORT DESCRIPTION	50th	75th	90th	MFS	RVU
68520	Remove tear sac	1072	1435	1763	554	15.31
68525	Biopsy tear sac	274	367	451	245	6.76
68530	Clearance tear duct	864	1157	1421	693	19.15
68540	Remove tear gland lesion	1750	2343	2878	753	20.79
68550	Remove tear gland lesion	1750	2343	2878	884	24.42
68700	Repair tear ducts	1320	1767	2171	497	13.74
68705	Revise tear duct opening	638	854	1050	379	10.47
68720	Create tear sac drain	2273	3044	3739	629	17.38
68745	Create tear duct drain	1923	2574	3163	609	16.83
68750	Create tear duct drain	2164	2897	3559	633	17.49
68760	Close tear duct opening	522	700	859	310	8.57
68761	Close tear duct opening	197	264	325	163	4.51
68770	Close tear system fistula	1526	2044	2511	906	25.04
68801	Dilate tear duct opening	170	228	280	67	1.86
68810	Probe nasolacrimal duct	231	310	380	161	4.46
68811	Probe nasolacrimal duct	397	532	653	178	4.91
68815	Probe nasolacrimal duct	1062	1422	1746	631	17.42
68840	Explore/irrigate tear ducts	198	265	325	106	2.92
68850	Inject for tear sac x-ray	983	1316	1616	584	16.12
68899	Tear duct system surgery	0	0	0	0	.00

CPT	SHORT DESCRIPTION	50th	75th	90th	MFS	RVU

NEW CODE CPT 2002 •

CPT	SHORT DESCRIPTION	50th	75th	90th	MFS	RVU

AUDITORY SYSTEM

EXTERNAL EAR

CPT	SHORT DESCRIPTION	50th	75th	90th	MFS	RVU
69000	Drain external ear lesion	152	186	224	134	3.69
69005	Drain external ear lesion	353	432	522	174	4.82
69020	Drain outer ear canal lesion	194	238	287	139	3.84
69090	Pierce earlobes	55	67	81	0	.00
69100	Biopsy external ear	121	148	179	83	2.29
69105	Biopsy external ear canal	133	162	196	88	2.42
69110	Remove external ear, partial	655	801	967	259	7.16
69120	Remove external ear	1213	1483	1791	327	9.04
69140	Remove ear canal lesion(s)	2068	2529	3055	607	16.77
69145	Remove ear canal lesion(s)	568	695	839	225	6.21
69150	Extensive ear canal surgery	1310	1602	1934	937	25.88
69155	Extensive ear/neck surgery	1939	2371	2864	1396	38.57
69200	Clear outer ear canal	107	130	157	82	2.27
69205	Clear outer ear canal	335	410	495	104	2.87
69210	Remove impacted ear wax	61	74	90	45	1.24
69220	Clean out mastoid cavity	103	126	152	88	2.42
69222	Clean out mastoid cavity	196	239	289	135	3.74
69300	Revise external ear	1140	1394	1683	404	11.17
69310	Rebuild outer ear canal	1740	2129	2571	775	21.42
69320	Rebuild outer ear canal	1651	2019	2438	1155	31.90
69399	Outer ear surgery procedure	0	0	0	0	.00

CPT	SHORT DESCRIPTION	50th	75th	90th	MFS	RVU
MIDDLE EAR						
69400	Inflate middle ear canal	106	137	189	87	2.40
69401	Inflate middle ear canal	80	102	141	75	2.08
69405	Catheterize middle ear canal	626	807	1113	214	5.90
69410	Inset middle ear (baffle)	91	117	162	63	1.74
69420	Incise eardrum	215	278	383	137	3.78
69421	Incise eardrum	346	446	615	161	4.44
69424	Remove ventilating tube	205	264	363	94	2.59
69433	Create eardrum opening	336	433	597	143	3.95
69436	Create eardrum opening	471	607	837	150	4.15
69440	Explore middle ear	1895	2442	3368	561	15.51
69450	Eardrum revise	1320	1701	2346	439	12.14
69501	Mastoidectomy	1710	2203	3039	649	17.94
69502	Mastoidectomy	2304	2968	4094	870	24.04
69505	Remove mastoid structures	2402	3094	4268	900	24.85
69511	Extensive mastoid surgery	2727	3512	4845	939	25.93
69530	Extensive mastoid surgery	3664	4720	6511	1288	35.57
69535	Remove part temporal bone	3711	4780	6594	2312	63.86
69540	Remove ear lesion	303	390	538	129	3.56
69550	Remove ear lesion	2274	2929	4040	788	21.76
69552	Remove ear lesion	2912	3751	5174	1290	35.63
69554	Remove ear lesion	3377	4350	6000	2073	57.27
69601	Mastoid surgery revise	1819	2343	3232	946	26.13
69602	Mastoid surgery revise	2743	3533	4873	944	26.07
69603	Mastoid surgery revise	2828	3644	5026	971	26.82
69604	Mastoid surgery revise	2811	3621	4995	969	26.76

NEW CODE CPT 2002 •

CPT	SHORT DESCRIPTION	50th	75th	90th	MFS	RVU
69605	Mastoid surgery revise	3195	4116	5678	1236	34.15
69610	Repair eardrum	391	504	695	326	9.01
69620	Repair eardrum	1831	2358	3253	477	13.19
69631	Repair eardrum structures	3064	3948	5445	721	19.93
69632	Rebuild eardrum structures	3383	4358	6011	918	25.37
69633	Rebuild eardrum structures	3590	4625	6380	880	24.30
69635	Repair eardrum structures	2719	3503	4831	927	25.61
69636	Rebuild eardrum structures	3097	3990	5503	1069	29.52
69637	Rebuild eardrum structures	3114	4011	5533	1062	29.33
69641	Revise middle ear & mastoid	3874	4991	6884	893	24.66
69642	Revise middle ear & mastoid	3387	4364	6019	1165	32.18
69643	Revise middle ear & mastoid	4236	5457	7527	1073	29.64
69644	Revise middle ear & mastoid	3412	4395	6062	1172	32.38
69645	Revise middle ear & mastoid	3303	4255	5869	1133	31.31
69646	Revise middle ear & mastoid	3294	4243	5853	1234	34.08
69650	Release middle ear bone	1570	2023	2791	683	18.87
69660	Revise middle ear bone	3510	4521	6237	818	22.60
69661	Revise middle ear bone	2484	3200	4414	1067	29.47
69662	Revise middle ear bone	3078	3965	5469	1053	29.08
69666	Repair middle ear structures	2143	2761	3808	691	19.08
69667	Repair middle ear structures	2145	2764	3812	690	19.06
69670	Remove mastoid air cells	2461	3171	4373	820	22.65
69676	Remove middle ear nerve	1772	2283	3149	700	19.35
69700	Close mastoid fistula	734	946	1304	527	14.55
69710	Implant/replace hearing aid	976	1257	1734	0	.00
69711	Remove/repair hearing aid	1414	1822	2513	749	20.68

CPT	SHORT DESCRIPTION	50th	75th	90th	MFS	RVU
69714	Implant temple bone w/stimul	1640	2113	2914	961	26.54
69715	Temple bone implant w/stimulat	2077	2676	3691	1217	33.62
69717	Temple bone implant revise	1689	2176	3002	996	27.52
69718	Revise temple bone implant	2102	2708	3735	1232	34.04
69720	Release facial nerve	2925	3768	5198	1023	28.26
69725	Release facial nerve	4550	5862	8085	1634	45.13
69740	Repair facial nerve	2971	3828	5280	1013	27.99
69745	Repair facial nerve	4333	5582	7700	1104	30.49
69799	Middle ear surgery procedure	0	0	0	0	.00

INNER EAR

CPT	SHORT DESCRIPTION	50th	75th	90th	MFS	RVU
69801	Incise inner ear	2156	2778	3831	620	17.12
69802	Incise inner ear	2695	3471	4788	919	25.38
69805	Explore inner ear	2685	3459	4771	930	25.70
69806	Explore inner ear	2972	3829	5282	870	24.03
69820	Establish inner ear window	2425	3124	4309	716	19.78
69840	Revise inner ear window	1412	1819	2509	720	19.90
69905	Remove inner ear	2258	2909	4013	790	21.81
69910	Remove inner ear & mastoid	2735	3523	4859	941	25.99
69915	Incise inner ear nerve	4103	5286	7291	1399	38.65
69930	Implant cochlear device	3285	4232	5837	1120	30.94
69949	Inner ear surgery procedure	0	0	0	0	.00

TEMPORAL BONE, MIDDLE FOSSA APPROACH

CPT	SHORT DESCRIPTION	50th	75th	90th	MFS	RVU
69950	Incise inner ear nerve	4625	5958	8219	1638	45.25
69955	Release facial nerve	4906	6321	8718	1713	47.32
69960	Release inner ear canal	4857	6256	8630	1733	47.87

NEW CODE CPT 2002 •

CPT	SHORT DESCRIPTION	50th	75th	90th	MFS	RVU
69970	Remove inner ear lesion	5467	7043	9715	1864	51.50
69979	Temporal bone surgery	0	0	0	0	.00
69990	Microsurgery add-on	601	774	1068	214	5.90

CPT	SHORT DESCRIPTION	50th	75th	90th	MFS	RVU

NEW CODE CPT 2002 •

DIAGNOSTIC RADIOLOGY

HEAD AND NECK

CPT	SHORT DESCRIPTION	50th	75th	90th	MFS	RVU
70010	Contrast x-ray brain	308	374	456	216	5.96
70010-26	Contrast x-ray brain	114	138	169	60	1.67
70015	Contrast x-ray brain	253	308	375	109	3.02
70015-26	Contrast x-ray brain	94	114	139	60	1.66
70030	X-ray eye for foreign body	90	109	133	24	.65
70030-26	X-ray eye for foreign body	31	38	47	9	.24
70100	X-ray exam jaw	104	127	154	28	.77
70100-26	X-ray exam jaw	34	42	51	9	.25
70110	X-ray exam jaw	123	150	183	35	.97
70110-26	X-ray exam jaw	46	55	68	13	.35
70120	X-ray exam mastoids	114	139	169	31	.87
70120-26	X-ray exam mastoids	41	50	61	9	.25
70130	X-ray exam mastoids	125	152	185	45	1.25
70130-26	X-ray exam mastoids	55	67	81	17	.47
70134	X-ray exam middle ear	130	158	192	44	1.21
70134-26	X-ray exam middle ear	58	71	87	17	.47
70140	X-ray exam facial bones	99	121	147	32	.89
70140-26	X-ray exam facial bones	36	43	53	10	.27
70150	X-ray exam facial bones	134	163	198	41	1.14
70150-26	X-ray exam facial bones	47	57	69	13	.36
70160	X-ray exam nasal bones	98	120	146	28	.76
70160-26	X-ray exam nasal bones	32	39	48	9	.24

CPT	SHORT DESCRIPTION	50th	75th	90th	MFS	RVU
70170	X-ray exam tear duct	115	140	171	50	1.37
70170-26	X-ray exam tear duct	43	52	63	15	.42
70190	X-ray exam eye sockets	122	149	181	33	.91
70190-26	X-ray exam eye sockets	40	49	60	10	.29
70200	X-ray exam eye sockets	137	167	203	42	1.17
70200-26	X-ray exam eye sockets	48	58	71	14	.39
70210	X-ray exam sinuses	73	89	109	31	.86
70210-26	X-ray exam sinuses	24	29	36	9	.24
70220	X-ray exam sinuses	122	149	181	41	1.13
70220-26	X-ray exam sinuses	47	57	69	13	.35
70240	X-ray exam pituitary saddle	82	100	122	25	.68
70240-26	X-ray exam pituitary saddle	35	42	51	10	.27
70250	X-ray exam skull	102	124	151	34	.95
70250-26	X-ray exam skull	43	52	63	12	.33
70260	X-ray exam skull	140	171	208	49	1.36
70260-26	X-ray exam skull	56	68	83	17	.47
70300	X-ray exam teeth	22	27	33	15	.42
70300-26	X-ray exam teeth	9	12	14	5	.15
70310	X-ray exam teeth	46	56	69	24	.65
70310-26	X-ray exam teeth	18	22	27	9	.24
70320	Full mouth x-ray teeth	109	132	161	39	1.09
70320-26	Full mouth x-ray teeth	39	48	58	11	.31
70328	X-ray exam jaw joint	98	119	145	27	.74
70328-26	X-ray exam jaw joint	37	45	55	9	.25
70330	X-ray exam jaw joints	140	170	207	42	1.17
70330-26	X-ray exam jaw joints	49	59	72	12	.33

    NEW CODE CPT 2002 •

CPT	SHORT DESCRIPTION	50th	75th	90th	MFS	RVU
70332	X-ray exam jaw joint	277	337	410	103	2.84
70332-26	X-ray exam jaw joint	94	114	139	27	.75
70336	Magnetic image jaw joint	1135	1380	1681	478	13.20
70336-26	Magnetic image jaw joint	204	248	303	75	2.07
70350	X-ray head for orthodontia	84	102	125	22	.62
70350-26	X-ray head for orthodontia	35	43	52	9	.24
70355	Panoramic x-ray jaws	77	94	115	31	.85
70355-26	Panoramic x-ray jaws	26	32	39	10	.28
70360	X-ray exam neck	75	91	111	24	.65
70360-26	X-ray exam neck	31	38	46	9	.24
70370	Throat x-ray & fluoroscopy	210	256	311	63	1.74
70370-26	Throat x-ray & fluoroscopy	65	79	97	16	.44
70371	Speech evaluation, complex	288	351	427	118	3.27
70371-26	Speech evaluation, complex	130	158	192	43	1.18
70373	Contrast x-ray larynx	203	247	301	87	2.39
70373-26	Contrast x-ray larynx	75	91	111	22	.61
70380	X-ray exam salivary gland	97	118	143	33	.90
70380-26	X-ray exam salivary gland	32	39	47	9	.24
70390	X-ray exam salivary duct	216	263	320	84	2.31
70390-26	X-ray exam salivary duct	67	81	99	19	.53
70450	CT head/brain w/o dye	690	814	954	213	5.88
70450-26	CT head/brain w/o dye	172	203	239	43	1.19
70460	CT head/brain w/dye	802	946	1110	261	7.20
70460-26	CT head/brain w/dye	208	246	288	57	1.58
70470	CT head/brain w/o&w dye	1001	1182	1385	319	8.80
70470-26	CT head/brain w/o&w dye	230	272	319	64	1.78

CPT	SHORT DESCRIPTION	50th	75th	90th	MFS	RVU
70480	CT orbit/ear/fossa w/o dye	646	762	894	235	6.48
70480-26	CT orbit/ear/fossa w/o dye	207	244	286	65	1.79
70481	CT orbit/ear/fossa w/dye	746	880	1032	273	7.54
70481-26	CT orbit/ear/fossa w/dye	224	264	310	70	1.92
70482	CT orbit/ear/fossa w/o&w dye	895	1056	1239	327	9.04
70482-26	CT orbit/ear/fossa w/o&w dye	233	275	322	73	2.02
70486	CT maxillofacial w/o dye	655	773	906	227	6.28
70486-26	CT maxillofacial w/o dye	190	224	263	58	1.59
70487	CT maxillofacial w/dye	790	933	1094	269	7.44
70487-26	CT maxillofacial w/dye	221	261	306	66	1.82
70488	CT maxillofacial w/o&w dye	957	1129	1324	326	9.00
70488-26	CT maxillofacial w/o&w dye	239	282	331	72	1.98
70490	CT soft tissue neck w/o dye	656	775	908	235	6.48
70490-26	CT soft tissue neck w/o dye	210	248	291	65	1.79
70491	CT soft tissue neck w/dye	768	906	1063	273	7.54
70491-26	CT soft tissue neck w/dye	230	272	319	70	1.92
70492	CT soft tissue neck w/o & w/dye	957	1130	1324	327	9.04
70492-26	CT soft tissue neck w/o & w/dye	249	294	344	73	2.02
70496	CT angiography head	675	796	934	352	9.72
70496-26	CT angiography head	175	207	243	92	2.53
70498	CT angiography neck	675	796	934	352	9.72
70498-26	CT angiography neck	175	207	243	92	2.53
70540	MRI orbit/face/neck w/o dye	1435	1693	1986	464	12.82
70540-26	MRI orbit/face/neck w/o dye	258	305	357	67	1.86
70542	MRI orbit/face/neck w/dye	1036	1223	1434	557	15.39
70542-26	MRI orbit/face/neck w/dye	197	232	273	81	2.24

NEW CODE CPT 2002 •

CPT	SHORT DESCRIPTION	50th	75th	90th	MFS	RVU
70543	MRI orbit/fac/neck w/o&w dye	1655	1953	2290	989	27.31
70543-26	MRI orbit/fac/neck w/o&w dye	348	410	481	108	2.97
70544	Mr angiography head w/o dye	1082	1278	1498	463	12.80
70544-26	Mr angiography head w/o dye	195	230	270	60	1.67
70545	Mr angiography head w/dye	899	1061	1244	463	12.80
70545-26	Mr angiography head w/dye	171	202	236	60	1.67
70546	Mr angiography head w/o&w dye	1704	2011	2358	879	24.29
70546-26	Mr angiography head w/o&w dye	358	422	495	91	2.51
70547	Mr angiography neck w/o dye	1078	1272	1491	463	12.80
70547-26	Mr angiography neck w/o dye	194	229	268	60	1.67
70548	Mr angiography neck w/dye	899	1061	1244	463	12.80
70548-26	Mr angiography neck w/dye	171	202	236	60	1.67
70549	Mr angiography neck w/o&w dye	1704	2011	2358	879	24.29
70549-26	Mr angiography neck w/o&w dye	358	422	495	91	2.51
70551	MRI brain w/o dye	1262	1490	1747	478	13.20
70551-26	MRI brain w/o dye	227	268	314	75	2.07
70552	MRI brain w/dye	1734	2046	2399	573	15.84
70552-26	MRI brain w/dye	329	389	456	90	2.50
70553	MRI brain w/o&w dye	1869	2206	2586	1014	28.02
70553-26	MRI brain w/o&w dye	392	463	543	119	3.29

CHEST

CPT	SHORT DESCRIPTION	50th	75th	90th	MFS	RVU
71010	Chest x-ray	75	87	99	26	.72
71010-26	Chest x-ray	31	36	41	9	.25
71015	Chest x-ray	83	97	110	29	.81
71015-26	Chest x-ray	33	39	44	10	.29
71020	Chest x-ray	92	107	121	34	.93

CPT	SHORT DESCRIPTION	50th	75th	90th	MFS	RVU
71020-26	Chest x-ray	38	44	50	11	.31
71021	Chest x-ray	111	129	147	40	1.11
71021-26	Chest x-ray	42	49	56	13	.37
71022	Chest x-ray	124	145	165	43	1.18
71022-26	Chest x-ray	52	61	69	16	.44
71023	Chest x-ray and fluoroscopy	148	172	196	48	1.32
71023-26	Chest x-ray and fluoroscopy	65	76	86	20	.54
71030	Chest x-ray	121	141	161	44	1.21
71030-26	Chest x-ray	51	59	68	16	.43
71034	Chest x-ray and fluoroscopy	184	214	244	76	2.09
71034-26	Chest x-ray and fluoroscopy	72	83	95	24	.65
71035	Chest x-ray	80	93	106	28	.77
71035-26	Chest x-ray	34	40	46	9	.25
71040	Contrast x-ray bronchi	188	219	249	82	2.27
71040-26	Contrast x-ray bronchi	83	96	110	29	.81
71060	Contrast x-ray bronchi	268	311	354	117	3.23
71060-26	Contrast x-ray bronchi	110	127	145	37	1.03
71090	X-ray & pacemaker insert	233	271	308	89	2.47
71090-26	X-ray & pacemaker insert	93	108	123	28	.78
71100	X-ray exam ribs	113	131	149	32	.88
71100-26	X-ray exam ribs	48	56	64	11	.31
71101	X-ray exam ribs/chest	109	127	145	37	1.03
71101-26	X-ray exam ribs/chest	47	55	62	13	.37
71110	X-ray exam ribs	128	149	170	42	1.15
71110-26	X-ray exam ribs	51	60	68	13	.37
71111	X-ray exam ribs/ chest	147	171	195	48	1.33

NEW CODE CPT 2002 •

CPT	SHORT DESCRIPTION	50th	75th	90th	MFS	RVU
71111-26	X-ray exam ribs/ chest	59	68	78	16	.44
71120	X-ray exam breastbone	102	118	135	34	.93
71120-26	X-ray exam breastbone	34	39	44	10	.28
71130	X-ray exam breastbone	102	118	135	37	1.01
71130-26	X-ray exam breastbone	39	45	51	11	.31
71250	CT thorax w/o dye	770	894	1019	271	7.49
71250-26	CT thorax w/o dye	208	242	275	59	1.62
71260	CT thorax w/dye	920	1069	1217	316	8.74
71260-26	CT thorax w/dye	230	267	304	62	1.72
71270	CT thorax w/o&w dye	1022	1187	1352	387	10.70
71270-26	CT thorax w/o&w dye	245	285	325	70	1.92
71275	CT angiography chest	734	854	972	415	11.47
71275-26	CT angiography chest	191	222	253	100	2.75
71550	MRI chest w/o dye	1675	1946	2216	471	13.02
71550-26	MRI chest w/o dye	301	350	399	73	2.01
71551	MRI chest w/dye	1057	1228	1399	564	15.58
71551-26	MRI chest w/dye	201	233	266	87	2.39
71552	MRI chest w/o&w dye	1875	2179	2481	989	27.33
71552-26	MRI chest w/o&w dye	394	458	521	113	3.13
71555	MRI angio chest w or w/o dye	1685	1958	2230	494	13.66
71555-26	MRI angio chest w or w/o dye	320	372	424	92	2.53

SPINE AND PELVIS

CPT	SHORT DESCRIPTION	50th	75th	90th	MFS	RVU
72010	X-ray exam spine	159	190	223	60	1.66
72010-26	X-ray exam spine	62	74	87	23	.64
72020	X-ray exam spine	70	84	99	22	.62
72020-26	X-ray exam spine	32	38	45	8	.21

CPT	SHORT DESCRIPTION	50th	75th	90th	MFS	RVU
72040	X-ray exam neck spine	105	126	148	33	.91
72040-26	X-ray exam neck spine	35	42	49	11	.31
72050	X-ray exam neck spine	141	169	199	48	1.33
72050-26	X-ray exam neck spine	50	59	70	16	.44
72052	X-ray exam neck spine	169	202	239	59	1.63
72052-26	X-ray exam neck spine	56	67	79	18	.51
72069	X-ray exam trunk spine	104	125	147	30	.82
72069-26	X-ray exam trunk spine	35	42	50	12	.33
72070	X-ray exam thoracic spine	105	125	147	35	.96
72070-26	X-ray exam thoracic spine	41	49	58	11	.31
72072	X-ray exam thoracic spine	116	139	164	38	1.05
72072-26	X-ray exam thoracic spine	42	50	59	11	.31
72074	X-ray exam thoracic spine	138	165	194	44	1.22
72074-26	X-ray exam thoracic spine	40	48	56	11	.31
72080	X-ray exam trunk spine	107	128	151	35	.98
72080-26	X-ray exam trunk spine	46	55	65	12	.32
72090	X-ray exam trunk spine	127	151	178	38	1.06
72090-26	X-ray exam trunk spine	56	67	78	14	.40
72100	X-ray exam lower spine	102	122	143	35	.98
72100-26	X-ray exam lower spine	40	47	56	12	.32
72110	X-ray exam lower spine	146	174	205	49	1.35
72110-26	X-ray exam lower spine	58	70	82	16	.44
72114	X-ray exam lower spine	191	229	269	62	1.70
72114-26	X-ray exam lower spine	71	85	100	19	.52
72120	X-ray exam lower spine	137	164	193	44	1.21
72120-26	X-ray exam lower spine	47	56	66	12	.32

NEW CODE CPT 2002 •

CPT	SHORT DESCRIPTION	50th	75th	90th	MFS	RVU
72125	CT neck spine w/o dye	830	988	1178	271	7.49
72125-26	CT neck spine w/o dye	216	257	306	59	1.62
72126	CT neck spine w/dye	1011	1204	1435	316	8.72
72126-26	CT neck spine w/dye	232	277	330	62	1.70
72127	CT neck spine w/o&w dye	1044	1244	1483	382	10.56
72127-26	CT neck spine w/o&w dye	209	249	297	64	1.78
72128	CT chest spine w/o dye	832	991	1181	271	7.49
72128-26	CT chest spine w/o dye	216	258	307	59	1.62
72129	CT chest spine w/dye	1006	1199	1430	316	8.72
72129-26	CT chest spine w/dye	231	276	329	62	1.70
72130	CT chest spine w/o&w dye	1044	1244	1483	382	10.56
72130-26	CT chest spine w/o&w dye	209	249	297	64	1.78
72131	CT lumbar spine w/o dye	825	983	1172	271	7.49
72131-26	CT lumbar spine w/o dye	215	256	305	59	1.62
72132	CT lumbar spine w/dye	1005	1198	1428	316	8.73
72132-26	CT lumbar spine w/dye	231	275	329	62	1.71
72133	CT lumbar spine w/o&w dye	1276	1519	1812	382	10.56
72133-26	CT lumbar spine w/o&w dye	255	304	362	64	1.78
72141	MRI neck spine w/o dye	1200	1430	1705	484	13.36
72141-26	MRI neck spine w/o dye	216	257	307	81	2.23
72142	MRI neck spine w/dye	1878	2238	2668	581	16.04
72142-26	MRI neck spine w/dye	357	425	507	98	2.70
72146	MRI chest spine w/o dye	1290	1537	1833	528	14.58
72146-26	MRI chest spine w/o dye	232	277	330	81	2.23
72147	MRI chest spine w/dye	1881	2241	2672	580	16.03
72147-26	MRI chest spine w/dye	357	426	508	97	2.69

CPT	SHORT DESCRIPTION	50th	75th	90th	MFS	RVU
72148	MRI lumbar spine w/o dye	1335	1591	1897	522	14.42
72148-26	MRI lumbar spine w/o dye	240	286	341	75	2.07
72149	MRI lumbar spine w/dye	1700	2025	2415	574	15.85
72149-26	MRI lumbar spine w/dye	323	385	459	91	2.51
72156	MRI neck spine w/o&w dye	2002	2385	2844	1025	28.32
72156-26	MRI neck spine w/o&w dye	420	501	597	130	3.59
72157	MRI chest spine w/o&w dye	2042	2432	2900	1025	28.31
72157-26	MRI chest spine w/o&w dye	429	511	609	130	3.58
72158	MRI lumbar spine w/o&w dye	1790	2133	2543	1015	28.03
72158-26	MRI lumbar spine w/o&w dye	376	448	534	119	3.30
72159	Mr angio spine w/o&w dye	1473	1755	2093	541	14.95
72159-26	Mr angio spine w/o&w dye	280	333	398	94	2.60
72170	X-ray exam pelvis	85	101	121	28	.76
72170-26	X-ray exam pelvis	28	33	40	9	.24
72190	X-ray exam pelvis	112	134	159	34	.95
72190-26	X-ray exam pelvis	40	48	57	10	.29
72191	CT angiography pelvis w/o&w dye	734	875	1043	397	10.97
72191-26	CT angiography pelvis w/o&w dye	191	227	271	94	2.59
72192	CT pelvis w/o dye	836	996	1187	268	7.39
72192-26	CT pelvis w/o dye	201	239	285	55	1.52
72193	CT pelvis w/dye	960	1143	1363	305	8.42
72193-26	CT pelvis w/dye	221	263	314	59	1.62
72194	CT pelvis w/o&w dye	1194	1423	1697	366	10.12
72194-26	CT pelvis w/o&w dye	239	285	339	62	1.70
72195	MRI pelvis w/o dye	1123	1338	1596	472	13.03
72195-26	MRI pelvis w/o dye	202	241	287	73	2.02

    NEW CODE CPT 2002 •

CPT	SHORT DESCRIPTION	50th	75th	90th	MFS	RVU
72196	MRI pelvis w/dye	1206	1437	1714	564	15.57
72196-26	MRI pelvis w/dye	229	273	326	86	2.38
72197	MRI pelvis w/o & w dye	1713	2040	2433	997	27.53
72197-26	MRI pelvis w/o & w dye	360	428	511	113	3.13
72198	Mr angio pelvis w/o&w dye	1730	2061	2457	497	13.73
72198-26	Mr angio pelvis w/o&w dye	329	392	467	94	2.60
72200	X-ray exam sacroiliac joints	86	103	122	28	.76
72200-26	X-ray exam sacroiliac joints	37	44	53	9	.24
72202	X-ray exam sacroiliac joints	103	123	147	32	.89
72202-26	X-ray exam sacroiliac joints	46	54	65	10	.27
72220	X-ray exam tailbone	92	110	131	29	.81
72220-26	X-ray exam tailbone	40	47	56	9	.24
72240	Contrast x-ray neck spine	381	453	541	216	5.98
72240-26	Contrast x-ray neck spine	160	190	227	46	1.26
72255	Contrast x-ray thorax spine	388	462	552	201	5.54
72255-26	Contrast x-ray thorax spine	159	190	226	45	1.25
72265	Contrast x-ray lower spine	358	427	509	188	5.20
72265-26	Contrast x-ray lower spine	147	175	209	42	1.15
72270	Contrast x-ray spine	579	690	823	287	7.92
72270-26	Contrast x-ray spine	220	262	313	67	1.86
72275	Epidurography	502	598	713	115	3.17
72275-26	Epidurography	191	227	271	36	1.00
72285	X-ray c/t spine disk	1107	1319	1572	359	9.93
72285-26	X-ray c/t spine disk	177	211	252	58	1.61
72295	X-ray lower spine disk	950	1132	1350	324	8.96
72295-26	X-ray lower spine disk	152	181	216	42	1.16

CPT	SHORT DESCRIPTION	50th	75th	90th	MFS	RVU

UPPER EXTREMITIES

CPT	SHORT DESCRIPTION	50th	75th	90th	MFS	RVU
73000	X-ray exam collar bone	80	94	111	27	.75
73000-26	X-ray exam collar bone	30	35	41	8	.23
73010	X-ray exam shoulder blade	92	109	128	28	.76
73010-26	X-ray exam shoulder blade	34	40	47	9	.24
73020	X-ray exam shoulder	79	93	109	25	.68
73020-26	X-ray exam shoulder	28	33	39	8	.21
73030	X-ray exam shoulder	94	111	131	30	.82
73030-26	X-ray exam shoulder	39	45	54	9	.25
73040	Contrast x-ray shoulder	263	310	365	103	2.85
73040-26	Contrast x-ray shoulder	97	115	135	28	.76
73050	X-ray exam shoulders	99	117	138	34	.95
73050-26	X-ray exam shoulders	33	39	46	10	.29
73060	X-ray exam humerus	86	101	120	29	.81
73060-26	X-ray exam humerus	31	37	43	9	.24
73070	X-ray exam elbow	77	91	108	26	.73
73070-26	X-ray exam elbow	24	28	33	8	.21
73080	X-ray exam elbow	91	107	126	29	.81
73080-26	X-ray exam elbow	34	40	47	9	.24
73085	Contrast x-ray elbow	281	331	390	104	2.86
73085-26	Contrast x-ray elbow	104	122	144	28	.77
73090	X-ray exam forearm	77	91	108	27	.75
73090-26	X-ray exam forearm	31	37	43	8	.23
73092	X-ray exam arm, infant	73	86	101	26	.72
73092-26	X-ray exam arm, infant	29	34	40	8	.23
73100	X-ray exam wrist	74	88	103	26	.73

NEW CODE CPT 2002 •

CPT	SHORT DESCRIPTION	50th	75th	90th	MFS	RVU
73100-26	X-ray exam wrist	30	35	41	9	.24
73110	X-ray exam wrist	83	98	115	28	.77
73110-26	X-ray exam wrist	34	40	47	9	.24
73115	Contrast x-ray wrist	226	266	314	85	2.35
73115-26	Contrast x-ray wrist	93	109	129	28	.77
73120	X-ray exam hand	71	84	99	26	.72
73120-26	X-ray exam hand	26	30	36	8	.23
73130	X-ray exam hand	85	100	118	28	.77
73130-26	X-ray exam hand	31	36	43	9	.24
73140	X-ray exam finger(s)	65	77	91	22	.60
73140-26	X-ray exam finger(s)	25	29	35	7	.19
73200	CT upper extremity w/o dye	756	892	1050	233	6.44
73200-26	CT upper extremity w/o dye	197	232	273	55	1.52
73201	CT upper extremity w/dye	841	992	1168	271	7.49
73201-26	CT upper extremity w/dye	210	248	292	59	1.62
73202	CT upper extremity w/o&w dye	894	1055	1242	329	9.08
73202-26	CT upper extremity w/o&w dye	197	232	273	62	1.71
73206	CT angio upper extrm w/o&w dye	657	775	912	361	9.96
73206-26	CT angio upper extrm w/o&w dye	171	201	237	94	2.59
73218	MRI upper extremity w/o dye	1116	1316	1551	464	12.82
73218-26	MRI upper extremity w/o dye	201	237	279	67	1.86
73219	MRI upper extremity w/dye	1071	1263	1488	557	15.39
73219-26	MRI upper extremity w/dye	203	240	283	81	2.24
73220	MRI upper extremity w/o&w dye	1339	1580	1861	989	27.32
73220-26	MRI upper extremity w/o&w dye	281	332	391	108	2.98
73221	MRI joint upper extrem w/o dye	1175	1386	1633	464	12.82

CPT	SHORT DESCRIPTION	50th	75th	90th	MFS	RVU
73221-26	MRI joint upper extrem w/o dye	212	250	294	67	1.86
73222	MRI joint upper extrem w/ dye	1359	1603	1888	557	15.39
73222-26	MRI joint upper extrem w/ dye	258	304	359	81	2.24
73223	MRI joint upper extr w/o&w dye	1925	2271	2675	989	27.31
73223-26	MRI joint upper extr w/o&w dye	404	477	562	108	2.97
73225	Mr angio upper extr w/o&w dye	1337	1577	1858	493	13.63
73225-26	Mr angio upper extr w/o&w dye	254	300	353	90	2.50

LOWER EXTREMITIES

CPT	SHORT DESCRIPTION	50th	75th	90th	MFS	RVU
73500	X-ray exam hip	77	92	109	26	.71
73500-26	X-ray exam hip	31	37	44	9	.24
73510	X-ray exam hip	98	117	138	31	.87
73510-26	X-ray exam hip	32	39	46	11	.30
73520	X-ray exam hips	132	156	186	37	1.03
73520-26	X-ray exam hips	53	63	74	13	.37
73525	Contrast x-ray hip	298	354	420	104	2.86
73525-26	Contrast x-ray hip	110	131	155	28	.77
73530	X-ray exam hip	114	136	161	33	.92
73530-26	X-ray exam hip	54	64	76	14	.40
73540	X-ray exam pelvis & hips	95	112	133	31	.86
73540-26	X-ray exam pelvis & hips	32	38	45	10	.29
73542	X-ray exam sacroiliac joint	512	607	720	104	2.88
73542-26	X-ray exam sacroiliac joint	195	231	274	29	.79
73550	X-ray exam thigh	92	109	129	29	.81
73550-26	X-ray exam thigh	33	39	47	9	.24
73560	X-ray exam knee, 1 or 2	82	98	116	28	.77
73560-26	X-ray exam knee, 1 or 2	30	35	42	9	.25

CPT	SHORT DESCRIPTION	50th	75th	90th	MFS	RVU
73562	X-ray exam knee, 3	96	114	136	30	.83
73562-26	X-ray exam knee, 3	35	41	49	9	.26
73564	X-ray exam knee, 4 or more	111	131	156	34	.94
73564-26	X-ray exam knee, 4 or more	44	52	62	12	.32
73565	X-ray exam knees	90	107	127	27	.75
73565-26	X-ray exam knees	33	39	46	9	.26
73580	Contrast x-ray knee joint	325	385	457	122	3.37
73580-26	Contrast x-ray knee joint	97	116	137	28	.76
73590	X-ray exam lower leg	86	102	120	28	.76
73590-26	X-ray exam lower leg	27	32	39	9	.24
73592	X-ray exam leg, infant	86	102	120	26	.72
73592-26	X-ray exam leg, infant	30	36	42	8	.23
73600	X-ray exam ankle	75	89	105	26	.72
73600-26	X-ray exam ankle	26	31	37	8	.23
73610	X-ray exam ankle	90	107	127	28	.77
73610-26	X-ray exam ankle	32	38	46	9	.24
73615	Contrast x-ray ankle	248	294	348	103	2.85
73615-26	Contrast x-ray ankle	92	109	129	28	.76
73620	X-ray exam foot	69	82	97	26	.72
73620-26	X-ray exam foot	27	32	38	8	.23
73630	X-ray exam foot	84	100	118	28	.77
73630-26	X-ray exam foot	34	41	48	9	.24
73650	X-ray exam heel	74	88	105	25	.70
73650-26	X-ray exam heel	26	31	37	8	.23
73660	X-ray exam toe(s)	67	79	94	22	.60
73660-26	X-ray exam toe(s)	23	28	33	7	.19

• NEW CODE CPT 2002   CPT codes and descriptions only copyright AMA

CPT	SHORT DESCRIPTION	50th	75th	90th	MFS	RVU
73700	CT lower extremity w/o dye	805	963	1148	233	6.44
73700-26	CT lower extremity w/o dye	209	250	299	55	1.52
73701	CT lower extremity w/dye	881	1054	1257	271	7.49
73701-26	CT lower extremity w/dye	220	264	314	59	1.62
73702	CT lower extr w/o&w dye	1057	1264	1507	328	9.07
73702-26	CT lower extr w/o&w dye	232	278	331	62	1.70
73706	CT angio low extr w/o&w dye	699	836	996	365	10.09
73706-26	CT angio low extr w/o&w dye	182	217	259	98	2.72
73718	MRI lower extremity w/o dye	1209	1446	1723	464	12.82
73718-26	MRI lower extremity w/o dye	218	260	310	67	1.86
73719	MRI lower extremity w/dye	1139	1363	1624	557	15.38
73719-26	MRI lower extremity w/dye	216	259	309	81	2.23
73720	MRI lower extr w/o&w dye	1267	1516	1806	989	27.32
73720-26	MRI lower extr w/o&w dye	266	318	379	108	2.98
73721	MRI joint lower extre w/o dye	1235	1478	1761	464	12.82
73721-26	MRI joint lower extre w/o dye	222	266	317	67	1.86
73722	MRI joint lower extr w/dye	1139	1363	1624	557	15.40
73722-26	MRI joint lower extr w/dye	216	259	309	81	2.25
73723	MRI joint low extr w/o&w dye	2048	2450	2920	989	27.31
73723-26	MRI joint low extr w/o&w dye	430	515	613	108	2.97
73725	Mr ang lower ext w or w/o dye	1761	2106	2510	495	13.67
73725-26	Mr ang lower ext w or w/o dye	334	400	477	92	2.54

ABDOMEN

CPT	SHORT DESCRIPTION	50th	75th	90th	MFS	RVU
74000	X-ray exam abdomen	86	100	115	28	.77
74000-26	X-ray exam abdomen	33	38	44	9	.25
74010	X-ray exam abdomen	105	123	141	32	.89

NEW CODE CPT 2002 •

CPT	SHORT DESCRIPTION	50th	75th	90th	MFS	RVU
74010-26	X-ray exam abdomen	43	50	58	12	.32
74020	X-ray exam abdomen	120	140	161	36	.99
74020-26	X-ray exam abdomen	47	55	63	13	.37
74022	X-ray exam series, abdomen	135	157	181	43	1.18
74022-26	X-ray exam series, abdomen	57	66	76	16	.44
74150	CT abdomen w/o dye	729	852	993	264	7.28
74150-26	CT abdomen w/o dye	204	238	278	60	1.66
74160	CT abdomen w/dye	910	1064	1240	310	8.57
74160-26	CT abdomen w/dye	228	266	310	64	1.77
74170	CT abdomen w/o&w dye	1138	1330	1550	375	10.37
74170-26	CT abdomen w/o&w dye	250	293	341	71	1.95
74175	CT angio abdom w/o&w dye	696	814	949	402	11.10
74175-26	CT angio abdom w/o&w dye	181	212	247	98	2.72
74181	MRI abdomen w/o dye	1627	1902	2217	471	13.02
74181-26	MRI abdomen w/o dye	293	342	399	73	2.01
74182	MRI abdomen w/dye	1036	1210	1411	564	15.58
74182-26	MRI abdomen w/dye	197	230	268	87	2.39
74183	MRI abdomen w/o&w dye	1608	1880	2191	997	27.53
74183-26	MRI abdomen w/o&w dye	338	395	460	113	3.13
74185	MRI angio, abdom w or w/o dye	1523	1780	2075	494	13.64
74185-26	MRI angio, abdom w or w/o dye	289	338	394	91	2.51
74190	X-ray exam peritoneum	133	155	181	71	1.97
74190-26	X-ray exam peritoneum	53	62	72	24	.67

GASTROINTESTINAL TRACT

CPT	SHORT DESCRIPTION	50th	75th	90th	MFS	RVU
74210	Contrast x-ray exam throat	194	230	267	61	1.69
74210-26	Contrast x-ray exam throat	72	85	99	18	.51

CPT	SHORT DESCRIPTION	50th	75th	90th	MFS	RVU
74220	Contrast x-ray esophagus	173	205	237	66	1.82
74220-26	Contrast x-ray esophagus	74	88	102	23	.64
74230	Cine/video x-ray throat/eso	207	245	284	74	2.04
74230-26	Cine/video x-ray throat/eso	91	108	125	27	.74
74235	Remove esophagus obstruction	411	487	564	154	4.26
74235-26	Remove esophagus obstruction	189	224	260	60	1.65
74240	X-ray exam upper gi tract	215	254	294	88	2.42
74240-26	X-ray exam upper gi tract	105	124	144	35	.96
74241	X-ray exam upper gi tract	224	265	307	88	2.44
74241-26	X-ray exam upper gi tract	110	130	150	35	.96
74245	X-ray exam upper gi tract	329	390	451	132	3.64
74245-26	X-ray exam upper gi tract	138	164	190	46	1.27
74246	Contrast x-ray upper gi tract	240	284	329	94	2.60
74246-26	Contrast x-ray upper gi tract	108	128	148	35	.96
74247	Contrast x-ray upper gi tract	264	312	362	96	2.65
74247-26	Contrast x-ray upper gi tract	121	144	166	35	.96
74249	Contrast x-ray upper gi tract	372	441	511	139	3.83
74249-26	Contrast x-ray upper gi tract	153	181	209	46	1.27
74250	X-ray exam small bowel	187	221	256	71	1.95
74250-26	X-ray exam small bowel	78	93	108	24	.65
74251	X-ray exam small bowel	252	298	345	82	2.26
74251-26	X-ray exam small bowel	96	113	131	35	.96
74260	X-ray exam small bowel	220	260	301	79	2.17
74260-26	X-ray exam small bowel	92	109	126	25	.69
74270	Contrast x-ray exam colon	243	288	333	97	2.67
74270-26	Contrast x-ray exam colon	107	127	147	35	.96

NEW CODE CPT 2002 •

CPT	SHORT DESCRIPTION	50th	75th	90th	MFS	RVU
74280	Contrast x-ray exam colon	327	387	448	131	3.61
74280-26	Contrast x-ray exam colon	150	178	206	50	1.38
74283	Contrast x-ray exam colon	397	470	545	194	5.37
74283-26	Contrast x-ray exam colon	250	296	343	102	2.82
74290	Contrast x-ray gallbladder	115	136	158	43	1.18
74290-26	Contrast x-ray gallbladder	52	61	71	16	.44
74291	Contrast x-rays gallbladder	79	94	109	25	.69
74291-26	Contrast x-rays gallbladder	38	45	52	10	.28
74300	X-ray bile ducts/pancreas	146	172	200	0	.00
74300-26	X-ray bile ducts/pancreas	64	76	88	18	.51
74301	X-rays at surgery add-on	85	101	117	0	.00
74301-26	X-rays at surgery add-on	37	44	51	10	.29
74305	X-ray bile ducts/pancreas	154	182	211	50	1.37
74305-26	X-ray bile ducts/pancreas	78	93	108	21	.59
74320	Contrast x-ray bile ducts	410	485	562	140	3.88
74320-26	Contrast x-ray bile ducts	107	126	146	27	.75
74327	X-ray bile stone remove	501	593	688	99	2.73
74327-26	X-ray bile stone remove	356	421	488	35	.97
74328	X-ray bile duct endoscopy	402	475	551	149	4.11
74328-26	X-ray bile duct endoscopy	120	143	165	35	.98
74329	X-ray for pancreas endoscopy	423	501	580	149	4.11
74329-26	X-ray for pancreas endoscopy	127	150	174	35	.98
74330	X-ray bile/panc endoscopy	467	553	641	159	4.39
74330-26	X-ray bile/panc endoscopy	140	166	192	46	1.26
74340	X-ray guide for gi tube	354	419	486	122	3.36
74340-26	X-ray guide for gi tube	106	126	146	27	.75

CPT	SHORT DESCRIPTION	50th	75th	90th	MFS	RVU
74350	X-ray guide stomach tube	373	441	512	152	4.19
74350-26	X-ray guide stomach tube	134	159	184	38	1.06
74355	X-ray guide intestinal tube	359	424	492	132	3.66
74355-26	X-ray guide intestinal tube	129	153	177	38	1.05
74360	X-ray guide gi dilation	379	448	519	140	3.88
74360-26	X-ray guide gi dilation	95	112	130	27	.75
74363	X-ray bile duct dilation	375	444	515	264	7.29
74363-26	X-ray bile duct dilation	225	267	309	45	1.23

URINARY TRACT

CPT	SHORT DESCRIPTION	50th	75th	90th	MFS	RVU
74400	Contrast x-ray urinary tract	233	276	329	86	2.37
74400-26	Contrast x-ray urinary tract	84	99	118	25	.68
74410	Contrast x-ray urinary tract	243	287	342	95	2.62
74410-26	Contrast x-ray urinary tract	87	103	123	25	.68
74415	Contrast x-ray urinary tract	300	355	422	101	2.79
74415-26	Contrast x-ray urinary tract	99	117	139	25	.68
74420	Contrast x-ray urinary tract	293	347	413	113	3.12
74420-26	Contrast x-ray urinary tract	62	73	87	18	.51
74425	Contrast x-ray urinary tract	207	245	291	66	1.81
74425-26	Contrast x-ray urinary tract	68	81	96	18	.51
74430	Contrast x-ray bladder	151	178	212	54	1.50
74430-26	Contrast x-ray bladder	60	71	85	16	.45
74440	X-ray male genital tract	157	186	221	60	1.65
74440-26	X-ray male genital tract	57	67	80	19	.53
74445	X-ray exam penis	188	222	265	98	2.70
74445-26	X-ray exam penis	122	145	172	57	1.58
74450	X-ray urethra/bladder	192	227	271	70	1.93

NEW CODE CPT 2002 •

CPT	SHORT DESCRIPTION	50th	75th	90th	MFS	RVU
74450-26	X-ray urethra/bladder	62	73	87	17	.47
74455	X-ray urethra/bladder	213	252	300	74	2.04
74455-26	X-ray urethra/bladder	68	81	96	17	.46
74470	X-ray exam kidney lesion	190	225	268	72	1.99
74470-26	X-ray exam kidney lesion	91	108	129	27	.75
74475	X-ray control, cath insert	503	595	709	174	4.80
74475-26	X-ray control, cath insert	116	137	163	27	.75
74480	X-ray control, cath insert	351	414	493	174	4.80
74480-26	X-ray control, cath insert	126	149	178	27	.75
74485	X-ray guide, gu dilation	423	500	595	141	3.89
74485-26	X-ray guide, gu dilation	110	130	155	28	.76

GYNECOLOGICAL AND OBSTETRICAL

CPT	SHORT DESCRIPTION	50th	75th	90th	MFS	RVU
74710	X-ray measurement pelvis	146	173	206	55	1.53
74710-26	X-ray measurement pelvis	56	66	78	17	.48
74740	X-ray female genital tract	207	245	292	66	1.83
74740-26	X-ray female genital tract	68	81	96	19	.53
74742	X-ray fallopian tube	202	239	285	145	4.00
74742-26	X-ray fallopian tube	57	67	80	31	.87

HEART

CPT	SHORT DESCRIPTION	50th	75th	90th	MFS	RVU
74775	X-ray exam perineum	222	263	313	85	2.34
74775-26	X-ray exam perineum	100	118	141	32	.88
75552	Heart MRI for morph w/o dye	1862	2266	2805	484	13.36
75552-26	Heart MRI for morph w/o dye	335	408	505	81	2.23
75553	Heart MRI for morph w/dye	1300	1582	1958	504	13.93
75553-26	Heart MRI for morph w/dye	247	301	372	101	2.80

CPT	SHORT DESCRIPTION	50th	75th	90th	MFS	RVU
75554	Cardiac MRI/function	1283	1561	1932	497	13.72
75554-26	Cardiac MRI/function	231	281	348	94	2.59
75555	Cardiac MRI/limited study	1273	1549	1918	493	13.62
75555-26	Cardiac MRI/limited study	216	263	326	90	2.49
75556	Cardiac MRI/flow mapping	639	778	963	0	.00
75556-26	Cardiac MRI/flow mapping	115	140	173	0	.00

AORTA AND ARTERIES

CPT	SHORT DESCRIPTION	50th	75th	90th	MFS	RVU
75600	Contrast x-ray exam aorta	680	828	1025	478	13.21
75600-26	Contrast x-ray exam aorta	191	232	287	26	.71
75605	Contrast x-ray exam aorta	741	902	1116	511	14.12
75605-26	Contrast x-ray exam aorta	193	234	290	59	1.62
75625	Contrast x-ray exam aorta	794	966	1196	510	14.10
75625-26	Contrast x-ray exam aorta	199	241	299	58	1.60
75630	X-ray aorta, leg arteries	1455	1770	2191	564	15.58
75630-26	X-ray aorta, leg arteries	698	850	1052	92	2.54
75635	Ct angio abdominal arteries	750	912	1129	428	11.83
75635-26	Ct angio abdominal arteries	195	237	294	125	3.45
75650	Artery x-rays head & neck	974	1186	1468	528	14.59
75650-26	Artery x-rays head & neck	244	296	367	76	2.09
75658	Artery x-rays arm	1502	1827	2262	519	14.35
75658-26	Artery x-rays arm	375	457	565	67	1.85
75660	Artery x-rays head & neck	910	1107	1370	519	14.35
75660-26	Artery x-rays head & neck	227	277	343	67	1.85
75662	Artery x-rays head & neck	961	1170	1448	539	14.88
75662-26	Artery x-rays head & neck	298	363	449	86	2.38
75665	Artery x-rays head & neck	921	1120	1386	519	14.35

NEW CODE CPT 2002 •

CPT	SHORT DESCRIPTION	50th	75th	90th	MFS	RVU
75665-26	Artery x-rays head & neck	230	280	347	67	1.85
75671	Artery x-rays head & neck	715	870	1077	537	14.83
75671-26	Artery x-rays head & neck	286	348	431	84	2.33
75676	Artery x-rays neck	879	1070	1325	519	14.35
75676-26	Artery x-rays neck	220	267	331	67	1.85
75680	Artery x-rays neck	953	1160	1436	537	14.83
75680-26	Artery x-rays neck	276	336	416	84	2.33
75685	Artery x-rays spine	890	1083	1340	519	14.34
75685-26	Artery x-rays spine	222	271	335	67	1.84
75705	Artery x-rays spine	1827	2222	2751	564	15.58
75705-26	Artery x-rays spine	365	444	550	111	3.08
75710	Artery x-rays arm/leg	743	904	1119	511	14.12
75710-26	Artery x-rays arm/leg	186	226	280	59	1.62
75716	Artery x-rays arms/legs	888	1080	1337	519	14.34
75716-26	Artery x-rays arms/legs	222	270	334	67	1.84
75722	Artery x-rays kidney	810	985	1220	511	14.12
75722-26	Artery x-rays kidney	203	246	305	59	1.62
75724	Artery x-rays kidneys	825	1004	1243	530	14.64
75724-26	Artery x-rays kidneys	248	301	373	77	2.14
75726	Artery x-rays abdomen	640	779	964	510	14.09
75726-26	Artery x-rays abdomen	218	265	328	58	1.59
75731	Artery x-rays adrenal gland	1323	1609	1992	510	14.09
75731-26	Artery x-rays adrenal gland	331	402	498	58	1.59
75733	Artery x-rays adrenals	1498	1822	2256	519	14.34
75733-26	Artery x-rays adrenals	419	510	632	67	1.84
75736	Artery x-rays pelvis	822	1000	1238	510	14.10

CPT	SHORT DESCRIPTION	50th	75th	90th	MFS	RVU
75736-26	Artery x-rays pelvis	205	250	309	58	1.60
75741	Artery x-rays lung	676	823	1018	519	14.33
75741-26	Artery x-rays lung	237	288	356	66	1.83
75743	Artery x-rays lungs	896	1091	1350	536	14.81
75743-26	Artery x-rays lungs	287	349	432	84	2.31
75746	Artery x-rays lung	1323	1609	1992	510	14.09
75746-26	Artery x-rays lung	661	805	996	58	1.59
75756	Artery x-rays chest	1327	1615	1999	513	14.16
75756-26	Artery x-rays chest	451	549	680	60	1.66
75774	Artery x-ray each vessel	972	1182	1463	471	13.01
75774-26	Artery x-ray each vessel	194	236	293	18	.51
75790	Visualize a-v shunt	749	911	1128	142	3.93
75790-26	Visualize a-v shunt	300	364	451	93	2.57

VEINS AND LYMPHATICS

CPT	SHORT DESCRIPTION	50th	75th	90th	MFS	RVU
75801	Lymph vessel x-ray arm/leg	545	694	868	236	6.52
75801-26	Lymph vessel x-ray arm/leg	164	208	260	41	1.14
75803	Lymph vessel x-ray,arms/legs	674	859	1073	254	7.01
75803-26	Lymph vessel x-ray,arms/legs	169	215	268	59	1.63
75805	Lymph vessel x-ray trunk	694	884	1105	261	7.20
75805-26	Lymph vessel x-ray trunk	201	256	321	41	1.14
75807	Lymph vessel x-ray trunk	740	943	1178	278	7.69
75807-26	Lymph vessel x-ray trunk	200	255	318	59	1.63
75809	Nonvascular shunt x-ray	266	339	424	52	1.44
75809-26	Nonvascular shunt x-ray	77	98	123	24	.66
75810	Vein x-ray spleen/liver	996	1268	1586	510	14.10
75810-26	Vein x-ray spleen/liver	269	342	428	58	1.60

  NEW CODE CPT 2002 •

CPT	SHORT DESCRIPTION	50th	75th	90th	MFS	RVU
75820	Vein x-ray arm/leg	413	526	657	70	1.93
75820-26	Vein x-ray arm/leg	120	152	191	35	.98
75822	Vein x-ray arms/legs	641	817	1021	107	2.95
75822-26	Vein x-ray arms/legs	180	229	286	54	1.48
75825	Vein x-ray trunk	734	935	1169	510	14.10
75825-26	Vein x-ray trunk	198	252	316	58	1.60
75827	Vein x-ray chest	697	888	1110	510	14.09
75827-26	Vein x-ray chest	188	240	300	58	1.59
75831	Vein x-ray kidney	995	1268	1585	510	14.09
75831-26	Vein x-ray kidney	269	342	428	58	1.59
75833	Vein x-ray kidneys	1220	1553	1942	528	14.59
75833-26	Vein x-ray kidneys	427	544	680	76	2.09
75840	Vein x-ray adrenal gland	561	714	893	511	14.13
75840-26	Vein x-ray adrenal gland	151	193	241	59	1.63
75842	Vein x-ray adrenal glands	1029	1310	1638	528	14.58
75842-26	Vein x-ray adrenal glands	360	459	573	75	2.08
75860	Vein x-ray neck	852	1085	1357	511	14.13
75860-26	Vein x-ray neck	230	293	366	59	1.63
75870	Vein x-ray skull	852	1085	1356	511	14.12
75870-26	Vein x-ray skull	230	293	366	59	1.62
75872	Vein x-ray skull	995	1268	1585	510	14.09
75872-26	Vein x-ray skull	269	342	428	58	1.59
75880	Vein x-ray eye socket	276	351	439	71	1.95
75880-26	Vein x-ray eye socket	58	74	92	36	1.00
75885	Vein x-ray liver	715	911	1139	525	14.50
75885-26	Vein x-ray liver	250	319	398	72	2.00

CPT	SHORT DESCRIPTION	50th	75th	90th	MFS	RVU
75887	Vein x-ray liver	576	734	918	525	14.50
75887-26	Vein x-ray liver	202	257	321	72	2.00
75889	Vein x-ray liver	751	957	1197	510	14.09
75889-26	Vein x-ray liver	203	258	323	58	1.59
75891	Vein x-ray liver	995	1268	1585	510	14.09
75891-26	Vein x-ray liver	269	342	428	58	1.59
75893	Venous sampling by catheter	1868	2379	2974	480	13.25
75893-26	Venous sampling by catheter	1046	1332	1666	27	.75
75894	X-rays transcath therapy	2264	2793	3727	934	25.81
75894-26	X-rays transcath therapy	566	698	932	67	1.84
75896	X-rays transcath therapy	1992	2457	3278	822	22.70
75896-26	X-rays transcath therapy	498	614	819	67	1.85
75898	Follow-up angiography	375	463	618	122	3.37
75898-26	Follow-up angiography	285	352	469	84	2.32
75900	Arterial catheter exchange	1888	2329	3107	779	21.52
75900-26	Arterial catheter exchange	661	815	1088	25	.68
75940	X-ray placement vein filter	1115	1376	1836	480	13.26
75940-26	X-ray placement vein filter	279	344	459	28	.76
75945	Intravascular us	368	454	606	185	5.11
75945-26	Intravascular us	63	77	103	21	.58
75946	Intravascular us add-on	206	254	339	104	2.86
75946-26	Intravascular us add-on	60	74	98	21	.57
75952	Endovasc repair abdom aorta	430	531	708	0	.00
75953	Abdom aneurysm endovas rpr	177	218	291	0	.00
75960	Transcatheter intro, stent	1399	1726	2303	577	15.95
75960-26	Transcatheter intro, stent	448	552	737	42	1.16

NEW CODE CPT 2002 •

CPT	SHORT DESCRIPTION	50th	75th	90th	MFS	RVU
75961	Retrieve broken catheter	929	1146	1529	592	16.35
75961-26	Retrieve broken catheter	678	836	1116	214	5.92
75962	Repair arterial blockage	1440	1776	2370	594	16.41
75962-26	Repair arterial blockage	576	710	948	28	.77
75964	Repair artery blockage, each	439	542	723	320	8.84
75964-26	Repair artery blockage, each	92	114	152	18	.51
75966	Repair arterial blockage	1536	1895	2529	634	17.51
75966-26	Repair arterial blockage	615	758	1011	68	1.87
75968	Repair artery blockage, each	776	957	1277	320	8.84
75968-26	Repair artery blockage, each	194	239	319	18	.51
75970	Vascular biopsy	625	771	1028	457	12.63
75970-26	Vascular biopsy	150	185	247	42	1.17
75978	Repair venous blockage	1720	2122	2831	593	16.39
75978-26	Repair venous blockage	637	785	1048	27	.75
75980	Contrast x-ray exam bile duct	631	779	1039	267	7.38
75980-26	Contrast x-ray exam bile duct	253	312	416	72	2.00
75982	Contrast x-ray exam bile duct	499	616	822	292	8.06
75982-26	Contrast x-ray exam bile duct	260	320	427	72	2.00
75984	X-ray control catheter change	320	395	527	106	2.94
75984-26	X-ray control catheter change	131	162	216	36	1.00
75989	Abscess drain under x-ray	292	360	481	173	4.79
75989-26	Abscess drain under x-ray	207	256	341	60	1.66
75992	Atherectomy x-ray exam	1869	2305	3075	594	16.40
75992-26	Atherectomy x-ray exam	112	138	184	28	.76
75993	Atherectomy x-ray exam	744	918	1225	320	8.84
75993-26	Atherectomy x-ray exam	45	55	73	18	.51

CPT	SHORT DESCRIPTION	50th	75th	90th	MFS	RVU
75994	Atherectomy x-ray exam	1241	1531	2042	634	17.51
75994-26	Atherectomy x-ray exam	136	168	225	68	1.87
75995	Atherectomy x-ray exam	1985	2449	3268	633	17.48
75995-26	Atherectomy x-ray exam	218	269	359	67	1.84
75996	Atherectomy x-ray exam	1104	1361	1816	319	8.82
75996-26	Atherectomy x-ray exam	66	82	109	18	.49
76000	Fluoroscope examination	350	439	548	56	1.55
76000-26	Fluoroscope examination	70	88	110	9	.25
76001	Fluoroscope exam, extensive	385	483	603	129	3.55
76001-26	Fluoroscope exam, extensive	127	160	199	34	.94
76003	Needle localization by x-ray	247	309	386	75	2.06
76003-26	Needle localization by x-ray	111	139	174	28	.76
76005	Fluoroguide for spine inject	238	298	372	76	2.10
76005-26	Fluoroguide for spine inject	121	152	190	29	.80
76006	X-ray stress view	66	83	104	24	.65
76010	X-ray nose to rectum	94	118	148	28	.77
76010-26	X-ray nose to rectum	38	47	59	9	.25
76012	Percut vertebroplasty fluor	221	277	346	0	.00
76013	Percut vertebroplasty, ct	182	228	284	0	.00
76020	X-rays for bone age	104	131	163	29	.79
76020-26	X-rays for bone age	32	41	51	10	.27
76040	X-rays bone evaluation	143	180	225	43	1.18
76040-26	X-rays bone evaluation	56	70	88	14	.40
76061	X-rays bone survey	210	263	328	59	1.63
76061-26	X-rays bone survey	98	124	154	23	.63
76062	X-rays bone survey	263	329	411	79	2.19

NEW CODE CPT 2002 •

CPT	SHORT DESCRIPTION	50th	75th	90th	MFS	RVU
76062-26	X-rays bone survey	116	145	181	27	.75
76065	X-rays bone evaluation	137	172	214	62	1.70
76065-26	X-rays bone evaluation	52	65	81	35	.96
76066	Joint survey, single view	155	194	242	56	1.55
76066-26	Joint survey, single view	54	68	85	16	.44
76070	CT scan bone density study	445	558	697	119	3.29
76070-26	CT scan bone density study	58	73	91	13	.36
76075	US exam abdom, limited	276	347	433	127	3.50
76075-26	US exam abdom, limited	36	45	56	15	.42
76076	Dual energy x-ray study	125	157	196	39	1.07
76076-26	Dual energy x-ray study	21	27	33	11	.31
76078	Radiographic absorptiometry	78	98	123	38	1.05
76078-26	Radiographic absorptiometry	26	32	41	10	.29
76080	X-ray exam fistula	203	254	317	65	1.80
76080-26	X-ray exam fistula	101	127	159	27	.75
• 76085	Computer mammogram add-on	42	53	67	14	.39
• 76085-26	Computer mammogram add-on	10	12	15	3	.09
76086	X-ray mammary duct	356	447	558	113	3.12
76086-26	X-ray mammary duct	71	89	112	18	.51
76088	X-ray mammary ducts	288	361	451	155	4.27
76088-26	X-ray mammary ducts	55	69	86	23	.63
76090	Mammogram one breast	125	156	195	73	2.03
76090-26	Mammogram one breast	39	48	60	35	.98
76091	Mammogram both breasts	178	224	279	90	2.50
76091-26	Mammogram both breasts	68	85	106	43	1.20
76092	Mammogram screening	131	164	205	81	2.23

CPT	SHORT DESCRIPTION	50th	75th	90th	MFS	RVU
76092-26	Mammogram screening	41	51	64	35	.98
76093	Magnetic image breast	1622	2035	2540	716	19.77
76093-26	Magnetic image breast	308	387	483	82	2.27
76094	Magnetic image both breasts	1783	2238	2793	942	26.01
76094-26	Magnetic image both breasts	375	470	586	82	2.27
76095	Stereotactic breast biopsy	808	1014	1265	338	9.35
76095-26	Stereotactic breast biopsy	275	345	430	81	2.24
76096	X-ray needle wire, breast	395	496	619	76	2.09
76096-26	X-ray needle wire, breast	131	164	204	29	.79
76098	X-ray exam breast specimen	104	131	163	23	.64
76098-26	X-ray exam breast specimen	42	52	65	8	.23
76100	X-ray exam body section	210	263	329	74	2.05
76100-26	X-ray exam body section	103	129	161	29	.81
76101	Complex body section x-ray	235	295	368	81	2.23
76101-26	Complex body section x-ray	108	136	170	29	.81
76102	Complex body section x-rays	321	403	503	92	2.54
76102-26	Complex body section x-rays	132	165	206	29	.81
76120	Cine/video x-rays	180	226	281	58	1.59
76120-26	Cine/video x-rays	75	95	118	20	.54
76125	Cine/ video x-rays add-on	132	166	207	42	1.16
76125-26	Cine/ video x-rays add-on	50	63	79	14	.38
76140	X-ray consultation	60	75	93	0	.00
76150	X-ray exam, dry process	76	95	118	15	.41
76350	Special x-ray contrast study	45	57	71	0	.00
76355	CAT scan for localization	1194	1499	1870	358	9.90
76355-26	CAT scan for localization	251	315	393	62	1.71

NEW CODE CPT 2002 •

CPT	SHORT DESCRIPTION	50th	75th	90th	MFS	RVU
76360	CAT scan for needle biopsy	1076	1350	1684	355	9.80
76360-26	CAT scan for needle biopsy	226	283	354	58	1.61
• **76362**	CAT scan for tissue ablation	1587	1992	2486	529	14.62
• **76362-26**	CAT scan for tissue ablation	603	757	945	202	5.57
76370	CAT scan for therapy guide	540	678	846	149	4.12
76370-26	CAT scan for therapy guide	178	224	279	43	1.19
76375	3D/holograph reconstr add-on	353	443	553	135	3.74
76375-26	3D/holograph reconstr add-on	28	35	44	8	.23
76380	CAT scan follow-up study	391	490	612	175	4.83
76380-26	CAT scan follow-up study	113	142	177	49	1.36
76390	Mr spectroscopy	1049	1316	1642	474	13.09
76390-26	Mr spectroscopy	168	211	263	71	1.96
76393	Mr guidance for needle place	1043	1309	1633	477	13.19
76393-26	Mr guidance for needle place	188	236	294	76	2.09
• **76394**	MRI for tissue ablation	1934	2426	3028	645	17.81
• **76394-26**	MRI for tissue ablation	638	801	999	213	5.88
76400	Magnetic image bone marrow	1451	1820	2272	484	13.36
76400-26	Magnetic image bone marrow	261	328	409	81	2.23
• **76490**	Us for tissue ablation	488	612	764	163	4.49
• **76490-26**	Us for tissue ablation	307	386	481	102	2.81
76499	Radiographic procedure	0	0	0	0	.00

CPT	SHORT DESCRIPTION	50th	75th	90th	MFS	RVU

NEW CODE CPT 2002 •

DIAGNOSTIC ULTRASOUND

HEAD AND NECK

CPT	SHORT DESCRIPTION	50th	75th	90th	MFS	RVU
76506	Echo exam head	254	311	391	85	2.34
76506-26	Echo exam head	125	152	192	33	.92
76511	Echo exam eye	313	383	483	123	3.39
76511-26	Echo exam eye	150	184	232	51	1.41
76512	Echo exam eye	266	326	410	117	3.24
76512-26	Echo exam eye	123	150	189	35	.98
76513	Echo exam eye, water bath	299	365	460	132	3.65
76513-26	Echo exam eye, water bath	137	168	212	36	.99
76516	Echo exam eye	220	269	338	96	2.65
76516-26	Echo exam eye	103	126	159	29	.81
76519	Echo exam eye	199	243	306	91	2.52
76519-26	Echo exam eye	93	114	144	29	.81
76529	Echo exam eye	242	296	373	121	3.35
76529-26	Echo exam eye	114	139	175	31	.85
76536	Us exam head and neck	232	284	358	80	2.20
76536-26	Us exam head and neck	107	131	164	28	.78

CHEST

CPT	SHORT DESCRIPTION	50th	75th	90th	MFS	RVU
76604	Us exam chest, b-scan	246	289	342	75	2.06
76604-26	Us exam chest, b-scan	106	124	147	28	.76
76645	Us exam breast(s)	188	220	261	66	1.81
76645-26	Us exam breast(s)	94	110	130	28	.76

ABDOMEN AND PERITONEUM

CPT	SHORT DESCRIPTION	50th	75th	90th	MFS	RVU
76700	Us exam abdom, complete	306	359	425	112	3.09

CPT	SHORT DESCRIPTION	50th	75th	90th	MFS	RVU
76700-26	Us exam abdom, complete	144	169	200	41	1.13
76705	Us exam abdom, limited	223	261	310	81	2.25
76705-26	Us exam abdom, limited	100	118	140	30	.83
76770	Us exam abdo back wall, comp	293	344	408	108	2.99
76770-26	Us exam abdo back wall, comp	129	151	179	37	1.03
76775	Us exam abdo back wall, lim	219	256	304	81	2.23
76775-26	Us exam abdo back wall, lim	98	115	137	29	.81
76778	Us exam kidney transplant	279	326	387	108	2.99
76778-26	Us exam kidney transplant	134	157	186	37	1.03

SPINAL CANAL

CPT	SHORT DESCRIPTION	50th	75th	90th	MFS	RVU
76800	Us exam spinal canal	355	430	517	108	2.97
76800-26	Us exam spinal canal	163	198	238	56	1.55

PELVIS

CPT	SHORT DESCRIPTION	50th	75th	90th	MFS	RVU
76805	Us exam pg uterus, compl	289	350	421	126	3.48
76805-26	Us exam pg uterus, compl	139	168	202	50	1.39
76810	Us exam pg uterus, mult	476	576	693	252	6.96
76810-26	Us exam pg uterus, mult	195	236	284	101	2.79
76815	Us exam pg uterus limit	204	247	297	85	2.34
76815-26	Us exam pg uterus limit	92	111	134	33	.92
76816	Us exam pg uterus repeat	191	232	279	70	1.92
76816-26	Us exam pg uterus repeat	97	118	142	29	.81
76818	Fetal biophy profile w/nst	289	350	421	113	3.11
76818-26	Fetal biophy profile w/nst	139	168	202	54	1.50
76819	Fetal biophys profile w/o nst	269	326	392	98	2.70
76819-26	Fetal biophys profile w/o nst	129	156	188	39	1.09

  NEW CODE CPT 2002 •

CPT	SHORT DESCRIPTION	50th	75th	90th	MFS	RVU
76825	Echo exam fetal heart	382	463	557	156	4.32
76825-26	Echo exam fetal heart	164	199	239	85	2.36
76826	Echo exam fetal heart	196	237	285	68	1.87
76826-26	Echo exam fetal heart	92	111	134	42	1.16
76827	Echo exam fetal heart	255	309	372	92	2.55
76827-26	Echo exam fetal heart	112	136	163	30	.82
76828	Echo exam fetal heart	220	266	320	70	1.94
76828-26	Echo exam fetal heart	103	125	150	29	.81
76830	Us exam transvaginal	267	323	389	90	2.48
76830-26	Us exam transvaginal	115	139	167	35	.96
76831	Echo exam uterus	281	340	409	92	2.53
76831-26	Echo exam uterus	121	146	176	37	1.01
76856	Us exam pelvic, complete	267	324	389	90	2.48
76856-26	Us exam pelvic, complete	118	142	171	35	.96
76857	Us exam pelvic, limited	158	192	231	57	1.58
76857-26	Us exam pelvic, limited	65	79	95	19	.53

GENITALIA

CPT	SHORT DESCRIPTION	50th	75th	90th	MFS	RVU
76870	Us exam scrotum	261	315	377	87	2.41
76870-26	Us exam scrotum	115	139	166	32	.89
76872	Echo exam transrectal	303	365	436	90	2.49
76872-26	Echo exam transrectal	148	179	214	35	.97
76873	Echograp trans r, pros study	417	503	601	155	4.29
76873-26	Echograp trans r, pros study	221	266	318	79	2.17
76880	Us exam extremity	235	284	339	81	2.25
76880-26	Us exam extremity	104	125	149	30	.83
76885	Us exam infant hips, dynamic	276	333	398	92	2.55

CPT	SHORT DESCRIPTION	50th	75th	90th	MFS	RVU
76885-26	Us exam infant hips, dynamic	121	147	175	37	1.03
76886	Us exam infant hips, static	262	317	378	83	2.29
76886-26	Us exam infant hips, static	115	139	166	31	.87

ULTRASONIC GUIDANCE PROCEDURES

CPT	SHORT DESCRIPTION	50th	75th	90th	MFS	RVU
76930	Echo guide cardiocentesis	206	262	342	90	2.48
76930-26	Echo guide cardiocentesis	95	120	157	35	.96
76932	Echo guide for heart biopsy	259	329	430	90	2.48
76932-26	Echo guide for heart biopsy	124	158	207	35	.96
76936	Echo guide for artery repair	502	639	835	328	9.06
76936-26	Echo guide for artery repair	291	370	484	101	2.80
76941	Echo guide for transfuse	202	258	337	125	3.45
76941-26	Echo guide for transfuse	97	124	162	70	1.93
76942	Echo guide for biopsy	275	350	457	89	2.46
76942-26	Echo guide for biopsy	129	164	215	34	.94
76945	Echo guide villus sampling	284	361	472	89	2.46
76945-26	Echo guide villus sampling	128	162	212	34	.94
76946	Echo guide for amniocentesis	226	288	376	75	2.06
76946-26	Echo guide for amniocentesis	81	104	135	20	.54
76948	Echo guide ova aspiration	340	432	565	74	2.05
76948-26	Echo guide ova aspiration	109	138	181	19	.53
76950	Echo guidance radiotherapy	222	283	369	77	2.12
76950-26	Echo guidance radiotherapy	102	130	170	30	.82
76965	Echo guidance radiotherapy	686	873	1141	268	7.40
76965-26	Echo guidance radiotherapy	329	419	548	68	1.87
76970	Ultrasound exam follow-up	133	169	221	58	1.61
76970-26	Ultrasound exam follow-up	57	73	95	20	.56

NEW CODE CPT 2002 •

CPT	SHORT DESCRIPTION	50th	75th	90th	MFS	RVU
76975	Gi endoscopic ultrasound	440	560	732	96	2.65
76975-26	Gi endoscopic ultrasound	198	252	329	41	1.13
76977	Us bone density measure	75	95	125	33	.90
76977-26	Us bone density measure	56	71	93	3	.08
76986	Ultrasound guide intraoper	506	644	842	156	4.30
76986-26	Ultrasound guide intraoper	233	296	387	61	1.69
76999	Echo examination procedure	0	0	0	0	.00

CPT	SHORT DESCRIPTION	50th	75th	90th	MFS	RVU

NEW CODE CPT 2002 •

CPT	SHORT DESCRIPTION	50th	75th	90th	MFS	RVU

RADIATION ONCOLOGY

PLANNING

CPT	SHORT DESCRIPTION	50th	75th	90th	MFS	RVU
77261	Radiation therapy planning	355	468	567	73	2.01
77262	Radiation therapy planning	509	671	814	109	3.02
77263	Radiation therapy planning	703	927	1124	163	4.50

SIMULATION

CPT	SHORT DESCRIPTION	50th	75th	90th	MFS	RVU
77280	Set radiation therapy field	566	746	905	160	4.43
77280-26	Set radiation therapy field	170	224	271	35	.98
77285	Set radiation therapy field	876	1154	1400	254	7.01
77285-26	Set radiation therapy field	263	346	420	53	1.47
77290	Set radiation therapy field	989	1304	1581	313	8.65
77290-26	Set radiation therapy field	346	456	553	79	2.18
77295	Set radiation therapy field	3412	4495	5452	1237	34.16
77295-26	Set radiation therapy field	716	944	1145	232	6.40
77299	Radiation therapy planning	0	0	0	0	.00

MEDICAL RADIATION PHYSICS, DOSIMETRY TREATMENT DEVICES, AND SPECIAL SERVICES

CPT	SHORT DESCRIPTION	50th	75th	90th	MFS	RVU
77300	Radiation therapy dose plan	274	330	423	80	2.21
77300-26	Radiation therapy dose plan	137	165	212	31	.87
• 77301	Radiotherapy dos plan, imrt	4485	5393	6919	1416	39.13
• 77301-26	Radiotherapy dos plan, imrt	1301	1564	2007	412	11.37
77305	Radiation therapy dose plan	342	412	528	102	2.83
77305-26	Radiation therapy dose plan	154	185	238	35	.98
77310	Radiation therapy dose plan	433	520	668	137	3.79
77310-26	Radiation therapy dose plan	216	260	334	53	1.47

CPT	SHORT DESCRIPTION	50th	75th	90th	MFS	RVU
77315	Radiation therapy dose plan	545	656	842	175	4.83
77315-26	Radiation therapy dose plan	305	367	471	79	2.18
77321	Radiation therapy port plan	627	754	967	193	5.34
77321-26	Radiation therapy port plan	213	256	329	48	1.33
77326	Radiation therapy dose plan	383	461	591	132	3.66
77326-26	Radiation therapy dose plan	172	207	266	47	1.31
77327	Radiation therapy dose plan	535	644	826	195	5.40
77327-26	Radiation therapy dose plan	268	322	413	71	1.95
77328	Radiation therapy dose plan	890	1070	1373	284	7.85
77328-26	Radiation therapy dose plan	427	513	659	106	2.93
77331	Special radiation dosimetry	204	245	315	62	1.72
77331-26	Special radiation dosimetry	161	194	249	44	1.22
77332	Radiation treat aid(s)	271	325	417	76	2.09
77332-26	Radiation treat aid(s)	130	156	200	27	.75
77333	Radiation treat aid(s)	369	444	569	111	3.07
77333-26	Radiation treat aid(s)	181	217	279	43	1.18
77334	Radiation treat aid(s)	575	692	887	180	4.97
77334-26	Radiation treat aid(s)	265	318	408	63	1.74
77336	Radiation physics consult	285	343	440	107	2.96
77370	Radiation physics consult	371	446	573	125	3.46
77399	External radiation dosimetry	0	0	0	0	.00

RADIATION TREATMENT DELIVERY

CPT	SHORT DESCRIPTION	50th	75th	90th	MFS	RVU
77401	Radiation treat delivery	97	126	141	64	1.77
77402	Radiation treat delivery	183	238	267	64	1.77
77403	Radiation treat delivery	198	257	288	64	1.77
77404	Radiation treat delivery	194	252	283	64	1.77

  NEW CODE CPT 2002 •

CPT	SHORT DESCRIPTION	50th	75th	90th	MFS	RVU
77406	Radiation treat delivery	126	164	184	64	1.77
77407	Radiation treat delivery	169	219	246	75	2.08
77408	Radiation treat delivery	210	272	305	75	2.08
77409	Radiation treat delivery	205	267	299	75	2.08
77411	Radiation treat delivery	126	163	183	75	2.08
77412	Radiation treat delivery	278	361	405	84	2.32
77413	Radiation treat delivery	276	359	402	84	2.32
77414	Radiation treat delivery	297	386	432	84	2.32
77416	Radiation treat delivery	259	336	377	84	2.32
77417	Radiology port film(s)	84	109	122	21	.59
• 77418	Radiation tx delivery, imrt	1984	2576	2887	586	16.18

RADIATION TREATMENT MANAGEMENT

CPT	SHORT DESCRIPTION	50th	75th	90th	MFS	RVU
77427	Radiation tx management, x5	677	863	1069	168	4.64
77431	Radiation therapy management	256	327	404	94	2.61
77432	Stereotactic radiation trmt	1982	2529	3131	417	11.51
77470	Special radiation treat	1547	1973	2443	507	14.01
77470-26	Special radiation treat	217	276	342	106	2.93
77499	Radiation therapy management	0	0	0	0	.00

PROTON BEAM TREATMENT DELIVERY

CPT	SHORT DESCRIPTION	50th	75th	90th	MFS	RVU
77520	Proton trmt, simple w/o comp	0	0	0	0	.00
77522	Proton trmt, simple w/comp	0	0	0	0	.00
77523	Proton trmt, intermediate	0	0	0	0	.00
77525	Proton treat, complex	0	0	0	0	.00

HYPERTHERMIA

CPT	SHORT DESCRIPTION	50th	75th	90th	MFS	RVU
77600	Hyperthermia treat	741	946	1171	189	5.21

CPT	SHORT DESCRIPTION	50th	75th	90th	MFS	RVU
77600-26	Hyperthermia treat	371	473	585	79	2.19
77605	Hyperthermia treat	999	1274	1577	254	7.02
77605-26	Hyperthermia treat	499	637	789	108	2.98
77610	Hyperthermia treat	571	729	902	188	5.20
77610-26	Hyperthermia treat	286	364	451	79	2.18
77615	Hyperthermia treat	763	973	1204	252	6.96
77615-26	Hyperthermia treat	381	486	602	106	2.92

CLINICAL INTRACAVITARY HYPERTHERMIA

CPT	SHORT DESCRIPTION	50th	75th	90th	MFS	RVU
77620	Hyperthermia treat	454	579	717	189	5.22
77620-26	Hyperthermia treat	227	290	358	80	2.20

CLINICAL BRACHYTHERAPY

CPT	SHORT DESCRIPTION	50th	75th	90th	MFS	RVU
77750	Infuse radioactive materials	837	1113	1529	296	8.18
77750-26	Infuse radioactive materials	728	968	1330	248	6.85
77761	Apply intrcav radiat simple	734	976	1340	275	7.60
77761-26	Apply intrcav radiat simple	573	761	1046	185	5.10
77762	Apply intrcav radiat interm	1095	1455	1999	417	11.52
77762-26	Apply intrcav radiat interm	843	1121	1540	287	7.93
77763	Apply intrcav radiat compl	1345	1787	2456	597	16.48
77763-26	Apply intrcav radiat compl	1076	1430	1964	435	12.03
77776	Apply interstit radiat simple	963	1280	1759	316	8.73
77776-26	Apply interstit radiat simple	780	1037	1424	237	6.55
77777	Apply interstit radiat inter	1514	2013	2765	519	14.35
77777-26	Apply interstit radiat inter	1151	1530	2102	367	10.15
77778	Apply iterstit radiat compl	2557	3398	4668	752	20.78
77778-26	Apply iterstit radiat compl	2071	2752	3782	568	15.68

NEW CODE CPT 2002 •

CPT	SHORT DESCRIPTION	50th	75th	90th	MFS	RVU
77781	High intensity brachytherapy	1590	2113	2903	814	22.49
77781-26	High intensity brachytherapy	159	211	290	84	2.33
77782	High intensity brachytherapy	1669	2218	3048	856	23.65
77782-26	High intensity brachytherapy	250	333	457	126	3.49
77783	High intensity brachytherapy	3145	4179	5742	919	25.38
77783-26	High intensity brachytherapy	629	836	1148	189	5.22
77784	High intensity brachytherapy	3750	4983	6847	1014	28.01
77784-26	High intensity brachytherapy	1050	1395	1917	284	7.85
77789	Apply surface radiation	164	218	300	73	2.01
77789-26	Apply surface radiation	135	179	246	56	1.56
77790	Radiation handling	250	332	456	71	1.97
77790-26	Radiation handling	205	272	374	53	1.47
77799	Radium/radioisotope therapy	0	0	0	0	.00

CPT	SHORT DESCRIPTION	50th	75th	90th	MFS	RVU

NEW CODE CPT 2002 •

CPT	SHORT DESCRIPTION	50th	75th	90th	MFS	RVU

NUCLEAR MEDICINE

DIAGNOSTIC NUCLEAR MEDICINE

CPT	SHORT DESCRIPTION	50th	75th	90th	MFS	RVU
78000	Thyroid, single uptake	139	168	218	45	1.24
78000-26	Thyroid, single uptake	35	42	54	10	.27
78001	Thyroid, multiple uptakes	234	282	366	60	1.66
78001-26	Thyroid, multiple uptakes	65	79	102	13	.36
78003	Thyroid suppress/stimul	176	213	276	52	1.43
78003-26	Thyroid suppress/stimul	69	83	107	17	.46
78006	Thyroid imaging with uptake	327	395	512	111	3.06
78006-26	Thyroid imaging with uptake	98	118	154	25	.69
78007	Thyroid image, mult uptakes	385	465	602	118	3.26
78007-26	Thyroid image, mult uptakes	108	130	169	25	.70
78010	Thyroid imaging	280	338	438	86	2.37
78010-26	Thyroid imaging	81	98	127	20	.55
78011	Thyroid imaging with flow	344	415	538	110	3.03
78011-26	Thyroid imaging with flow	93	112	145	23	.63
78015	Thyroid met imaging	434	525	680	127	3.50
78015-26	Thyroid met imaging	148	178	231	34	.94
78016	Thyroid met imaging/studies	485	586	760	167	4.62
78016-26	Thyroid met imaging/studies	155	187	243	42	1.16
78018	Thyroid met imaging, body	666	804	1043	239	6.60
78018-26	Thyroid met imaging, body	180	217	282	44	1.21
78020	Thyroid met uptake	152	184	238	80	2.21
78070	Parathyroid nuclear imaging	247	299	387	108	2.97
78070-26	Parathyroid nuclear imaging	119	143	186	42	1.15

CPT	SHORT DESCRIPTION	50th	75th	90th	MFS	RVU
78075	Adrenal nuclear imaging	329	397	515	233	6.45
78075-26	Adrenal nuclear imaging	72	87	113	38	1.06
78099	Endocrine nuclear procedure	0	0	0	0	.00
78102	Bone marrow imaging, ltd	315	410	504	102	2.82
78102-26	Bone marrow imaging, ltd	113	147	181	28	.78
78103	Bone marrow imaging, mult	515	670	824	152	4.20
78103-26	Bone marrow imaging, mult	165	214	264	38	1.05
78104	Bone marrow imaging, body	578	751	924	187	5.17
78104-26	Bone marrow imaging, body	168	218	268	41	1.12
78110	Plasma volume, single	184	240	295	44	1.22
78110-26	Plasma volume, single	48	62	77	10	.27
78111	Plasma volume, multiple	267	347	427	104	2.87
78111-26	Plasma volume, multiple	40	52	64	11	.31
78120	Red cell mass, single	213	277	340	75	2.06
78120-26	Red cell mass, single	45	58	71	12	.33
78121	Red cell mass, multiple	343	446	549	121	3.33
78121-26	Red cell mass, multiple	55	71	88	16	.45
78122	Blood volume	537	698	858	189	5.21
78122-26	Blood volume	86	112	137	23	.64
78130	Red cell survival study	413	537	661	134	3.69
78130-26	Red cell survival study	120	156	192	31	.86
78135	Red cell survival kinetics	486	632	776	208	5.74
78135-26	Red cell survival kinetics	102	133	163	33	.90
78140	Red cell sequestration	404	525	645	172	4.76
78140-26	Red cell sequestration	101	131	161	31	.85
78160	Plasma iron turnover	290	377	463	149	4.12

 NEW CODE CPT 2002 •

CPT	SHORT DESCRIPTION	50th	75th	90th	MFS	RVU
78160-26	Plasma iron turnover	41	53	65	17	.48
78162	Iron absorption exam	427	555	683	138	3.82
78162-26	Iron absorption exam	90	117	143	23	.64
78170	Red cell iron utilization	447	582	715	212	5.87
78170-26	Red cell iron utilization	72	93	114	22	.60
78172	Total body iron estimation	152	198	244	0	.00
78172-26	Total body iron estimation	59	77	95	27	.75
78185	Spleen imaging	327	425	523	106	2.92
78185-26	Spleen imaging	92	119	146	21	.57
78190	Platelet survival, kinetics	551	717	881	262	7.23
78190-26	Platelet survival, kinetics	105	136	167	56	1.55
78191	Platelet survival	620	807	992	295	8.14
78191-26	Platelet survival	87	113	139	31	.86
78195	Lymph system imaging	638	830	1020	208	5.74
78195-26	Lymph system imaging	160	207	255	61	1.69
78199	Blood/lymph nuclear exam	0	0	0	0	.00
78201	Liver imaging	292	348	413	108	2.97
78201-26	Liver imaging	79	94	112	22	.62
78202	Liver imaging with flow	345	410	488	130	3.58
78202-26	Liver imaging with flow	93	111	132	26	.72
78205	Liver imaging (3d)	774	920	1094	249	6.87
78205-26	Liver imaging (3d)	147	175	208	36	1.00
78206	Liver image (3d) w/flow	694	826	982	255	7.05
78206-26	Liver image (3d) w/flow	160	190	226	49	1.35
78215	Liver and spleen imaging	471	560	666	130	3.60
78215-26	Liver and spleen imaging	118	140	167	25	.69

CPT	SHORT DESCRIPTION	50th	75th	90th	MFS	RVU
78216	Liver & spleen image/flow	542	645	767	154	4.26
78216-26	Liver & spleen image/flow	136	161	192	29	.80
78220	Liver function study	535	636	756	159	4.39
78220-26	Liver function study	118	140	166	25	.69
78223	Hepatobiliary imaging	456	542	644	174	4.82
78223-26	Hepatobiliary imaging	146	173	206	43	1.18
78230	Salivary gland imaging	271	322	383	102	2.81
78230-26	Salivary gland imaging	76	90	107	23	.63
78231	Serial salivary imaging	275	327	388	141	3.89
78231-26	Serial salivary imaging	66	78	93	27	.74
78232	Salivary gland function exam	296	352	418	151	4.17
78232-26	Salivary gland function exam	62	74	88	24	.66
78258	Esophageal motility study	384	457	543	141	3.90
78258-26	Esophageal motility study	131	155	185	38	1.04
78261	Gastric mucosa imaging	357	425	505	183	5.05
78261-26	Gastric mucosa imaging	89	106	126	35	.98
78262	Gastroesophageal reflux exam	516	613	729	188	5.18
78262-26	Gastroesophageal reflux exam	129	153	182	35	.96
78264	Gastric emptying study	511	608	723	188	5.19
78264-26	Gastric emptying study	138	164	195	39	1.09
78267	Breath test attain/anal c-14	52	62	74	0	.00
78268	Breath test analysis, c-14	214	254	302	0	.00
78270	Vit b-12 absorption exam	186	221	263	66	1.83
78270-26	Vit b-12 absorption exam	41	49	58	10	.28
78271	Vit b-12 absorp exam, if	186	221	263	70	1.92
78271-26	Vit b-12 absorp exam, if	43	51	61	10	.28

NEW CODE CPT 2002 •

CPT	SHORT DESCRIPTION	50th	75th	90th	MFS	RVU
78272	Vit b-12 absorp, combined	226	269	319	97	2.69
78272-26	Vit b-12 absorp, combined	52	62	73	14	.38
78278	Acute gi blood loss imaging	592	703	836	225	6.22
78278-26	Acute gi blood loss imaging	166	197	234	50	1.38
78282	Gi protein loss exam	297	353	420	0	.00
78282-26	Gi protein loss exam	119	141	168	19	.53
78290	Meckel's divert exam	403	479	570	144	3.97
78290-26	Meckel's divert exam	125	149	177	34	.95
78291	Leveen/shunt patency exam	302	359	427	155	4.28
78291-26	Leveen/shunt patency exam	109	129	154	45	1.24
78299	Gi nuclear procedure	0	0	0	0	.00
78300	Bone imaging limited area	358	423	495	121	3.35
78300-26	Bone imaging limited area	107	127	149	31	.87
78305	Bone imaging multiple areas	460	543	637	174	4.80
78305-26	Bone imaging multiple areas	133	158	185	42	1.16
78306	Bone imaging whole body	597	705	825	197	5.45
78306-26	Bone imaging whole body	155	183	215	44	1.21
78315	Bone imaging 3 phase	670	792	927	224	6.18
78315-26	Bone imaging 3 phase	181	214	250	52	1.43
78320	Bone imaging (3d)	759	896	1050	266	7.34
78320-26	Bone imaging (3d)	190	224	262	53	1.47
78350	Bone mineral single photon	187	221	258	39	1.07
78350-26	Bone mineral single photon	65	77	90	11	.31
78351	Bone mineral dual photon	232	274	321	71	1.95
78351-26	Bone mineral dual photon	51	60	71	0	.00
78399	Musculoskeletal nuclear exam	0	0	0	0	.00

• NEW CODE CPT 2002   CPT codes and descriptions only copyright AMA

CPT	SHORT DESCRIPTION	50th	75th	90th	MFS	RVU
78414	Non-imaging heart function	384	492	611	0	.00
78414-26	Non-imaging heart function	77	98	122	23	.63
78428	Cardiac shunt imaging	311	398	494	122	3.38
78428-26	Cardiac shunt imaging	127	163	203	41	1.13
78445	Vascular flow imaging	326	418	519	92	2.54
78445-26	Vascular flow imaging	114	146	182	25	.69
78455	Venous thrombosis study	388	497	617	180	4.97
78455-26	Venous thrombosis study	109	139	173	37	1.02
78456	Acute venous thrombus image	424	543	674	197	5.43
78456-26	Acute venous thrombus image	169	217	269	51	1.41
78457	Venous thrombosis imaging	290	371	461	135	3.73
78457-26	Venous thrombosis imaging	110	141	175	39	1.08
78458	Ven thrombosis images bilat	484	620	770	191	5.27
78458-26	Ven thrombosis images bilat	145	186	231	46	1.28
78459	Heart muscle imaging (pet)	0	0	0	0	.00
78460	Heart muscle blood single	426	545	677	129	3.55
78460-26	Heart muscle blood single	175	224	278	43	1.20
78461	Heart muscle blood multiple	824	1055	1310	233	6.43
78461-26	Heart muscle blood multiple	272	348	432	63	1.74
78464	Heart image (3d) single	719	921	1144	310	8.56
78464-26	Heart image (3d) single	165	212	263	56	1.54
78465	Heart image (3d) multiple	1217	1558	1935	499	13.78
78465-26	Heart image (3d) multiple	231	296	368	75	2.07
78466	Heart infarct image	926	1186	1473	130	3.59
78466-26	Heart infarct image	315	403	501	35	.98
78468	Heart infarct image (ef)	439	563	699	173	4.77

NEW CODE CPT 2002 •

CPT	SHORT DESCRIPTION	50th	75th	90th	MFS	RVU
78468-26	Heart infarct image (ef)	132	169	210	41	1.13
78469	Heart infarct image (3d)	617	790	981	235	6.49
78469-26	Heart infarct image (3d)	154	198	245	47	1.30
78472	Gated heart planar, single	812	1040	1291	249	6.87
78472-26	Gated heart planar, single	211	270	336	50	1.39
78473	Gated heart, multiple	1292	1655	2055	372	10.27
78473-26	Gated heart, multiple	271	347	432	75	2.08
78478	Heart wall motion add-on	228	292	362	88	2.44
78478-26	Heart wall motion add-on	84	108	134	32	.88
78480	Heart function add-on	224	287	356	88	2.44
78480-26	Heart function add-on	83	106	132	32	.88
78481	Heart first pass, single	581	744	924	239	6.59
78481-26	Heart first pass, single	157	201	249	51	1.40
78483	Heart first pass, multiple	1207	1546	1919	359	9.91
78483-26	Heart first pass, multiple	265	340	422	76	2.10
78491	Heart image (pet), single	0	0	0	0	.00
78492	Heart image (pet), multiple	0	0	0	0	.00
78494	Heart image, spect	787	1008	1252	312	8.63
78494-26	Heart image, spect	173	222	275	60	1.67
78496	Heart first pass add-on	364	467	579	278	7.68
78496-26	Heart first pass add-on	106	135	168	26	.72
78499	Cardiovascular nuclear exam	0	0	0	0	.00
78580	Lung perfuse imaging	444	539	649	161	4.45
78580-26	Lung perfuse imaging	138	167	201	38	1.04
78584	Lung v/q image single breath	459	557	671	165	4.56
78584-26	Lung v/q image single breath	170	206	248	50	1.38

CPT	SHORT DESCRIPTION	50th	75th	90th	MFS	RVU
78585	Lung v/q imaging	745	904	1090	258	7.13
78585-26	Lung v/q imaging	201	244	294	55	1.53
78586	Aerosol lung image, single	388	471	567	114	3.14
78586-26	Aerosol lung image, single	97	118	142	20	.56
78587	Aerosol lung image, multiple	507	615	741	126	3.47
78587-26	Aerosol lung image, multiple	127	154	185	25	.69
78588	Perfuse lung image	562	682	823	171	4.72
78588-26	Perfuse lung image	163	198	239	55	1.53
78591	Vent image, 1 breath, 1 proj	412	500	603	123	3.40
78591-26	Vent image, 1 breath, 1 proj	91	110	133	21	.57
78593	Vent image, 1 proj, gas	557	675	814	149	4.12
78593-26	Vent image, 1 proj, gas	117	142	171	25	.69
78594	Vent image, mult proj, gas	773	938	1131	206	5.68
78594-26	Vent image, mult proj, gas	131	159	192	27	.74
78596	Lung differential function	486	590	711	319	8.80
78596-26	Lung differential function	190	230	277	64	1.78
78599	Respiratory nuclear exam	0	0	0	0	.00
78600	Brain imaging, ltd static	356	439	533	126	3.48
78600-26	Brain imaging, ltd static	82	101	123	22	.62
78601	Brain imaging, ltd w/ flow	458	565	686	148	4.09
78601-26	Brain imaging, ltd w/ flow	105	130	158	26	.71
78605	Brain imaging, complete	461	568	690	149	4.12
78605-26	Brain imaging, complete	106	131	159	27	.74
78606	Brain imaging, compl w/flow	528	651	791	172	4.74
78606-26	Brain imaging, compl w/flow	121	150	182	33	.90
78607	Brain imaging (3d)	808	996	1209	299	8.27

    NEW CODE CPT 2002 •

CPT	SHORT DESCRIPTION	50th	75th	90th	MFS	RVU
78607-26	Brain imaging (3d)	218	269	327	63	1.75
78608	Brain imaging (pet)	1922	2369	2877	0	.00
78609	Brain imaging (pet)	2248	2772	3366	0	.00
78610	Brain flow imaging only	205	253	307	72	2.00
78610-26	Brain flow imaging only	53	66	80	15	.42
78615	Cerebral vascular flow image	453	558	678	160	4.42
78615-26	Cerebral vascular flow image	82	100	122	22	.60
78630	Cerebrospinal fluid scan	694	856	1040	215	5.95
78630-26	Cerebrospinal fluid scan	146	180	218	34	.95
78635	Csf ventriculography	436	538	653	124	3.42
78635-26	Csf ventriculography	140	172	209	32	.88
78645	Csf shunt evaluation	528	651	791	152	4.21
78645-26	Csf shunt evaluation	137	169	206	29	.80
78647	Cerebrospinal fluid scan	656	809	982	258	7.13
78647-26	Cerebrospinal fluid scan	157	194	236	46	1.26
78650	Csf leakage imaging	610	752	913	198	5.46
78650-26	Csf leakage imaging	128	158	192	31	.85
78660	Nuclear exam tear flow	291	359	436	103	2.85
78660-26	Nuclear exam tear flow	96	118	144	27	.74
78699	Nervous system nuclear exam	0	0	0	0	.00
78700	Kidney imaging, static	536	666	787	132	3.65
78700-26	Kidney imaging, static	118	146	173	23	.63
78701	Kidney imaging with flow	612	760	898	152	4.21
78701-26	Kidney imaging with flow	128	160	189	25	.68
78704	Imaging renogram	504	625	739	180	4.97
78704-26	Imaging renogram	136	169	200	38	1.04

CPT	SHORT DESCRIPTION	50th	75th	90th	MFS	RVU
78707	Kidney flow/function image	611	759	897	209	5.78
78707-26	Kidney flow/function image	177	220	260	49	1.35
78708	Kidney flow/function image	524	651	769	222	6.13
78708-26	Kidney flow/function image	183	228	269	62	1.70
78709	Kidney flow/function image	556	691	817	232	6.41
78709-26	Kidney flow/function image	195	242	286	72	1.98
78710	Kidney imaging (3d)	711	883	1044	246	6.79
78710-26	Kidney imaging (3d)	128	159	188	33	.92
78715	Renal vascular flow exam	209	260	307	72	2.00
78715-26	Renal vascular flow exam	65	81	95	15	.42
78725	Kidney function study	312	388	458	84	2.31
78725-26	Kidney function study	84	105	124	19	.53
78730	Urinary bladder retention	196	244	288	71	1.97
78730-26	Urinary bladder retention	73	90	107	18	.51
78740	Ureteral reflux study	329	409	483	105	2.91
78740-26	Ureteral reflux study	115	143	169	29	.80
78760	Testicular imaging	375	465	550	130	3.58
78760-26	Testicular imaging	131	163	193	33	.92
78761	Testicular imaging/flow	417	518	613	151	4.18
78761-26	Testicular imaging/flow	129	161	190	36	1.00
78799	Genitourinary nuclear exam	0	0	0	0	.00
78800	Tumor imaging, limited area	478	734	1028	156	4.30
78800-26	Tumor imaging, limited area	129	198	277	33	.92
78801	Tumor imaging, mult areas	618	949	1329	192	5.30
78801-26	Tumor imaging, mult areas	161	247	345	40	1.11
78802	Tumor imaging, whole body	809	1241	1738	243	6.71

NEW CODE CPT 2002 •

CPT	SHORT DESCRIPTION	50th	75th	90th	MFS	RVU
78802-26	Tumor imaging, whole body	194	298	417	44	1.21
78803	Tumor imaging (3d)	978	1501	2101	292	8.06
78803-26	Tumor imaging (3d)	235	360	504	56	1.54
78805	Abscess imaging, ltd area	493	756	1059	160	4.41
78805-26	Abscess imaging, ltd area	143	219	307	37	1.03
78806	Abscess imaging, whole body	845	1298	1817	275	7.61
78806-26	Abscess imaging, whole body	186	286	400	44	1.21
78807	Nuclear localization/abscess	518	795	1113	292	8.08
78807-26	Nuclear localization/abscess	140	215	301	56	1.56
78810	Tumor imaging (pet)	3045	4674	6543	0	.00
78810-26	Tumor imaging (pet)	518	795	1112	101	2.79
78890	Nuclear medicine data proc	112	171	240	50	1.37
78890-26	Nuclear medicine data proc	9	14	19	3	.08
78891	Nuclear med data proc	225	345	483	100	2.75
78891-26	Nuclear med data proc	22	35	48	5	.15
78990	Provide diag radionuclide(s)	85	131	183	0	.00
78999	Nuclear diagnostic exam	0	0	0	0	.00

THERAPEUTIC

CPT	SHORT DESCRIPTION	50th	75th	90th	MFS	RVU
79000	Init hyperthyroid therapy	547	647	795	186	5.13
79000-26	Init hyperthyroid therapy	323	382	469	91	2.52
79001	Repeat hyperthyroid therapy	233	276	339	101	2.78
79001-26	Repeat hyperthyroid therapy	140	166	203	54	1.48
79020	Thyroid ablation	393	466	572	186	5.13
79020-26	Thyroid ablation	228	270	332	91	2.52
79030	Thyroid ablation, carcinoma	649	769	944	201	5.56
79030-26	Thyroid ablation, carcinoma	396	469	576	107	2.95

CPT	SHORT DESCRIPTION	50th	75th	90th	MFS	RVU
79035	Thyroid metastatic therapy	684	810	995	223	6.16
79035-26	Thyroid metastatic therapy	452	535	657	129	3.55
79100	Hematopoetic nuclear therapy	311	369	453	163	4.49
79100-26	Hematopoetic nuclear therapy	156	184	226	68	1.88
79200	Intracavitary nuclear trmt	415	491	603	196	5.41
79200-26	Intracavitary nuclear trmt	253	300	368	101	2.80
79300	Interstitial nuclear therapy	252	298	366	0	.00
79300-26	Interstitial nuclear therapy	194	230	282	85	2.35
79400	Nonhemato nuclear therapy	373	442	542	195	5.38
79400-26	Nonhemato nuclear therapy	220	261	320	100	2.77
79420	Intravascular nuclear ther	187	221	272	0	.00
79420-26	Intravascular nuclear ther	114	135	166	76	2.11
79440	Nuclear joint therapy	460	544	668	198	5.48
79440-26	Nuclear joint therapy	280	332	408	104	2.87
79900	Provide ther radiopharm(s)	0	0	0	0	.00
79999	Nuclear medicine therapy	0	0	0	0	.00

NEW CODE CPT 2002 •

PATHOLOGY & LABORATORY

CPT	SHORT DESCRIPTION	50th	75th	90th	MFS	RVU
	ORGAN OR DISEASE ORIENTED PANELS					
80048	Basic metabolic panel	37	46	62	0	.00
80048-26	Basic metabolic panel	7	8	11	0	.00
80050	General health panel	141	176	238	0	.00
80050-26	General health panel	58	72	98	0	.00
80051	Electrolyte panel	24	30	40	0	.00
80051-26	Electrolyte panel	10	12	16	0	.00
80053	Comprehensive metabolic panel	46	57	77	0	.00
80053-26	Comprehensive metabolic panel	13	17	22	0	.00
80055	Obstetric panel	138	173	233	0	.00
80055-26	Obstetric panel	46	57	77	0	.00
80061	Lipid panel	62	78	105	0	.00
80061-26	Lipid panel	22	28	38	0	.00
80069	Renal function panel	39	48	65	0	.00
80069-26	Renal function panel	9	12	16	0	.00
80074	Acute hepatitis panel	286	357	482	0	.00
80074-26	Acute hepatitis panel	117	146	198	0	.00
80076	Hepatic function panel	38	48	64	0	.00
80076-26	Hepatic function panel	16	19	26	0	.00
80090	Torch antibody panel	155	193	261	0	.00
80090-26	Torch antibody panel	65	81	110	0	.00

CPT	SHORT DESCRIPTION	50th	75th	90th	MFS	RVU
DRUG TESTING						
80100	Drug screen, qualitate/multi	68	85	115	0	.00
80100-26	Drug screen, qualitate/multi	20	25	33	0	.00
80101	Drug screen, single	40	50	68	0	.00
80101-26	Drug screen, single	11	14	19	0	.00
80102	Drug confirmation	78	97	131	0	.00
80102-26	Drug confirmation	23	28	38	0	.00
80103	Drug analysis, tissue prep	35	44	59	0	.00
80103-26	Drug analysis, tissue prep	13	16	21	0	.00
THERAPEUTIC DRUG ASSAYS						
80150	Assay amikacin	43	54	73	0	.00
80150-26	Assay amikacin	14	17	23	0	.00
80152	Assay amitriptyline	91	114	154	0	.00
80152-26	Assay amitriptyline	29	37	49	0	.00
80154	Assay benzodiazepines	102	128	173	0	.00
80154-26	Assay benzodiazepines	32	40	54	0	.00
80156	Assay carbamazepine, total	77	96	130	0	.00
80156-26	Assay carbamazepine, total	24	30	40	0	.00
80157	Assay carbamazepine, free	0	0	0	0	.00
80158	Assay cyclosporine	118	147	199	0	.00
80158-26	Assay cyclosporine	40	50	68	0	.00
80160	Assay desipramine	93	117	158	0	.00
80160-26	Assay desipramine	32	40	54	0	.00
80162	Assay digoxin	67	83	112	0	.00
80162-26	Assay digoxin	20	25	34	0	.00

      NEW CODE CPT 2002 •

CPT	SHORT DESCRIPTION	50th	75th	90th	MFS	RVU
80164	Assay dipropylacetic acid	81	101	137	0	.00
80164-26	Assay dipropylacetic acid	26	32	44	0	.00
80166	Assay doxepin	42	52	71	0	.00
80166-26	Assay doxepin	12	15	20	0	.00
80168	Assay ethosuximide	90	112	152	0	.00
80168-26	Assay ethosuximide	36	45	61	0	.00
80170	Assay gentamicin	61	76	103	0	.00
80170-26	Assay gentamicin	21	26	35	0	.00
80172	Assay gold	63	79	107	0	.00
80172-26	Assay gold	18	23	31	0	.00
80173	Assay haloperidol	0	0	0	0	.00
80174	Assay imipramine	90	112	152	0	.00
80174-26	Assay imipramine	26	33	44	0	.00
80176	Assay lidocaine	52	65	88	0	.00
80176-26	Assay lidocaine	16	20	27	0	.00
80178	Assay lithium	43	53	72	0	.00
80178-26	Assay lithium	16	20	27	0	.00
80182	Assay nortriptyline	106	132	178	0	.00
80182-26	Assay nortriptyline	34	42	57	0	.00
80184	Assay phenobarbital	78	98	132	0	.00
80184-26	Assay phenobarbital	23	28	38	0	.00
80185	Assay phenytoin, total	77	96	130	0	.00
80185-26	Assay phenytoin, total	21	26	35	0	.00
80186	Assay phenytoin, free	76	95	128	0	.00
80186-26	Assay phenytoin, free	22	28	37	0	.00
80188	Assay primidone	60	75	102	0	.00

CPT	SHORT DESCRIPTION	50th	75th	90th	MFS	RVU
80188-26	Assay primidone	19	23	32	0	.00
80190	Assay procainamide	67	84	113	0	.00
80190-26	Assay procainamide	21	27	36	0	.00
80192	Assay procainamide	100	125	169	0	.00
80192-26	Assay procainamide	39	49	66	0	.00
80194	Assay quinidine	81	101	136	0	.00
80194-26	Assay quinidine	24	30	41	0	.00
80196	Assay salicylate	40	50	68	0	.00
80196-26	Assay salicylate	12	15	20	0	.00
80197	Assay tacrolimus	72	90	122	0	.00
80197-26	Assay tacrolimus	23	29	39	0	.00
80198	Assay theophylline	72	91	122	0	.00
80198-26	Assay theophylline	17	22	29	0	.00
80200	Assay tobramycin	58	72	98	0	.00
80200-26	Assay tobramycin	19	24	32	0	.00
80201	Assay topiramate	91	113	153	0	.00
80201-26	Assay topiramate	30	37	51	0	.00
80202	Assay vancomycin	62	77	104	0	.00
80202-26	Assay vancomycin	20	25	34	0	.00
80299	Quantitative assay drug	0	0	0	0	.00

EVOCATIVE/SUPPRESSION TESTING

CPT	SHORT DESCRIPTION	50th	75th	90th	MFS	RVU
80400	ACTH stimulation panel	132	164	222	0	.00
80400-26	ACTH stimulation panel	45	56	76	0	.00
80402	ACTH stimulation panel	247	308	417	0	.00
80402-26	ACTH stimulation panel	77	96	129	0	.00
80406	ACTH stimulation panel	227	283	383	0	.00

CPT	SHORT DESCRIPTION	50th	75th	90th	MFS	RVU
80406-26	ACTH stimulation panel	70	88	119	0	.00
80408	Aldosterone suppression eval	329	410	555	0	.00
80408-26	Aldosterone suppression eval	118	148	200	0	.00
80410	Calcitonin stimul panel	307	384	518	0	.00
80410-26	Calcitonin stimul panel	101	127	171	0	.00
80412	Crh stimulation panel	808	1009	1363	0	.00
80412-26	Crh stimulation panel	267	333	450	0	.00
80414	Testosterone response	117	146	197	0	.00
80414-26	Testosterone response	36	45	61	0	.00
80415	Estradiol response panel	122	153	207	0	.00
80415-26	Estradiol response panel	38	47	64	0	.00
80416	Renin stimulation panel	387	484	654	0	.00
80416-26	Renin stimulation panel	136	169	229	0	.00
80417	Renin stimulation panel	159	199	269	0	.00
80417-26	Renin stimulation panel	56	70	94	0	.00
80418	Pituitary evaluation panel	1909	2385	3223	0	.00
80418-26	Pituitary evaluation panel	554	692	935	0	.00
80420	Dexamethasone panel	245	305	413	0	.00
80420-26	Dexamethasone panel	76	95	128	0	.00
80422	Glucagon tolerance panel	152	190	257	0	.00
80422-26	Glucagon tolerance panel	46	57	77	0	.00
80424	Glucagon tolerance panel	154	193	260	0	.00
80424-26	Glucagon tolerance panel	45	56	75	0	.00
80426	Gonadotropin hormone panel	359	448	606	0	.00
80426-26	Gonadotropin hormone panel	86	108	145	0	.00
80428	Growth hormone panel	175	219	296	0	.00

CPT	SHORT DESCRIPTION	50th	75th	90th	MFS	RVU
80428-26	Growth hormone panel	37	46	62	0	.00
80430	Growth hormone panel	217	271	366	0	.00
80430-26	Growth hormone panel	56	70	95	0	.00
80432	Insulin suppression panel	400	500	675	0	.00
80432-26	Insulin suppression panel	96	120	162	0	.00
80434	Insulin tolerance panel	263	329	444	0	.00
80434-26	Insulin tolerance panel	82	102	138	0	.00
80435	Insulin tolerance panel	272	340	459	0	.00
80435-26	Insulin tolerance panel	82	102	138	0	.00
80436	Metyrapone panel	249	311	420	0	.00
80436-26	Metyrapone panel	72	90	122	0	.00
80438	Trh stimulation panel	160	200	270	0	.00
80438-26	Trh stimulation panel	50	62	84	0	.00
80439	Trh stimulation panel	168	210	284	0	.00
80439-26	Trh stimulation panel	32	40	54	0	.00
80440	Trh stimulation panel	152	190	256	0	.00
80440-26	Trh stimulation panel	29	36	49	0	.00

CONSULTATIONS (CLINICAL PATHOLOGY)

CPT	SHORT DESCRIPTION	50th	75th	90th	MFS	RVU
80500	Lab pathology consultation	67	78	89	21	.59
80502	Lab pathology consultation	154	178	203	73	2.01

URINALYSIS

CPT	SHORT DESCRIPTION	50th	75th	90th	MFS	RVU
81000	Urinalysis, nonauto w/scope	17	21	26	0	.00
81000-26	Urinalysis, nonauto w/scope	7	9	11	0	.00
81001	Urinalysis, auto w/scope	22	28	34	0	.00
81002	Urinalysis nonauto w/o scope	13	16	20	0	.00

NEW CODE CPT 2002 •

CPT	SHORT DESCRIPTION	50th	75th	90th	MFS	RVU
81002-26	Urinalysis nonauto w/o scope	6	8	10	0	.00
81003	Urinalysis, auto, w/o scope	16	21	26	0	.00
81003-26	Urinalysis, auto, w/o scope	5	7	8	0	.00
81005	Urinalysis	11	14	17	0	.00
81005-26	Urinalysis	4	5	6	0	.00
81007	Urine screen for bacteria	18	23	29	0	.00
81007-26	Urine screen for bacteria	6	8	9	0	.00
81015	Microscopic exam urine	15	19	24	0	.00
81015-26	Microscopic exam urine	6	8	9	0	.00
81020	Urinalysis, glass test	17	21	26	0	.00
81020-26	Urinalysis, glass test	6	8	10	0	.00
81025	Urine pregnancy test	23	30	36	0	.00
81025-26	Urine pregnancy test	12	15	18	0	.00
81050	Urinalysis, volume measure	92	116	143	0	.00
81050-26	Urinalysis, volume measure	30	38	47	0	.00
81099	Urinalysis test procedure	0	0	0	0	.00

CHEMISTRY

CPT	SHORT DESCRIPTION	50th	75th	90th	MFS	RVU
82000	Assay blood acetaldehyde	47	65	90	0	.00
82000-26	Assay blood acetaldehyde	14	20	27	0	.00
82003	Assay acetaminophen	58	80	110	0	.00
82003-26	Assay acetaminophen	16	22	30	0	.00
82009	Test for acetone/ketones	18	24	33	0	.00
82009-26	Test for acetone/ketones	6	8	11	0	.00
82010	Acetone assay	22	30	41	0	.00
82010-26	Acetone assay	7	10	14	0	.00
82013	Acetylcholinesterase assay	79	109	149	0	.00

CPT	SHORT DESCRIPTION	50th	75th	90th	MFS	RVU
82013-26	Acetylcholinesterase assay	24	33	45	0	.00
82016	Acylcarnitines, qual	0	0	0	0	.00
82017	Acylcarnitines, quant	0	0	0	0	.00
82024	Assay ACTH	184	253	348	0	.00
82024-26	Assay ACTH	55	76	104	0	.00
82030	Assay adp & amp	78	107	147	0	.00
82030-26	Assay adp & amp	31	43	59	0	.00
82040	Assay serum albumin	15	20	28	0	.00
82040-26	Assay serum albumin	4	6	8	0	.00
82042	Assay urine albumin	16	22	30	0	.00
82042-26	Assay urine albumin	4	6	8	0	.00
82043	Microalbumin, quantitative	49	67	92	0	.00
82043-26	Microalbumin, quantitative	15	21	29	0	.00
82044	Microalbumin, semiquant	19	26	36	0	.00
82044-26	Microalbumin, semiquant	5	8	10	0	.00
82055	Assay ethanol	43	59	81	0	.00
82055-26	Assay ethanol	13	18	24	0	.00
82075	Assay breath ethanol	20	28	38	0	.00
82075-26	Assay breath ethanol	6	9	12	0	.00
82085	Assay aldolase	55	76	105	0	.00
82085-26	Assay aldolase	17	23	31	0	.00
82088	Assay aldosterone	175	241	332	0	.00
82088-26	Assay aldosterone	54	75	103	0	.00
82101	Assay urine alkaloids	49	68	93	0	.00
82101-26	Assay urine alkaloids	15	21	29	0	.00
82103	Alpha-1-antitrypsin, total	74	102	140	0	.00

  NEW CODE CPT 2002 •

CPT	SHORT DESCRIPTION	50th	75th	90th	MFS	RVU
82103-26	Alpha-1-antitrypsin, total	26	36	49	0	.00
82104	Alpha-1-antitrypsin, pheno	102	141	194	0	.00
82104-26	Alpha-1-antitrypsin, pheno	34	47	64	0	.00
82105	Alpha-fetoprotein, serum	64	88	121	0	.00
82105-26	Alpha-fetoprotein, serum	20	28	39	0	.00
82106	Alpha-fetoprotein, amniotic	63	88	120	0	.00
82106-26	Alpha-fetoprotein, amniotic	20	28	38	0	.00
82108	Assay aluminum	94	130	179	0	.00
82108-26	Assay aluminum	29	40	55	0	.00
82120	Amines, vaginal fluid qual	15	21	29	0	.00
82127	Amino acid, single qual	150	207	285	0	.00
82127-26	Amino acid, single qual	50	68	94	0	.00
82128	Amino acids, mult qual	58	80	110	0	.00
82128-26	Amino acids, mult qual	19	26	36	0	.00
82131	Amino acids, single quant	147	203	279	0	.00
82131-26	Amino acids, single quant	34	47	64	0	.00
82135	Assay aminolevulinic acid	47	65	89	0	.00
82135-26	Assay aminolevulinic acid	15	21	28	0	.00
82136	Amino acids, quant, 2-5	178	246	338	0	.00
82136-26	Amino acids, quant, 2-5	66	91	125	0	.00
82139	Amino acids, quant, 6 or more	266	366	504	0	.00
82139-26	Amino acids, quant, 6 or more	98	136	186	0	.00
82140	Assay ammonia	36	50	69	0	.00
82140-26	Assay ammonia	11	15	21	0	.00
82143	Amniotic fluid scan	50	69	95	0	.00
82143-26	Amniotic fluid scan	16	21	30	0	.00

CPT	SHORT DESCRIPTION	50th	75th	90th	MFS	RVU
82145	Assay amphetamines	27	37	51	0	.00
82145-26	Assay amphetamines	7	10	14	0	.00
82150	Assay amylase	28	39	54	0	.00
82150-26	Assay amylase	9	13	18	0	.00
82154	Androstanediol glucuronide	63	87	119	0	.00
82154-26	Androstanediol glucuronide	23	31	43	0	.00
82157	Assay androstenedione	163	224	308	0	.00
82157-26	Assay androstenedione	49	67	93	0	.00
82160	Assay androsterone	70	97	133	0	.00
82160-26	Assay androsterone	23	32	44	0	.00
82163	Assay angiotensin ii	66	91	124	0	.00
82163-26	Assay angiotensin ii	18	25	35	0	.00
82164	Angiotensin I enzyme test	94	130	179	0	.00
82164-26	Angiotensin I enzyme test	29	40	55	0	.00
82172	Assay apolipoprotein	49	68	93	0	.00
82172-26	Assay apolipoprotein	15	21	29	0	.00
82175	Assay arsenic	54	75	103	0	.00
82175-26	Assay arsenic	17	24	33	0	.00
82180	Assay ascorbic acid	64	88	121	0	.00
82180-26	Assay ascorbic acid	21	29	40	0	.00
82190	Atomic absorption	57	79	108	0	.00
82190-26	Atomic absorption	20	28	38	0	.00
82205	Assay barbiturates	62	85	117	0	.00
82205-26	Assay barbiturates	18	25	34	0	.00
82232	Assay beta-2 protein	90	125	171	0	.00
82232-26	Assay beta-2 protein	29	40	55	0	.00

NEW CODE CPT 2002 •

CPT	SHORT DESCRIPTION	50th	75th	90th	MFS	RVU
82239	Bile acids, total	35	48	65	0	.00
82239-26	Bile acids, total	12	17	24	0	.00
82240	Bile acids, cholylglycine	76	105	145	0	.00
82240-26	Bile acids, cholylglycine	24	33	45	0	.00
82247	Bilirubin, total	17	24	33	0	.00
82247-26	Bilirubin, total	5	7	10	0	.00
82248	Bilirubin, direct	16	22	30	0	.00
82248-26	Bilirubin, direct	5	7	9	0	.00
82252	Fecal bilirubin test	15	21	29	0	.00
82252-26	Fecal bilirubin test	5	6	9	0	.00
82261	Assay biotinidase	174	240	330	0	.00
82261-26	Assay biotinidase	59	82	112	0	.00
82270	Test for blood, feces	14	19	26	0	.00
82270-26	Test for blood, feces	6	8	10	0	.00
82273	Test for blood, other source	16	22	30	0	.00
82273-26	Test for blood, other source	4	5	7	0	.00
• 82274	Assay test for blood, fecal	0	0	0	0	.00
82286	Assay bradykinin	51	70	96	0	.00
82286-26	Assay bradykinin	14	19	26	0	.00
82300	Assay cadmium	39	53	73	0	.00
82300-26	Assay cadmium	12	17	23	0	.00
82306	Assay vitamin d	191	264	363	0	.00
82306-26	Assay vitamin d	63	87	120	0	.00
82307	Assay vitamin d	66	91	124	0	.00
82307-26	Assay vitamin d	22	31	42	0	.00
82308	Assay calcitonin	146	201	277	0	.00

CPT	SHORT DESCRIPTION	50th	75th	90th	MFS	RVU
82308-26	Assay calcitonin	44	60	83	0	.00
82310	Assay calcium	18	25	35	0	.00
82310-26	Assay calcium	5	8	10	0	.00
82330	Assay calcium	36	49	68	0	.00
82330-26	Assay calcium	10	14	20	0	.00
82331	Calcium infuse test	14	19	26	0	.00
82331-26	Calcium infuse test	4	6	8	0	.00
82340	Assay calcium in urine	25	35	48	0	.00
82340-26	Assay calcium in urine	8	12	16	0	.00
82355	Calculus analysis, qual	77	106	145	0	.00
82355-26	Calculus analysis, qual	25	34	46	0	.00
82360	Calculus assay, quant	52	71	98	0	.00
82360-26	Calculus assay, quant	17	23	31	0	.00
82365	Calculus spectroscopy	74	103	141	0	.00
82365-26	Calculus spectroscopy	22	30	41	0	.00
82370	X-ray assay, calculus	57	78	108	0	.00
82370-26	X-ray assay, calculus	19	26	36	0	.00
82373	Assay c-d transfer measure	0	0	0	0	.00
82374	Assay blood carbon dioxide	10	14	20	0	.00
82374-26	Assay blood carbon dioxide	3	5	6	0	.00
82375	Assay blood carbon monoxide	63	88	120	0	.00
82375-26	Assay blood carbon monoxide	18	25	35	0	.00
82376	Test for carbon monoxide	11	15	20	0	.00
82376-26	Test for carbon monoxide	3	4	6	0	.00
82378	Carcinoembryonic antigen	93	129	177	0	.00
82378-26	Carcinoembryonic antigen	27	37	51	0	.00

NEW CODE CPT 2002 •

CPT	SHORT DESCRIPTION	50th	75th	90th	MFS	RVU
82379	Assay carnitine	154	212	291	0	.00
82379-26	Assay carnitine	52	72	99	0	.00
82380	Assay carotene	60	83	114	0	.00
82380-26	Assay carotene	18	25	34	0	.00
82382	Assay urine catecholamines	76	105	145	0	.00
82382-26	Assay urine catecholamines	24	33	45	0	.00
82383	Assay blood catecholamines	71	97	134	0	.00
82383-26	Assay blood catecholamines	21	29	40	0	.00
82384	Assay three catecholamines	150	207	284	0	.00
82384-26	Assay three catecholamines	45	62	85	0	.00
82387	Assay cathepsin-d	66	91	124	0	.00
82387-26	Assay cathepsin-d	19	26	36	0	.00
82390	Assay ceruloplasmin	63	87	119	0	.00
82390-26	Assay ceruloplasmin	19	26	36	0	.00
82397	Chemiluminescent assay	39	54	74	0	.00
82397-26	Chemiluminescent assay	13	18	24	0	.00
82415	Assay chloramphenicol	48	67	92	0	.00
82415-26	Assay chloramphenicol	15	21	28	0	.00
82435	Assay blood chloride	11	15	20	0	.00
82435-26	Assay blood chloride	3	4	5	0	.00
82436	Assay urine chloride	19	26	36	0	.00
82436-26	Assay urine chloride	6	8	11	0	.00
82438	Assay other fluid chlorides	21	29	39	0	.00
82438-26	Assay other fluid chlorides	7	9	13	0	.00
82441	Test for chlorohydrocarbons	34	47	64	0	.00
82441-26	Test for chlorohydrocarbons	11	15	21	0	.00

CPT	SHORT DESCRIPTION	50th	75th	90th	MFS	RVU
82465	Assay blood/serum cholesterol	18	25	35	0	.00
82465-26	Assay blood/serum cholesterol	5	6	9	0	.00
82480	Assay serum cholinesterase	23	32	44	0	.00
82480-26	Assay serum cholinesterase	6	9	12	0	.00
82482	Assay rbc cholinesterase	32	45	61	0	.00
82482-26	Assay rbc cholinesterase	10	14	19	0	.00
82485	Assay chondroitin sulfate	58	80	110	0	.00
82485-26	Assay chondroitin sulfate	14	19	26	0	.00
82486	Gas/liquid chromatography	77	106	146	0	.00
82486-26	Gas/liquid chromatography	25	35	48	0	.00
82487	Paper chromatography	42	58	80	0	.00
82487-26	Paper chromatography	13	19	26	0	.00
82488	Paper chromatography	56	77	106	0	.00
82488-26	Paper chromatography	19	26	36	0	.00
82489	Thin layer chromatography	39	53	73	0	.00
82489-26	Thin layer chromatography	13	18	24	0	.00
82491	Chromotography, quant, sing	70	97	133	0	.00
82491-26	Chromotography, quant, sing	21	29	40	0	.00
82492	Chromotography, quant, mult	54	75	103	0	.00
82492-26	Chromotography, quant, mult	17	24	33	0	.00
82495	Assay chromium	43	59	81	0	.00
82495-26	Assay chromium	15	20	28	0	.00
82507	Assay citrate	93	128	176	0	.00
82507-26	Assay citrate	27	37	51	0	.00
82520	Assay cocaine	27	37	51	0	.00
82520-26	Assay cocaine	9	12	16	0	.00

NEW CODE CPT 2002 •

CPT	SHORT DESCRIPTION	50th	75th	90th	MFS	RVU
82523	Collagen crosslinks	78	108	148	0	.00
82523-26	Collagen crosslinks	31	43	59	0	.00
82525	Assay copper	65	90	124	0	.00
82525-26	Assay copper	19	26	36	0	.00
82528	Assay corticosterone	55	75	104	0	.00
82528-26	Assay corticosterone	17	24	33	0	.00
82530	Cortisol, free	88	121	167	0	.00
82530-26	Cortisol, free	27	38	52	0	.00
82533	Total cortisol	85	117	161	0	.00
82533-26	Total cortisol	24	33	45	0	.00
82540	Assay creatine	20	28	39	0	.00
82540-26	Assay creatine	7	9	13	0	.00
82541	Column chromotography, qual	190	262	360	0	.00
82541-26	Column chromotography, qual	61	84	115	0	.00
82542	Column chromotography, quant	146	201	277	0	.00
82542-26	Column chromotography, quant	47	64	89	0	.00
82543	Column chromotography/isotope	190	262	360	0	.00
82543-26	Column chromotography/isotope	61	84	115	0	.00
82544	Column chromotography/isotope	190	262	360	0	.00
82544-26	Column chromotography/isotope	61	84	115	0	.00
82550	Assay ck (cpk)	22	30	42	0	.00
82550-26	Assay ck (cpk)	6	8	11	0	.00
82552	Assay cpk in blood	33	45	63	0	.00
82552-26	Assay cpk in blood	10	14	19	0	.00
82553	Creatine, mb fraction	46	63	87	0	.00
82553-26	Creatine, mb fraction	15	21	29	0	.00

• NEW CODE CPT 2002   CPT codes and descriptions only copyright AMA

CPT	SHORT DESCRIPTION	50th	75th	90th	MFS	RVU
82554	Creatine, isoforms	32	44	61	0	.00
82554-26	Creatine, isoforms	11	15	20	0	.00
82565	Assay creatinine	21	29	40	0	.00
82565-26	Assay creatinine	4	5	7	0	.00
82570	Assay urine creatinine	27	37	51	0	.00
82570-26	Assay urine creatinine	7	9	13	0	.00
82575	Creatinine clearance test	51	70	96	0	.00
82575-26	Creatinine clearance test	17	23	32	0	.00
82585	Assay cryofibrinogen	40	55	76	0	.00
82585-26	Assay cryofibrinogen	8	12	16	0	.00
82595	Assay cryoglobulin	37	51	70	0	.00
82595-26	Assay cryoglobulin	11	16	22	0	.00
82600	Assay cyanide	39	54	74	0	.00
82600-26	Assay cyanide	12	16	22	0	.00
82607	Vitamin b-12	71	98	135	0	.00
82607-26	Vitamin b-12	21	29	39	0	.00
82608	B-12 binding capacity	63	88	120	0	.00
82608-26	B-12 binding capacity	20	28	38	0	.00
82615	Test for urine cystines	23	32	44	0	.00
82615-26	Test for urine cystines	7	10	14	0	.00
82626	Dehydroepiandrosterone	183	235	294	0	.00
82626-26	Dehydroepiandrosterone	60	77	97	0	.00
82627	Dehydroepiandrosterone	132	169	213	0	.00
82627-26	Dehydroepiandrosterone	42	54	68	0	.00
82633	Desoxycorticosterone	93	120	150	0	.00
82633-26	Desoxycorticosterone	28	36	45	0	.00

    NEW CODE CPT 2002 •

CPT	SHORT DESCRIPTION	50th	75th	90th	MFS	RVU
82634	Deoxycortisol	80	102	129	0	.00
82634-26	Deoxycortisol	24	31	39	0	.00
82638	Assay dibucaine number	29	38	47	0	.00
82638-26	Assay dibucaine number	9	12	15	0	.00
82646	Assay dihydrocodeinone	54	69	86	0	.00
82646-26	Assay dihydrocodeinone	16	20	25	0	.00
82649	Assay dihydromorphinone	59	76	95	0	.00
82649-26	Assay dihydromorphinone	24	30	38	0	.00
82651	Assay dihydrotestosterone	167	214	269	0	.00
82651-26	Assay dihydrotestosterone	67	86	108	0	.00
82652	Assay dihydroxyvitamin d	229	293	368	0	.00
82652-26	Assay dihydroxyvitamin d	69	88	110	0	.00
82654	Assay dimethadione	54	69	86	0	.00
82654-26	Assay dimethadione	16	20	25	0	.00
82657	Enzyme cell activity	204	261	328	0	.00
82657-26	Enzyme cell activity	65	84	105	0	.00
82658	Enzyme cell activity, ra	204	261	328	0	.00
82658-26	Enzyme cell activity, ra	65	84	105	0	.00
82664	Electrophoretic test	50	64	80	0	.00
82664-26	Electrophoretic test	16	20	26	0	.00
82666	Assay epiandrosterone	68	87	109	0	.00
82666-26	Assay epiandrosterone	20	26	33	0	.00
82668	Assay erythropoietin	133	171	214	0	.00
82668-26	Assay erythropoietin	41	53	66	0	.00
82670	Assay estradiol	112	144	181	0	.00
82670-26	Assay estradiol	34	43	54	0	.00

CPT	SHORT DESCRIPTION	50th	75th	90th	MFS	RVU
82671	Assay estrogens	126	162	203	0	.00
82671-26	Assay estrogens	37	47	59	0	.00
82672	Assay estrogen	135	173	217	0	.00
82672-26	Assay estrogen	38	48	61	0	.00
82677	Assay estriol	71	91	114	0	.00
82677-26	Assay estriol	23	30	38	0	.00
82679	Assay estrone	141	181	227	0	.00
82679-26	Assay estrone	42	54	68	0	.00
82690	Assay ethchlorvynol	34	44	55	0	.00
82690-26	Assay ethchlorvynol	14	18	23	0	.00
82693	Assay ethylene glycol	55	70	88	0	.00
82693-26	Assay ethylene glycol	17	22	28	0	.00
82696	Assay etiocholanolone	70	90	113	0	.00
82696-26	Assay etiocholanolone	24	31	39	0	.00
82705	Fats/lipids, feces, qual	47	61	76	0	.00
82705-26	Fats/lipids, feces, qual	18	23	29	0	.00
82710	Fats/lipids, feces, quant	52	66	83	0	.00
82710-26	Fats/lipids, feces, quant	16	20	26	0	.00
82715	Assay fecal fat	32	41	52	0	.00
82715-26	Assay fecal fat	11	14	17	0	.00
82725	Assay blood fatty acids	32	41	52	0	.00
82725-26	Assay blood fatty acids	10	13	16	0	.00
82726	Long chain fatty acids	106	135	170	0	.00
82726-26	Long chain fatty acids	34	43	54	0	.00
82728	Assay ferritin	64	82	103	0	.00
82728-26	Assay ferritin	19	25	31	0	.00

NEW CODE CPT 2002 •

CPT	SHORT DESCRIPTION	50th	75th	90th	MFS	RVU
82731	Assay fetal fibronectin	253	325	408	0	.00
82731-26	Assay fetal fibronectin	84	107	135	0	.00
82735	Assay fluoride	44	56	70	0	.00
82735-26	Assay fluoride	14	19	23	0	.00
82742	Assay flurazepam	52	66	83	0	.00
82742-26	Assay flurazepam	16	20	26	0	.00
82746	Blood folic acid serum	76	98	123	0	.00
82746-26	Blood folic acid serum	25	32	40	0	.00
82747	Assay folic acid, rbc	91	117	146	0	.00
82747-26	Assay folic acid, rbc	30	39	48	0	.00
82757	Assay semen fructose	32	41	51	0	.00
82757-26	Assay semen fructose	10	12	15	0	.00
82759	Assay rbc galactokinase	34	43	54	0	.00
82759-26	Assay rbc galactokinase	10	13	17	0	.00
82760	Assay galactose	26	33	41	0	.00
82760-26	Assay galactose	8	11	13	0	.00
82775	Assay galactose transferase	37	47	59	0	.00
82775-26	Assay galactose transferase	11	14	18	0	.00
82776	Galactose transferase test	25	32	40	0	.00
82776-26	Galactose transferase test	6	7	9	0	.00
82784	Assay gammaglobulin igm	48	61	77	0	.00
82784-26	Assay gammaglobulin igm	14	18	22	0	.00
82785	Assay gammaglobulin ige	74	95	119	0	.00
82785-26	Assay gammaglobulin ige	24	31	39	0	.00
82787	Igg 1, 2, 3 or 4, each	134	172	216	0	.00
82787-26	Igg 1, 2, 3 or 4, each	39	50	63	0	.00

CPT	SHORT DESCRIPTION	50th	75th	90th	MFS	RVU
82800	Blood pH	106	135	170	0	.00
82800-26	Blood pH	31	39	49	0	.00
82803	Blood gases: pH, pO_2 & pCO_2	72	93	117	0	.00
82803-26	Blood gases: pH, pO_2 & pCO_2	22	29	36	0	.00
82805	Blood gases w/O_2 saturation	49	63	79	0	.00
82805-26	Blood gases w/O_2 saturation	21	27	33	0	.00
82810	Blood gases, O_2 sat only	36	46	58	0	.00
82810-26	Blood gases, O_2 sat only	11	14	18	0	.00
82820	Hemoglobin-oxygen affinity	37	48	60	0	.00
82820-26	Hemoglobin-oxygen affinity	12	16	20	0	.00
82926	Assay gastric acid	18	23	29	0	.00
82926-26	Assay gastric acid	5	6	8	0	.00
82928	Assay gastric acid	59	76	95	0	.00
82928-26	Assay gastric acid	21	27	34	0	.00
82938	Gastrin test	55	70	88	0	.00
82938-26	Gastrin test	19	24	30	0	.00
82941	Assay gastrin	96	123	154	0	.00
82941-26	Assay gastrin	32	41	51	0	.00
82943	Assay glucagon	64	82	102	0	.00
82943-26	Assay glucagon	20	25	32	0	.00
82945	Glucose other fluid	27	34	43	0	.00
82946	Glucagon tolerance test	40	51	64	0	.00
82946-26	Glucagon tolerance test	10	13	17	0	.00
82947	Assay glucose, blood quant	19	25	31	0	.00
82947-26	Assay glucose, blood quant	6	7	9	0	.00
82948	Reagent strip/blood glucose	15	19	24	0	.00

NEW CODE CPT 2002 •

CPT	SHORT DESCRIPTION	50th	75th	90th	MFS	RVU
82948-26	Reagent strip/blood glucose	6	8	10	0	.00
82950	Glucose test	27	35	44	0	.00
82950-26	Glucose test	10	13	16	0	.00
82951	Glucose tolerance test (gtt)	46	59	74	0	.00
82951-26	Glucose tolerance test (gtt)	15	20	25	0	.00
82952	Gtt-added samples	14	18	22	0	.00
82952-26	Gtt-added samples	4	5	7	0	.00
82953	Glucose-tolbutamide test	50	64	81	0	.00
82953-26	Glucose-tolbutamide test	17	22	27	0	.00
82955	Assay g6pd enzyme	77	98	123	0	.00
82955-26	Assay g6pd enzyme	22	28	36	0	.00
82960	Test for g6pd enzyme	29	38	47	0	.00
82960-26	Test for g6pd enzyme	9	12	15	0	.00
82962	Glucose blood test	14	19	23	0	.00
82962-26	Glucose blood test	3	4	5	0	.00
82963	Assay glucosidase	54	69	86	0	.00
82963-26	Assay glucosidase	17	22	28	0	.00
82965	Assay gdh enzyme	17	22	28	0	.00
82965-26	Assay gdh enzyme	6	7	9	0	.00
82975	Assay glutamine	35	45	56	0	.00
82975-26	Assay glutamine	11	14	17	0	.00
82977	Assay ggt	19	25	31	0	.00
82977-26	Assay ggt	5	7	8	0	.00
82978	Assay glutathione	38	49	61	0	.00
82978-26	Assay glutathione	11	14	18	0	.00
82979	Assay rbc glutathione	26	34	42	0	.00

CPT	SHORT DESCRIPTION	50th	75th	90th	MFS	RVU
82979-26	Assay rbc glutathione	8	10	12	0	.00
82980	Assay glutethimide	52	66	83	0	.00
82980-26	Assay glutethimide	12	15	19	0	.00
82985	Glycated protein	43	55	69	0	.00
82985-26	Glycated protein	12	16	20	0	.00
83001	Gonadotropin (fsh)	90	115	144	0	.00
83001-26	Gonadotropin (fsh)	27	34	43	0	.00
83002	Gonadotropin (lh)	94	121	152	0	.00
83002-26	Gonadotropin (lh)	29	38	47	0	.00
83003	Assay growth hormone (hgh)	89	114	143	0	.00
83003-26	Assay growth hormone (hgh)	24	31	39	0	.00
83008	Assay guanosine	68	88	110	0	.00
83008-26	Assay guanosine	20	25	32	0	.00
83010	Assay haptoglobin, quant	77	99	124	0	.00
83010-26	Assay haptoglobin, quant	25	32	40	0	.00
83012	Assay haptoglobins	52	67	84	0	.00
83012-26	Assay haptoglobins	20	26	33	0	.00
83013	H pylori analysis	233	299	375	0	.00
83013-26	H pylori analysis	68	87	109	0	.00
83014	H pylori drug admin/collect	44	56	70	0	.00
83014-26	H pylori drug admin/collect	14	19	23	0	.00
83015	Heavy metal screen	88	113	142	0	.00
83015-26	Heavy metal screen	26	34	42	0	.00
83018	Quantitative screen, metals	39	51	63	0	.00
83018-26	Quantitative screen, metals	11	15	18	0	.00
83020	Hemoglobin electrophoresis	71	92	115	0	.00

NEW CODE CPT 2002 •

CPT	SHORT DESCRIPTION	50th	75th	90th	MFS	RVU
83020-26	Hemoglobin electrophoresis	19	24	30	20	.55
83021	Hemoglobin chromotography	97	124	156	0	.00
83021-26	Hemoglobin chromotography	32	41	52	0	.00
83026	Hemoglobin copper sulfate	17	22	27	0	.00
83026-26	Hemoglobin copper sulfate	10	13	17	0	.00
83030	Fetal hemoglobin, chemical	35	45	56	0	.00
83030-26	Fetal hemoglobin, chemical	12	16	20	0	.00
83033	Fetal hemoglobin assay, qual	19	24	30	0	.00
83033-26	Fetal hemoglobin assay, qual	5	7	9	0	.00
83036	Glycated hemoglobin test	53	68	86	0	.00
83036-26	Glycated hemoglobin test	19	25	31	0	.00
83045	Blood methemoglobin test	14	18	22	0	.00
83045-26	Blood methemoglobin test	5	6	7	0	.00
83050	Blood methemoglobin assay	47	61	76	0	.00
83050-26	Blood methemoglobin assay	16	20	25	0	.00
83051	Assay plasma hemoglobin	22	28	35	0	.00
83051-26	Assay plasma hemoglobin	7	9	11	0	.00
83055	Blood sulfhemoglobin test	22	28	35	0	.00
83055-26	Blood sulfhemoglobin test	7	9	12	0	.00
83060	Blood sulfhemoglobin assay	28	36	45	0	.00
83060-26	Blood sulfhemoglobin assay	8	10	13	0	.00
83065	Assay hemoglobin heat	12	16	20	0	.00
83065-26	Assay hemoglobin heat	4	6	7	0	.00
83068	Hemoglobin stability screen	14	18	23	0	.00
83068-26	Hemoglobin stability screen	4	5	6	0	.00
83069	Assay urine hemoglobin	11	15	18	0	.00

CPT	SHORT DESCRIPTION	50th	75th	90th	MFS	RVU
83069-26	Assay urine hemoglobin	3	4	6	0	.00
83070	Assay hemosiderin, qual	16	21	26	0	.00
83070-26	Assay hemosiderin, qual	5	7	9	0	.00
83071	Assay hemosiderin, quant	16	21	26	0	.00
83071-26	Assay hemosiderin, quant	5	6	8	0	.00
83080	Assay b hexosaminidase	233	299	375	0	.00
83080-26	Assay b hexosaminidase	68	87	109	0	.00
83088	Assay histamine	193	248	311	0	.00
83088-26	Assay histamine	60	77	96	0	.00
83090	Assay homocystine	160	205	257	0	.00
83150	Assay for hva	48	62	78	0	.00
83150-26	Assay for hva	16	20	26	0	.00
83491	Assay corticosteroids	100	128	161	0	.00
83491-26	Assay corticosteroids	29	37	47	0	.00
83497	Assay 5-hiaa	85	109	137	0	.00
83497-26	Assay 5-hiaa	26	34	43	0	.00
83498	Assay progesterone	147	189	237	0	.00
83498-26	Assay progesterone	49	62	78	0	.00
83499	Assay progesterone	74	95	119	0	.00
83499-26	Assay progesterone	22	29	36	0	.00
83500	Assay free hydroxyproline	67	86	107	0	.00
83500-26	Assay free hydroxyproline	21	27	34	0	.00
83505	Assay total hydroxyproline	88	112	141	0	.00
83505-26	Assay total hydroxyproline	25	33	41	0	.00
83516	Immunoassay, nonantibody	79	106	137	0	.00
83516-26	Immunoassay, nonantibody	25	34	44	0	.00

NEW CODE CPT 2002 •

CPT	SHORT DESCRIPTION	50th	75th	90th	MFS	RVU
83518	Immunoassay, dipstick	33	45	58	0	.00
83518-26	Immunoassay, dipstick	12	16	20	0	.00
83519	Immunoassay, nonantibody	83	112	145	0	.00
83519-26	Immunoassay, nonantibody	29	39	51	0	.00
83520	Immunoassay, ria	61	82	107	0	.00
83520-26	Immunoassay, ria	20	26	34	0	.00
83525	Assay insulin	67	90	117	0	.00
83525-26	Assay insulin	19	26	34	0	.00
83527	Assay insulin	84	113	146	0	.00
83527-26	Assay insulin	26	35	45	0	.00
83528	Assay intrinsic factor	74	100	129	0	.00
83528-26	Assay intrinsic factor	24	32	41	0	.00
83540	Assay iron	25	34	44	0	.00
83540-26	Assay iron	6	8	11	0	.00
83550	Iron binding test	28	38	49	0	.00
83550-26	Iron binding test	7	10	13	0	.00
83570	Assay idh enzyme	30	40	52	0	.00
83570-26	Assay idh enzyme	10	13	17	0	.00
83582	Assay ketogenic steroids	57	77	100	0	.00
83582-26	Assay ketogenic steroids	15	20	26	0	.00
83586	Assay 17- ketosteroids	71	96	124	0	.00
83586-26	Assay 17- ketosteroids	24	33	42	0	.00
83593	Fractionation, ketosteroids	110	148	192	0	.00
83593-26	Fractionation, ketosteroids	34	46	59	0	.00
83605	Assay lactic acid	51	68	89	0	.00
83605-26	Assay lactic acid	17	23	29	0	.00

CPT	SHORT DESCRIPTION	50th	75th	90th	MFS	RVU
83615	Lactate (ld) (ldh) enzyme	20	27	35	0	.00
83615-26	Lactate (ld) (ldh) enzyme	7	9	12	0	.00
83625	Assay ldh enzymes	115	156	201	0	.00
83625-26	Assay ldh enzymes	31	42	54	0	.00
83632	Placental lactogen	77	104	135	0	.00
83632-26	Placental lactogen	25	34	44	0	.00
83633	Test urine for lactose	16	22	29	0	.00
83633-26	Test urine for lactose	5	6	8	0	.00
83634	Assay urine for lactose	28	38	49	0	.00
83634-26	Assay urine for lactose	9	12	15	0	.00
83655	Assay lead	66	89	116	0	.00
83655-26	Assay lead	19	26	34	0	.00
83661	L/s ratio, fetal lung	104	140	181	0	.00
83661-26	L/s ratio, fetal lung	32	43	56	0	.00
83662	Foam stability, fetal lung	33	45	58	0	.00
83662-26	Foam stability, fetal lung	12	16	20	0	.00
83663	Fluoro polarize, fetal lung	0	0	0	0	.00
83664	Lamellar body, fetal lung	0	0	0	0	.00
83670	Assay lap enzyme	42	56	73	0	.00
83670-26	Assay lap enzyme	12	16	21	0	.00
83690	Assay lipase	29	39	50	0	.00
83690-26	Assay lipase	10	14	18	0	.00
83715	Assay blood lipoproteins	47	63	81	0	.00
83715-26	Assay blood lipoproteins	12	16	20	0	.00
83716	Assay blood lipoproteins	128	173	223	0	.00
83716-26	Assay blood lipoproteins	46	62	80	0	.00

NEW CODE CPT 2002 •

CPT	SHORT DESCRIPTION	50th	75th	90th	MFS	RVU
83718	Assay lipoprotein	32	44	56	0	.00
83718-26	Assay lipoprotein	9	12	16	0	.00
83719	Assay blood lipoprotein	33	45	58	0	.00
83719-26	Assay blood lipoprotein	11	15	19	0	.00
83721	Assay blood lipoprotein	34	46	59	0	.00
83721-26	Assay blood lipoprotein	11	15	20	0	.00
83727	Assay lrh hormone	74	100	129	0	.00
83727-26	Assay lrh hormone	24	32	41	0	.00
83735	Assay magnesium	26	36	46	0	.00
83735-26	Assay magnesium	10	13	17	0	.00
83775	Assay md enzyme	26	35	46	0	.00
83775-26	Assay md enzyme	8	11	14	0	.00
83785	Assay manganese	49	66	85	0	.00
83785-26	Assay manganese	15	20	26	0	.00
83788	Mass spectrometry qual	102	137	177	0	.00
83788-26	Mass spectrometry qual	34	45	59	0	.00
83789	Mass spectrometry quant	102	137	177	0	.00
83789-26	Mass spectrometry quant	34	45	59	0	.00
83805	Assay meprobamate	55	75	96	0	.00
83805-26	Assay meprobamate	19	25	33	0	.00
83825	Assay mercury	63	85	110	0	.00
83825-26	Assay mercury	20	27	35	0	.00
83835	Assay metanephrines	126	170	220	0	.00
83835-26	Assay metanephrines	37	49	64	0	.00
83840	Assay methadone	53	71	92	0	.00
83840-26	Assay methadone	17	23	30	0	.00

CPT	SHORT DESCRIPTION	50th	75th	90th	MFS	RVU
83857	Assay methemalbumin	34	46	59	0	.00
83857-26	Assay methemalbumin	11	15	19	0	.00
83858	Assay methsuximide	55	74	95	0	.00
83858-26	Assay methsuximide	17	24	30	0	.00
83864	Mucopolysaccharides	33	45	58	0	.00
83864-26	Mucopolysaccharides	9	13	16	0	.00
83866	Mucopolysaccharides screen	19	26	34	0	.00
83866-26	Mucopolysaccharides screen	5	7	9	0	.00
83872	Assay synovial fluid mucin	25	34	44	0	.00
83872-26	Assay synovial fluid mucin	8	11	15	0	.00
83873	Assay csf protein	85	115	149	0	.00
83873-26	Assay csf protein	29	39	51	0	.00
83874	Assay myoglobin	45	60	78	0	.00
83874-26	Assay myoglobin	15	20	26	0	.00
83883	Assay nephelometry not spec	35	49	67	0	.00
83883-26	Assay nephelometry not spec	11	15	20	0	.00
83885	Assay nickel	52	72	98	0	.00
83885-26	Assay nickel	16	22	30	0	.00
83887	Assay nicotine	46	63	86	0	.00
83887-26	Assay nicotine	14	19	26	0	.00
83890	Molecule isolate	32	44	60	0	.00
83890-26	Molecule isolate	9	13	17	0	.00
83891	Molecule isolate nucleic	76	105	144	0	.00
83891-26	Molecule isolate nucleic	22	30	42	0	.00
83892	Molecular diagnostics	31	42	58	0	.00
83892-26	Molecular diagnostics	9	12	17	0	.00

NEW CODE CPT 2002 •

CPT	SHORT DESCRIPTION	50th	75th	90th	MFS	RVU
83893	Molecule dot/slot/blot	28	39	54	0	.00
83893-26	Molecule dot/slot/blot	8	11	16	0	.00
83894	Molecule gel electrophor	43	60	82	0	.00
83894-26	Molecule gel electrophor	13	17	24	0	.00
83896	Molecular diagnostics	22	31	42	0	.00
83896-26	Molecular diagnostics	6	9	12	0	.00
83897	Molecule nucleic transfer	23	32	43	0	.00
83898	Molecule nucleic ampli	61	84	115	0	.00
83898-26	Molecule nucleic ampli	19	27	37	0	.00
83901	Molecule nucleic ampli	74	102	140	0	.00
83901-26	Molecule nucleic ampli	24	33	45	0	.00
83902	Molecular diagnostics	52	71	98	0	.00
83902-26	Molecular diagnostics	18	24	33	0	.00
83903	Molecule mutation scan	104	143	197	0	.00
83903-26	Molecule mutation scan	33	46	63	0	.00
83904	Molecule mutation identify	63	87	120	0	.00
83904-26	Molecule mutation identify	20	28	38	0	.00
83905	Molecule mutation identify	104	143	197	0	.00
83905-26	Molecule mutation identify	33	46	63	0	.00
83906	Molecule mutation identify	104	143	197	0	.00
83906-26	Molecule mutation identify	33	46	63	0	.00
83912	Genetic examination	48	66	90	0	.00
83912-26	Genetic examination	13	18	25	20	.55
83915	Assay nucleotidase	53	73	101	0	.00
83915-26	Assay nucleotidase	17	24	32	0	.00
83916	Oligoclonal bands	85	118	161	0	.00

CPT	SHORT DESCRIPTION	50th	75th	90th	MFS	RVU
83916-26	Oligoclonal bands	29	40	55	0	.00
83918	Organic acids, total, quant	153	211	290	0	.00
83918-26	Organic acids, total, quant	44	61	84	0	.00
83919	Organic acids, qual, each	140	193	265	0	.00
83919-26	Organic acids, qual, each	41	56	77	0	.00
83921	Organic acid, single, quant	177	244	335	0	.00
83925	Assay opiates	32	44	61	0	.00
83925-26	Assay opiates	13	18	24	0	.00
83930	Assay blood osmolality	27	37	51	0	.00
83930-26	Assay blood osmolality	8	12	16	0	.00
83935	Assay urine osmolality	29	40	55	0	.00
83935-26	Assay urine osmolality	9	13	17	0	.00
83937	Assay osteocalcin	78	107	147	0	.00
83937-26	Assay osteocalcin	25	34	47	0	.00
83945	Assay oxalate	62	86	117	0	.00
83945-26	Assay oxalate	21	29	40	0	.00
• 83950	Oncorprotein, her-2/neu	0	0	0	0	.00
83970	Assay parathormone	167	230	315	0	.00
83970-26	Assay parathormone	55	76	104	0	.00
83986	Assay body fluid acidity	16	22	30	0	.00
83986-26	Assay body fluid acidity	6	8	12	0	.00
83992	Assay for phencyclidine	74	102	139	0	.00
83992-26	Assay for phencyclidine	22	31	42	0	.00
84022	Assay phenothiazine	40	55	76	0	.00
84022-26	Assay phenothiazine	13	18	24	0	.00
84030	Assay blood pku	18	25	34	0	.00

NEW CODE CPT 2002 •

CPT	SHORT DESCRIPTION	50th	75th	90th	MFS	RVU
84030-26	Assay blood pku	5	7	10	0	.00
84035	Assay phenylketones	10	13	18	0	.00
84035-26	Assay phenylketones	3	4	5	0	.00
84060	Assay acid phosphatase	55	75	103	0	.00
84060-26	Assay acid phosphatase	18	25	34	0	.00
84061	Phosphatase, forensic exam	24	33	45	0	.00
84061-26	Phosphatase, forensic exam	7	10	14	0	.00
84066	Assay prostate phosphatase	55	77	105	0	.00
84066-26	Assay prostate phosphatase	19	27	37	0	.00
84075	Assay alkaline phosphatase	16	23	31	0	.00
84075-26	Assay alkaline phosphatase	4	6	8	0	.00
84078	Assay alkaline phosphatase	24	33	45	0	.00
84078-26	Assay alkaline phosphatase	7	9	13	0	.00
84080	Assay alkaline phosphatases	62	86	117	0	.00
84080-26	Assay alkaline phosphatases	19	26	35	0	.00
84081	Amniotic fluid enzyme test	73	101	138	0	.00
84081-26	Amniotic fluid enzyme test	24	33	46	0	.00
84085	Assay rbc pg6d enzyme	23	32	44	0	.00
84085-26	Assay rbc pg6d enzyme	8	12	16	0	.00
84087	Assay phosphohexose enzymes	26	35	48	0	.00
84087-26	Assay phosphohexose enzymes	7	10	14	0	.00
84100	Assay phosphorus	13	17	24	0	.00
84100-26	Assay phosphorus	4	5	7	0	.00
84105	Assay urine phosphorus	19	26	36	0	.00
84105-26	Assay urine phosphorus	6	8	11	0	.00
84106	Test for porphobilinogen	16	23	31	0	.00

CPT	SHORT DESCRIPTION	50th	75th	90th	MFS	RVU
84106-26	Test for porphobilinogen	4	5	7	0	.00
84110	Assay porphobilinogen	47	65	89	0	.00
84110-26	Assay porphobilinogen	14	20	27	0	.00
84119	Test urine for porphyrins	25	34	47	0	.00
84119-26	Test urine for porphyrins	7	10	14	0	.00
84120	Assay urine porphyrins	102	141	193	0	.00
84120-26	Assay urine porphyrins	30	41	56	0	.00
84126	Assay feces porphyrins	45	62	85	0	.00
84126-26	Assay feces porphyrins	13	19	25	0	.00
84127	Assay feces porphyrins	15	20	27	0	.00
84127-26	Assay feces porphyrins	5	7	10	0	.00
84132	Assay serum potassium	18	25	35	0	.00
84132-26	Assay serum potassium	5	8	10	0	.00
84133	Assay urine potassium	19	26	36	0	.00
84133-26	Assay urine potassium	6	8	11	0	.00
84134	Assay prealbumin	41	57	78	0	.00
84134-26	Assay prealbumin	12	17	23	0	.00
84135	Assay pregnanediol	48	66	90	0	.00
84135-26	Assay pregnanediol	16	22	31	0	.00
84138	Assay pregnanetriol	47	64	88	0	.00
84138-26	Assay pregnanetriol	15	21	29	0	.00
84140	Assay pregnenolone	109	150	206	0	.00
84140-26	Assay pregnenolone	23	32	43	0	.00
84143	Assay 17-hydroxypregneno	114	158	216	0	.00
84143-26	Assay 17-hydroxypregneno	38	52	71	0	.00
84144	Assay progesterone	87	120	164	0	.00

NEW CODE CPT 2002 •

CPT	SHORT DESCRIPTION	50th	75th	90th	MFS	RVU
84144-26	Assay progesterone	17	24	33	0	.00
84146	Assay prolactin	104	143	197	0	.00
84146-26	Assay prolactin	34	47	65	0	.00
84150	Assay prostaglandin	56	77	105	0	.00
84150-26	Assay prostaglandin	17	24	33	0	.00
84152	Assay psa, complexed	61	83	114	0	.00
84153	Assay psa, total	79	110	150	0	.00
84153-26	Assay psa, total	26	36	50	0	.00
84154	Assay psa, free	61	83	114	0	.00
84154-26	Assay psa, free	20	28	38	0	.00
84155	Assay protein	16	23	31	0	.00
84155-26	Assay protein	6	8	11	0	.00
84160	Assay serum protein	9	13	17	0	.00
84160-26	Assay serum protein	3	5	6	0	.00
84165	Assay serum proteins	55	77	105	0	.00
84165-26	Assay serum proteins	19	27	37	20	.55
84181	Western blot test	81	111	152	0	.00
84181-26	Western blot test	27	37	50	19	.53
84182	Protein, western blot test	136	187	257	0	.00
84182-26	Protein, western blot test	45	62	85	19	.53
84202	Assay rbc protoporphyrin	60	83	114	0	.00
84202-26	Assay rbc protoporphyrin	20	27	38	0	.00
84203	Test rbc protoporphyrin	15	21	29	0	.00
84203-26	Test rbc protoporphyrin	5	7	10	0	.00
84206	Assay proinsulin	66	91	125	0	.00
84206-26	Assay proinsulin	21	28	39	0	.00

CPT	SHORT DESCRIPTION	50th	75th	90th	MFS	RVU
84207	Assay vitamin b-6	177	243	334	0	.00
84207-26	Assay vitamin b-6	53	73	100	0	.00
84210	Assay pyruvate	29	40	55	0	.00
84210-26	Assay pyruvate	11	16	22	0	.00
84220	Assay pyruvate kinase	30	41	57	0	.00
84220-26	Assay pyruvate kinase	10	14	19	0	.00
84228	Assay quinine	43	59	80	0	.00
84228-26	Assay quinine	13	18	25	0	.00
84233	Assay estrogen	70	97	132	0	.00
84233-26	Assay estrogen	21	29	40	0	.00
84234	Assay progesterone	81	111	152	0	.00
84234-26	Assay progesterone	24	33	46	0	.00
84235	Assay endocrine hormone	172	238	326	0	.00
84235-26	Assay endocrine hormone	52	71	98	0	.00
84238	Assay nonendocrine receptor	197	272	372	0	.00
84238-26	Assay nonendocrine receptor	65	90	123	0	.00
84244	Assay renin	118	163	223	0	.00
84244-26	Assay renin	40	55	76	0	.00
84252	Assay vitamin b-2	145	200	273	0	.00
84252-26	Assay vitamin b-2	43	60	82	0	.00
84255	Assay selenium	38	52	64	0	.00
84255-26	Assay selenium	11	16	19	0	.00
84260	Assay serotonin	267	363	451	0	.00
84260-26	Assay serotonin	80	109	135	0	.00
84270	Assay sex hormone globul	90	122	152	0	.00
84270-26	Assay sex hormone globul	27	37	46	0	.00

NEW CODE CPT 2002 •

CPT	SHORT DESCRIPTION	50th	75th	90th	MFS	RVU
84275	Assay sialic acid	87	118	146	0	.00
84275-26	Assay sialic acid	25	34	42	0	.00
84285	Assay silica	67	91	113	0	.00
84285-26	Assay silica	19	26	33	0	.00
84295	Assay serum sodium	10	14	17	0	.00
84295-26	Assay serum sodium	3	5	6	0	.00
84300	Assay urine sodium	20	27	33	0	.00
84300-26	Assay urine sodium	6	9	11	0	.00
84305	Assay somatomedin	190	258	321	0	.00
84305-26	Assay somatomedin	61	83	103	0	.00
84307	Assay somatostatin	55	74	92	0	.00
84307-26	Assay somatostatin	18	24	30	0	.00
84311	Spectrophotometry	32	44	54	0	.00
84311-26	Spectrophotometry	10	13	16	0	.00
84315	Body fluid specific gravity	7	9	12	0	.00
84315-26	Body fluid specific gravity	3	4	5	0	.00
84375	Chromatogram assay, sugars	32	43	53	0	.00
84375-26	Chromatogram assay, sugars	9	12	15	0	.00
84376	Sugars, single, qual	27	36	45	0	.00
84376-26	Sugars, single, qual	8	11	14	0	.00
84377	Sugars, multiple, qual	27	36	45	0	.00
84377-26	Sugars, multiple, qual	8	11	14	0	.00
84378	Sugars single quant	64	87	108	0	.00
84378-26	Sugars single quant	21	29	36	0	.00
84379	Sugars multiple quant	64	87	108	0	.00
84379-26	Sugars multiple quant	21	29	36	0	.00

• NEW CODE CPT 2002   CPT codes and descriptions only copyright AMA

CPT	SHORT DESCRIPTION	50th	75th	90th	MFS	RVU
84392	Assay urine sulfate	39	53	66	0	.00
84392-26	Assay urine sulfate	10	13	17	0	.00
84402	Assay testosterone	116	158	196	0	.00
84402-26	Assay testosterone	36	49	61	0	.00
84403	Assay total testosterone	122	166	206	0	.00
84403-26	Assay total testosterone	37	50	62	0	.00
84425	Assay vitamin b-1	122	166	206	0	.00
84425-26	Assay vitamin b-1	39	53	66	0	.00
84430	Assay thiocyanate	42	58	72	0	.00
84430-26	Assay thiocyanate	14	18	23	0	.00
84432	Assay thyroglobulin	89	121	150	0	.00
84432-26	Assay thyroglobulin	28	38	47	0	.00
84436	Assay total thyroxine	31	43	53	0	.00
84436-26	Assay total thyroxine	7	10	12	0	.00
84437	Assay neonatal thyroxine	17	23	29	0	.00
84437-26	Assay neonatal thyroxine	6	8	9	0	.00
84439	Assay free thyroxine	61	82	102	0	.00
84439-26	Assay free thyroxine	16	22	28	0	.00
84442	Assay thyroid activity	65	89	110	0	.00
84442-26	Assay thyroid activity	16	22	28	0	.00
84443	Assay thyroid stim hormone	73	99	123	0	.00
84443-26	Assay thyroid stim hormone	18	24	30	0	.00
84445	Assay tsi	256	348	432	0	.00
84445-26	Assay tsi	77	104	130	0	.00
84446	Assay vitamin e	86	117	145	0	.00
84446-26	Assay vitamin e	27	36	45	0	.00

NEW CODE CPT 2002 •

CPT	SHORT DESCRIPTION	50th	75th	90th	MFS	RVU
84449	Assay transcortin	28	38	47	0	.00
84449-26	Assay transcortin	9	13	16	0	.00
84450	Transferase (ast) (sgot)	20	27	34	0	.00
84450-26	Transferase (ast) (sgot)	6	8	10	0	.00
84460	Alanine amino (alt) (sgpt)	20	27	34	0	.00
84460-26	Alanine amino (alt) (sgpt)	7	9	11	0	.00
84466	Assay transferrin	73	100	124	0	.00
84466-26	Assay transferrin	24	33	41	0	.00
84478	Assay triglycerides	18	24	30	0	.00
84478-26	Assay triglycerides	5	7	8	0	.00
84479	Assay thyroid (t3 or t4)	28	39	48	0	.00
84479-26	Assay thyroid (t3 or t4)	10	14	17	0	.00
84480	Assay, triiodothyronine (t3)	85	116	144	0	.00
84480-26	Assay, triiodothyronine (t3)	30	40	50	0	.00
84481	Free assay (ft-3)	117	159	197	0	.00
84481-26	Free assay (ft-3)	39	53	65	0	.00
84482	Reverse assay (t3)	185	251	311	0	.00
84482-26	Reverse assay (t3)	61	83	103	0	.00
84484	Assay troponin, quant	62	84	105	0	.00
84484-26	Assay troponin, quant	19	25	31	0	.00
84485	Assay duodenal fluid trypsin	25	34	42	0	.00
84485-26	Assay duodenal fluid trypsin	7	10	12	0	.00
84488	Test feces for trypsin	16	21	26	0	.00
84488-26	Test feces for trypsin	5	6	8	0	.00
84490	Assay feces for trypsin	19	26	32	0	.00
84490-26	Assay feces for trypsin	6	8	9	0	.00

CPT	SHORT DESCRIPTION	50th	75th	90th	MFS	RVU
84510	Assay tyrosine	32	44	54	0	.00
84510-26	Assay tyrosine	10	14	17	0	.00
84512	Assay troponin, qual	47	64	79	0	.00
84512-26	Assay troponin, qual	15	20	25	0	.00
84520	Assay urea nitrogen	17	23	29	0	.00
84520-26	Assay urea nitrogen	5	6	8	0	.00
84525	Urea nitrogen semi-quant	16	22	28	0	.00
84525-26	Urea nitrogen semi-quant	5	6	8	0	.00
84540	Assay urine/urea-n	21	29	36	0	.00
84540-26	Assay urine/urea-n	7	10	12	0	.00
84545	Urea-n clearance test	47	63	79	0	.00
84545-26	Urea-n clearance test	14	18	23	0	.00
84550	Assay blood/uric acid	17	23	29	0	.00
84550-26	Assay blood/uric acid	6	8	10	0	.00
84560	Assay urine/uric acid	21	28	35	0	.00
84560-26	Assay urine/uric acid	6	8	9	0	.00
84577	Assay feces/urobilinogen	22	31	38	0	.00
84577-26	Assay feces/urobilinogen	7	10	12	0	.00
84578	Test urine urobilinogen	10	14	18	0	.00
84578-26	Test urine urobilinogen	3	4	5	0	.00
84580	Assay urine urobilinogen	25	34	42	0	.00
84580-26	Assay urine urobilinogen	8	10	13	0	.00
84583	Assay urine urobilinogen	11	15	19	0	.00
84583-26	Assay urine urobilinogen	3	5	6	0	.00
84585	Assay urine vma	91	123	153	0	.00
84585-26	Assay urine vma	27	37	46	0	.00

NEW CODE CPT 2002 •

CPT	SHORT DESCRIPTION	50th	75th	90th	MFS	RVU
84586	Assay vip	81	110	136	0	.00
84586-26	Assay vip	27	36	45	0	.00
84588	Assay vasopressin	102	138	172	0	.00
84588-26	Assay vasopressin	34	46	57	0	.00
84590	Assay vitamin a	91	123	153	0	.00
84590-26	Assay vitamin a	30	41	50	0	.00
84591	Assay nos vitamin	0	0	0	0	.00
84597	Assay vitamin k	60	82	101	0	.00
84597-26	Assay vitamin k	17	24	29	0	.00
84600	Assay volatiles	41	56	69	0	.00
84600-26	Assay volatiles	12	17	21	0	.00
84620	Xylose tolerance test	51	70	86	0	.00
84620-26	Xylose tolerance test	15	21	26	0	.00
84630	Assay zinc	64	87	108	0	.00
84630-26	Assay zinc	21	28	35	0	.00
84681	Assay c-peptide	112	152	189	0	.00
84681-26	Assay c-peptide	37	50	62	0	.00
84702	Chorionic gonadotropin test	72	98	121	0	.00
84702-26	Chorionic gonadotropin test	23	31	39	0	.00
84703	Chorionic gonadotropin assay	38	52	65	0	.00
84703-26	Chorionic gonadotropin assay	12	16	20	0	.00
84830	Ovulation tests	31	43	53	0	.00
84830-26	Ovulation tests	10	13	16	0	.00
84999	Clinical chemistry test	0	0	0	0	.000

HEMATOLOGY AND COAGULATION

CPT	SHORT DESCRIPTION	50th	75th	90th	MFS	RVU
85002	Bleeding time test	27	32	40	0	.00

CPT	SHORT DESCRIPTION	50th	75th	90th	MFS	RVU
85002-26	Bleeding time test	9	10	13	0	.00
85007	Differential wbc count	16	18	23	0	.00
85007-26	Differential wbc count	5	6	8	0	.00
85008	Nondifferential wbc count	13	15	19	0	.00
85008-26	Nondifferential wbc count	5	6	8	0	.00
85009	Differential wbc count	11	13	16	0	.00
85009-26	Differential wbc count	4	5	6	0	.00
85013	Hematocrit	13	15	19	0	.00
85013-26	Hematocrit	3	4	5	0	.00
85014	Hematocrit	14	17	21	0	.00
85014-26	Hematocrit	4	4	5	0	.00
85018	Hemoglobin	14	17	21	0	.00
85018-26	Hemoglobin	6	7	8	0	.00
85021	Automated hemogram	24	28	35	0	.00
85021-26	Automated hemogram	7	8	10	0	.00
85022	Automated hemogram	27	31	39	0	.00
85022-26	Automated hemogram	8	9	11	0	.00
85023	Automated hemogram	34	39	49	0	.00
85023-26	Automated hemogram	11	13	16	0	.00
85024	Automated hemogram	30	35	44	0	.00
85024-26	Automated hemogram	9	11	13	0	.00
85025	Automated hemogram	32	38	47	0	.00
85025-26	Automated hemogram	10	11	14	0	.00
85027	Automated hemogram	27	31	39	0	.00
85027-26	Automated hemogram	9	10	13	0	.00
85031	Manual hemogram, cbc	27	32	40	0	.00

  NEW CODE CPT 2002 •

CPT	SHORT DESCRIPTION	50th	75th	90th	MFS	RVU
85031-26	Manual hemogram, cbc	7	9	11	0	.00
85041	Red blood cell (rbc) count	12	14	18	0	.00
85041-26	Red blood cell (rbc) count	5	6	8	0	.00
85044	Reticulocyte count	26	30	38	0	.00
85044-26	Reticulocyte count	9	10	12	0	.00
85045	Reticulocyte count	29	33	41	0	.00
85045-26	Reticulocyte count	9	11	14	0	.00
85046	Reticyte/hgb concentrate	32	38	47	0	.00
85048	White blood cell (wbc) count	16	18	23	0	.00
85048-26	White blood cell (wbc) count	7	8	10	0	.00
85060	Blood smear interpretation	56	65	82	24	.66
85060-26	Blood smear interpretation	16	19	24	0	.00
85097	Bone marrow interpretation	151	176	220	98	2.72
85130	Chromogenic substrate assay	31	41	55	0	.00
85130-26	Chromogenic substrate assay	10	14	18	0	.00
85170	Blood clot retraction	10	13	18	0	.00
85170-26	Blood clot retraction	3	4	6	0	.00
85175	Blood clot lysis time	19	26	34	0	.00
85175-26	Blood clot lysis time	6	8	11	0	.00
85210	Blood clot factor ii test	116	152	202	0	.00
85210-26	Blood clot factor ii test	33	44	59	0	.00
85220	Blood clot factor v test	173	228	304	0	.00
85220-26	Blood clot factor v test	57	75	100	0	.00
85230	Blood clot factor vii test	57	75	99	0	.00
85230-26	Blood clot factor vii test	17	22	30	0	.00
85240	Blood clot factor viii test	148	196	260	0	.00

CPT	SHORT DESCRIPTION	50th	75th	90th	MFS	RVU
85240-26	Blood clot factor viii test	47	63	83	0	.00
85244	Blood clot factor viii test	84	111	147	0	.00
85244-26	Blood clot factor viii test	26	34	46	0	.00
85245	Blood clot factor viii test	146	192	255	0	.00
85245-26	Blood clot factor viii test	50	65	87	0	.00
85246	Blood clot factor viii test	167	220	292	0	.00
85246-26	Blood clot factor viii test	57	75	99	0	.00
85247	Blood clot factor viii test	221	291	387	0	.00
85247-26	Blood clot factor viii test	75	99	131	0	.00
85250	Blood clot factor ix test	174	229	304	0	.00
85250-26	Blood clot factor ix test	50	66	88	0	.00
85260	Blood clot factor x test	60	79	105	0	.00
85260-26	Blood clot factor x test	17	23	30	0	.00
85270	Blood clot factor xi test	172	227	302	0	.00
85270-26	Blood clot factor xi test	50	66	88	0	.00
85280	Blood clot factor xii test	71	93	124	0	.00
85280-26	Blood clot factor xii test	21	27	36	0	.00
85290	Blood clot factor xiii test	64	85	112	0	.00
85290-26	Blood clot factor xiii test	19	25	33	0	.00
85291	Blood clot factor xiii test	30	39	52	0	.00
85291-26	Blood clot factor xiii test	9	12	17	0	.00
85292	Blood clot factor assay	58	77	102	0	.00
85292-26	Blood clot factor assay	20	26	35	0	.00
85293	Blood clot factor assay	58	77	102	0	.00
85293-26	Blood clot factor assay	20	26	35	0	.00
85300	Antithrombin iii test	120	158	210	0	.00

   NEW CODE CPT 2002 •

CPT	SHORT DESCRIPTION	50th	75th	90th	MFS	RVU
85300-26	Antithrombin iii test	39	52	69	0	.00
85301	Antithrombin iii test	139	183	243	0	.00
85301-26	Antithrombin iii test	46	60	80	0	.00
85302	Blood clot inhibitor antigen	151	200	265	0	.00
85302-26	Blood clot inhibitor antigen	50	66	88	0	.00
85303	Blood clot inhibitor test	165	218	290	0	.00
85303-26	Blood clot inhibitor test	53	70	93	0	.00
85305	Blood clot inhibitor assay	117	154	205	0	.00
85305-26	Blood clot inhibitor assay	41	54	72	0	.00
85306	Blood clot inhibitor test	152	201	267	0	.00
85306-26	Blood clot inhibitor test	50	66	88	0	.00
85307	Assay activated protein c	0	0	0	0	.00
85335	Factor inhibitor test	96	126	168	0	.00
85335-26	Factor inhibitor test	33	44	59	0	.00
85337	Thrombomodulin	53	69	92	0	.00
85337-26	Thrombomodulin	17	23	30	0	.00
85345	Coagulation time	10	14	18	0	.00
85345-26	Coagulation time	3	4	5	0	.00
85347	Coagulation time	22	30	39	0	.00
85347-26	Coagulation time	6	7	10	0	.00
85348	Coagulation time	16	21	28	0	.00
85348-26	Coagulation time	5	7	9	0	.00
85360	Euglobulin lysis	34	44	59	0	.00
85360-26	Euglobulin lysis	9	12	16	0	.00
85362	Fibrin degradation products	30	39	52	0	.00
85362-26	Fibrin degradation products	12	16	21	0	.00

CPT	SHORT DESCRIPTION	50th	75th	90th	MFS	RVU
85366	Fibrinogen test	34	44	59	0	.00
85366-26	Fibrinogen test	8	11	15	0	.00
85370	Fibrinogen test	32	42	56	0	.00
85370-26	Fibrinogen test	8	11	15	0	.00
85378	Fibrin degradation	36	47	62	0	.00
85378-26	Fibrin degradation	12	15	21	0	.00
85379	Fibrin degradation	40	53	70	0	.00
85379-26	Fibrin degradation	14	18	25	0	.00
85384	Fibrinogen	35	46	62	0	.00
85384-26	Fibrinogen	12	15	20	0	.00
85385	Fibrinogen	43	57	75	0	.00
85385-26	Fibrinogen	14	19	25	0	.00
85390	Fibrinolysins screen	206	272	361	0	.00
85390-26	Fibrinolysins screen	45	60	80	18	.50
85400	Fibrinolytic plasmin	54	72	95	0	.00
85400-26	Fibrinolytic plasmin	15	19	26	0	.00
85410	Fibrinolytic antiplasmin	54	72	95	0	.00
85410-26	Fibrinolytic antiplasmin	15	19	26	0	.00
85415	Fibrinolytic plasminogen	39	51	68	0	.00
85415-26	Fibrinolytic plasminogen	14	18	24	0	.00
85420	Fibrinolytic plasminogen	98	130	172	0	.00
85420-26	Fibrinolytic plasminogen	25	32	43	0	.00
85421	Fibrinolytic plasminogen	65	86	115	0	.00
85421-26	Fibrinolytic plasminogen	20	27	36	0	.00
85441	Heinz bodies, direct	9	11	14	0	.00
85441-26	Heinz bodies, direct	3	3	4	0	.00

NEW CODE CPT 2002 •

CPT	SHORT DESCRIPTION	50th	75th	90th	MFS	RVU
85445	Heinz bodies, induced	14	18	22	0	.00
85445-26	Heinz bodies, induced	5	6	7	0	.00
85460	Hemoglobin, fetal	41	51	62	0	.00
85460-26	Hemoglobin, fetal	12	15	18	0	.00
85461	Hemoglobin, fetal	42	53	64	0	.00
85461-26	Hemoglobin, fetal	11	14	17	0	.00
85475	Hemolysin	34	43	52	0	.00
85475-26	Hemolysin	10	12	15	0	.00
85520	Heparin assay	35	44	53	0	.00
85520-26	Heparin assay	10	13	15	0	.00
85525	Heparin	40	50	60	0	.00
85525-26	Heparin	13	16	19	0	.00
85530	Heparin-protamine tolerance	40	51	61	0	.00
85530-26	Heparin-protamine tolerance	13	16	19	0	.00
85536	Iron stain peripheral blood	0	0	0	0	.00
85540	Wbc alkaline phosphatase	74	94	113	0	.00
85540-26	Wbc alkaline phosphatase	22	27	33	0	.00
85547	Rbc mechanical fragility	25	31	37	0	.00
85547-26	Rbc mechanical fragility	7	8	10	0	.00
85549	Muramidase	89	112	135	0	.00
85549-26	Muramidase	29	37	45	0	.00
85555	Rbc osmotic fragility	25	32	38	0	.00
85555-26	Rbc osmotic fragility	8	10	12	0	.00
85557	Rbc osmotic fragility	48	60	73	0	.00
85557-26	Rbc osmotic fragility	14	17	21	0	.00
85576	Blood platelet aggregation	170	214	258	0	.00

CPT	SHORT DESCRIPTION	50th	75th	90th	MFS	RVU
85576-26	Blood platelet aggregation	42	54	65	20	.54
85585	Blood platelet estimation	15	19	23	0	.00
85585-26	Blood platelet estimation	4	5	6	0	.00
85590	Platelet count, manual	25	31	38	0	.00
85590-26	Platelet count, manual	7	9	11	0	.00
85595	Platelet count, automated	17	21	26	0	.00
85595-26	Platelet count, automated	6	8	10	0	.00
85597	Platelet neutralization	72	91	109	0	.00
85597-26	Platelet neutralization	22	28	34	0	.00
85610	Prothrombin time	23	28	34	0	.00
85610-26	Prothrombin time	7	9	11	0	.00
85611	Prothrombin test	22	28	34	0	.00
85611-26	Prothrombin test	7	9	11	0	.00
85612	Viper venom prothrombin time	28	35	42	0	.00
85612-26	Viper venom prothrombin time	8	10	12	0	.00
85613	Russell viper venom, diluted	83	105	126	0	.00
85613-26	Russell viper venom, diluted	24	30	37	0	.00
85635	Reptilase test	19	23	28	0	.00
85635-26	Reptilase test	6	7	9	0	.00
85651	Rbc sed rate, nonautomated	22	27	33	0	.00
85651-26	Rbc sed rate, nonautomated	5	7	8	0	.00
85652	Rbc sed rate, automated	26	32	39	0	.00
85660	Rbc sickle cell test	33	42	50	0	.00
85660-26	Rbc sickle cell test	11	14	17	0	.00
85670	Thrombin time, plasma	31	39	47	0	.00
85670-26	Thrombin time, plasma	8	10	12	0	.00

   CPT codes and descriptions only copyright AMA   NEW CODE CPT 2002 •

CPT	SHORT DESCRIPTION	50th	75th	90th	MFS	RVU
85675	Thrombin time, titer	22	27	33	0	.00
85675-26	Thrombin time, titer	7	9	11	0	.00
85705	Thromboplastin inhibition	45	57	69	0	.00
85705-26	Thromboplastin inhibition	15	19	23	0	.00
85730	Thromboplastin time, partial	28	35	43	0	.00
85730-26	Thromboplastin time, partial	8	11	13	0	.00
85732	Thromboplastin time, partial	60	76	92	0	.00
85732-26	Thromboplastin time, partial	19	24	28	0	.00
85810	Blood viscosity examination	49	62	75	0	.00
85810-26	Blood viscosity examination	11	14	16	0	.00
85999	Hematology procedure	0	0	0	0	.00

IMMUNOLOGY

CPT	SHORT DESCRIPTION	50th	75th	90th	MFS	RVU
86000	Agglutinins, febrile	32	39	47	0	.00
86000-26	Agglutinins, febrile	11	14	17	0	.00
86001	Allergen specific igg	2	3	3	0	.00
86003	Allergen specific ige	29	35	43	0	.00
86003-26	Allergen specific ige	9	12	14	0	.00
86005	Allergen specific ige	62	76	93	0	.00
86005-26	Allergen specific ige	25	30	37	0	.00
86021	Wbc antibody identification	101	123	151	0	.00
86021-26	Wbc antibody identification	29	36	44	0	.00
86022	Platelet antibodies	161	197	242	0	.00
86022-26	Platelet antibodies	52	63	77	0	.00
86023	Immunoglobulin assay	140	171	210	0	.00
86023-26	Immunoglobulin assay	49	60	74	0	.00
86038	Antinuclear antibodies	66	81	99	0	.00

CPT	SHORT DESCRIPTION	50th	75th	90th	MFS	RVU
86038-26	Antinuclear antibodies	22	27	33	0	.00
86039	Antinuclear antibodies (ana)	46	56	69	0	.00
86039-26	Antinuclear antibodies (ana)	15	19	23	0	.00
86060	Antistreptolysin o, titer	47	57	70	0	.00
86060-26	Antistreptolysin o, titer	12	14	18	0	.00
86063	Antistreptolysin o, screen	37	45	55	0	.00
86063-26	Antistreptolysin o, screen	11	13	16	0	.00
86077	Physician blood bank service	96	118	145	52	1.45
86077-26	Physician blood bank service	29	35	43	0	.00
86078	Physician blood bank service	119	145	178	54	1.48
86078-26	Physician blood bank service	36	44	53	0	.00
86079	Physician blood bank service	320	391	479	53	1.47
86079-26	Physician blood bank service	106	129	158	0	.00
86140	C-reactive protein	42	52	63	0	.00
86140-26	C-reactive protein	13	16	20	0	.00
• 86141	C-reactive protein, hs	0	0	0	0	.00
86146	Glycoprotein antibody	0	0	0	0	.00
86147	Cardiolipin antibody	95	116	143	0	.00
86147-26	Cardiolipin antibody	36	44	54	0	.00
86148	Phospholipid antibody	80	97	119	0	.00
86148-26	Phospholipid antibody	29	35	43	0	.00
86155	Chemotaxis assay	33	40	49	0	.00
86155-26	Chemotaxis assay	10	13	16	0	.00
86156	Cold agglutinin, screen	28	35	42	0	.00
86156-26	Cold agglutinin, screen	8	10	13	0	.00
86157	Cold agglutinin, titer	41	51	62	0	.00

  NEW CODE CPT 2002 •

CPT	SHORT DESCRIPTION	50th	75th	90th	MFS	RVU
86157-26	Cold agglutinin, titer	14	17	21	0	.00
86160	Complement, antigen	73	90	110	0	.00
86160-26	Complement, antigen	18	22	28	0	.00
86161	Complement/function activity	64	78	96	0	.00
86161-26	Complement/function activity	16	20	24	0	.00
86162	Complement, total (ch50)	126	155	189	0	.00
86162-26	Complement, total (ch50)	43	53	64	0	.00
86171	Complement fixation, each	32	39	48	0	.00
86171-26	Complement fixation, each	9	11	14	0	.00
86185	Counterimmunoelectrophoresis	35	42	52	0	.00
86185-26	Counterimmunoelectrophoresis	11	14	17	0	.00
86215	Deoxyribonuclease, antibody	81	99	122	0	.00
86215-26	Deoxyribonuclease, antibody	27	33	40	0	.00
86225	Dna antibody	74	91	112	0	.00
86225-26	Dna antibody	22	27	33	0	.00
86226	Dna antibody, single strand	104	127	156	0	.00
86226-26	Dna antibody, single strand	36	45	55	0	.00
86235	Nuclear antigen antibody	65	79	97	0	.00
86235-26	Nuclear antigen antibody	19	24	29	0	.00
86243	Fc receptor	60	73	90	0	.00
86243-26	Fc receptor	18	22	27	0	.00
86255	Fluorescent antibody, screen	67	82	100	0	.00
86255-26	Fluorescent antibody, screen	22	27	33	20	.55
86256	Fluorescent antibody, titer	63	77	95	0	.00
86256-26	Fluorescent antibody, titer	21	26	31	20	.55
86277	Growth hormone antibody	42	51	63	0	.00

CPT	SHORT DESCRIPTION	50th	75th	90th	MFS	RVU
86277-26	Growth hormone antibody	14	17	21	0	.00
86280	Hemagglutination inhibition	30	37	45	0	.00
86280-26	Hemagglutination inhibition	6	8	9	0	.00
86294	Immunoassay, tumor qual	0	0	0	0	.00
86300	Immunoassay, tumor ca 15-3	107	131	161	0	.00
86301	Immunoassay, tumor ca 19-9	114	139	171	0	.00
86304	Immunoassay, tumor, ca 125	113	138	170	0	.00
86308	Heterophile antibodies	27	33	41	0	.00
86308-26	Heterophile antibodies	10	13	16	0	.00
86309	Heterophile antibodies	32	39	48	0	.00
86309-26	Heterophile antibodies	9	11	13	0	.00
86310	Heterophile antibodies	32	39	48	0	.00
86310-26	Heterophile antibodies	11	13	16	0	.00
86316	Immunoassay, tumor other	104	127	156	0	.00
86316-26	Immunoassay, tumor other	30	37	45	0	.00
86317	Immunoassay,infectious agent	28	34	41	0	.00
86317-26	Immunoassay,infectious agent	9	11	13	0	.00
86318	Immunoassay,infectious agent	33	40	49	0	.00
86318-26	Immunoassay,infectious agent	13	16	20	0	.00
86320	Serum immunoelectrophoresis	104	128	156	0	.00
86320-26	Serum immunoelectrophoresis	42	51	63	20	.55
86325	Other immunoelectrophoresis	119	145	178	0	.00
86325-26	Other immunoelectrophoresis	39	48	59	20	.55
86327	Immunoelectrophoresis assay	59	72	88	0	.00
86327-26	Immunoelectrophoresis assay	19	23	28	23	.63
86329	Immunodiffuse	59	72	88	0	.00

NEW CODE CPT 2002 •

CPT	SHORT DESCRIPTION	50th	75th	90th	MFS	RVU
86329-26	Immunodiffuse	19	23	28	0	.00
86331	Immunodiffuse ouchterlony	46	57	70	0	.00
86331-26	Immunodiffuse ouchterlony	14	17	21	0	.00
86332	Immune complex assay	99	121	148	0	.00
86332-26	Immune complex assay	34	41	50	0	.00
86334	Immunofixation procedure	103	126	155	0	.00
86334-26	Immunofixation procedure	30	37	45	20	.55
• 86336	Inhibin a	0	0	0	0	.00
86337	Insulin antibodies	103	126	154	0	.00
86337-26	Insulin antibodies	35	43	52	0	.00
86340	Intrinsic factor antibody	100	123	150	0	.00
86340-26	Intrinsic factor antibody	33	41	50	0	.00
86341	Islet cell antibody	114	139	170	0	.00
86341-26	Islet cell antibody	39	47	58	0	.00
86343	Leukocyte histamine release	58	71	87	0	.00
86343-26	Leukocyte histamine release	19	23	29	0	.00
86344	Leukocyte phagocytosis	35	43	53	0	.00
86344-26	Leukocyte phagocytosis	12	15	18	0	.00
86353	Lymphocyte transformation	167	205	251	0	.00
86353-26	Lymphocyte transformation	50	61	75	0	.00
86359	T cells, total count	102	124	152	0	.00
86359-26	T cells, total count	34	41	50	0	.00
86360	T cell, absolute count/ratio	187	228	280	0	.00
86360-26	T cell, absolute count/ratio	62	75	92	0	.00
86361	T cell, absolute count	113	138	169	0	.00
86361-26	T cell, absolute count	37	46	56	0	.00

CPT	SHORT DESCRIPTION	50th	75th	90th	MFS	RVU
86376	Microsomal antibody	83	101	124	0	.00
86376-26	Microsomal antibody	26	31	38	0	.00
86378	Migration inhibitory factor	65	79	97	0	.00
86378-26	Migration inhibitory factor	21	26	32	0	.00
86382	Neutralization test, viral	58	71	87	0	.00
86382-26	Neutralization test, viral	18	22	27	0	.00
86384	Nitroblue tetrazolium dye	50	61	75	0	.00
86384-26	Nitroblue tetrazolium dye	17	21	26	0	.00
86403	Particle agglutination test	25	31	37	0	.00
86403-26	Particle agglutination test	5	6	8	0	.00
86406	Particle agglutination test	41	50	61	0	.00
86406-26	Particle agglutination test	10	12	15	0	.00
86430	Rheumatoid factor test	27	33	41	0	.00
86430-26	Rheumatoid factor test	9	11	14	0	.00
86431	Rheumatoid factor, quant	40	49	60	0	.00
86431-26	Rheumatoid factor, quant	15	19	23	0	.00
86485	Skin test, candida	27	33	40	0	.00
86485-26	Skin test, candida	9	11	13	0	.00
86490	Coccidioidomycosis skin test	18	22	27	11	.30
86490-26	Coccidioidomycosis skin test	6	7	8	0	.00
86510	Histoplasmosis skin test	20	24	30	12	.32
86510-26	Histoplasmosis skin test	7	8	10	0	.00
86580	Tb intradermal test	21	26	32	9	.26
86580-26	Tb intradermal test	7	9	10	0	.00
86585	Tb tine test	16	19	24	7	.20
86585-26	Tb tine test	5	6	8	0	.00

NEW CODE CPT 2002 •

CPT	SHORT DESCRIPTION	50th	75th	90th	MFS	RVU
86586	Skin test, unlisted	0	0	0	0	.00
86590	Streptokinase, antibody	27	33	40	0	.00
86590-26	Streptokinase, antibody	9	12	14	0	.00
86592	Blood serology, qualitative	23	28	34	0	.00
86592-26	Blood serology, qualitative	6	7	9	0	.00
86593	Blood serology, quantitative	21	26	32	0	.00
86593-26	Blood serology, quantitative	6	8	9	0	.00
86602	Antinomyces antibody	46	57	71	0	.00
86602-26	Antinomyces antibody	14	18	22	0	.00
86603	Adenovirus antibody	48	59	73	0	.00
86603-26	Adenovirus antibody	15	19	23	0	.00
86606	Aspergillus antibody	86	107	133	0	.00
86606-26	Aspergillus antibody	30	38	47	0	.00
86609	Bacterium antibody	190	236	294	0	.00
86609-26	Bacterium antibody	61	76	94	0	.00
86611	Bartonella antibody	0	0	0	0	.00
86612	Blastomyces antibody	68	84	105	0	.00
86612-26	Blastomyces antibody	20	25	31	0	.00
86615	Bordetella antibody	58	72	90	0	.00
86615-26	Bordetella antibody	17	22	27	0	.00
86617	Lyme disease antibody	106	131	163	0	.00
86617-26	Lyme disease antibody	35	43	54	0	.00
86618	Lyme disease antibody	88	109	135	0	.00
86618-26	Lyme disease antibody	28	35	43	0	.002
86619	Borrelia antibody	46	56	70	0	.00
86619-26	Borrelia antibody	14	17	21	0	.00

CPT	SHORT DESCRIPTION	50th	75th	90th	MFS	RVU
86622	Brucella antibody	54	67	83	0	.00
86622-26	Brucella antibody	18	22	28	0	.00
86625	Campylobacter antibody	58	72	90	0	.00
86625-26	Campylobacter antibody	17	22	27	0	.00
86628	Candida antibody	85	106	132	0	.00
86628-26	Candida antibody	27	34	42	0	.00
86631	Chlamydia antibody	42	52	64	0	.00
86631-26	Chlamydia antibody	13	17	21	0	.00
86632	Chlamydia igm antibody	143	177	220	0	.00
86632-26	Chlamydia igm antibody	46	57	70	0	.00
86635	Coccidioides antibody	77	96	119	0	.00
86635-26	Coccidioides antibody	22	28	35	0	.00
86638	Q fever antibody	48	59	73	0	.00
86638-26	Q fever antibody	15	19	23	0	.00
86641	Cryptococcus antibody	39	48	60	0	.00
86641-26	Cryptococcus antibody	14	17	21	0	.00
86644	Cmv antibody	86	107	133	0	.00
86644-26	Cmv antibody	29	35	44	0	.00
86645	Cmv antibody, igm	96	119	148	0	.00
86645-26	Cmv antibody, igm	33	42	52	0	.00
86648	Diphtheria antibody	88	109	135	0	.00
86648-26	Diphtheria antibody	31	38	47	0	.00
86651	Encephalitis antibody	46	56	70	0	.00
86651-26	Encephalitis antibody	16	20	25	0	.00
86652	Encephalitis antibody	46	56	70	0	.00
86652-26	Encephalitis antibody	16	20	25	0	.00

  NEW CODE CPT 2002 •

CPT	SHORT DESCRIPTION	50th	75th	90th	MFS	RVU
86653	Encephalitis antibody	46	56	70	0	.00
86653-26	Encephalitis antibody	16	20	25	0	.00
86654	Encephalitis antibody	46	56	70	0	.00
86654-26	Encephalitis antibody	16	20	25	0	.00
86658	Enterovirus antibody	131	163	202	0	.00
86658-26	Enterovirus antibody	46	57	71	0	.00
86663	Epstein-Barr antibody	67	84	104	0	.00
86663-26	Epstein-Barr antibody	24	29	36	0	.00
86664	Epstein-Barr antibody	66	82	102	0	.00
86664-26	Epstein-Barr antibody	22	27	34	0	.00
86665	Epstein-Barr antibody	89	111	137	0	.00
86665-26	Epstein-Barr antibody	29	36	45	0	.00
86666	Ehrlichia antibody	0	0	0	0	.00
86668	Francisella tularensis	35	43	53	0	.00
86668-26	Francisella tularensis	11	13	17	0	.00
86671	Fungus antibody	62	77	95	0	.00
86671-26	Fungus antibody	20	24	30	0	.00
86674	Giardia lamblia antibody	58	72	89	0	.00
86674-26	Giardia lamblia antibody	18	23	28	0	.00
86677	Helicobacter pylori	94	116	144	0	.00
86677-26	Helicobacter pylori	33	41	51	0	.00
86682	Helminth antibody	61	76	94	0	.00
86682-26	Helminth antibody	21	27	33	0	.00
86684	Hemophilus influenza	112	139	172	0	.00
86684-26	Hemophilus influenza	39	49	60	MFS	.00
86687	HTLV-I antibody	55	68	84	0	.00

CPT	SHORT DESCRIPTION	50th	75th	90th	MFS	RVU
86687-26	HTLV-I antibody	16	20	25	0	.00
86688	HTLV-II antibody	49	61	75	0	.00
86688-26	HTLV-II antibody	16	19	24	0	.00
86689	HTLV/HIV confirmatory test	94	116	144	0	.00
86689-26	HTLV/HIV confirmatory test	31	38	48	0	.00
86692	Hepatitis, delta agent	105	130	161	0	.00
86692-26	Hepatitis, delta agent	35	43	53	0	.00
86694	Herpes simplex test	83	103	128	0	.00
86694-26	Herpes simplex test	27	34	42	0	.00
86695	Herpes simplex test	69	86	107	0	.00
86695-26	Herpes simplex test	24	30	37	0	.00
86696	Herpes simplex type 2	92	114	142	0	.00
86698	Histoplasma	71	88	109	0	.00
86698-26	Histoplasma	23	28	35	0	.00
86701	HIV-1	79	98	122	0	.00
86701-26	HIV-1	24	30	38	0	.00
86702	HIV-2	91	113	140	0	.00
86702-26	HIV-2	32	39	49	0	.00
86703	HIV-1/hiv-2, single assay	52	65	80	0	.00
86703-26	HIV-1/hiv-2, single assay	17	21	27	0	.00
86704	Hepatitis B core antibody, total	59	73	91	0	.00
86704-26	Hepatitis B core antibody, total	19	24	30	0	.00
86705	Hepatitis B core antibody, igm	67	83	103	0	.00
86705-26	Hepatitis B core antibody, igm	21	26	32	0	.00
86706	Hepatitis B surface antibody	58	72	90	0	.00
86706-26	Hepatitis B surface antibody	20	25	31	0	.00

NEW CODE CPT 2002 •

CPT	SHORT DESCRIPTION	50th	75th	90th	MFS	RVU
86707	Hepatitis Be antibody	58	72	90	0	.00
86707-26	Hepatitis Be antibody	19	23	29	0	.00
86708	Hepatitis A antibody, total	63	79	98	0	.00
86708-26	Hepatitis A antibody, total	20	24	30	0	.00
86709	Hepatitis A antibody, igm	71	88	110	0	.00
86709-26	Hepatitis A antibody, igm	24	29	36	0	.00
86710	Influenza virus antibody	50	62	77	0	.00
86710-26	Influenza virus antibody	16	20	25	0	.00
86713	Legionella antibody	69	86	107	0	.00
86713-26	Legionella antibody	22	28	34	0	.00
86717	Leishmania antibody	48	59	73	0	.00
86717-26	Leishmania antibody	15	19	23	0	.00
86720	Leptospira antibody	46	56	70	0	.00
86720-26	Leptospira antibody	16	20	25	0	.00
86723	Listeria monocytogenes ab	46	56	70	0	.00
86723-26	Listeria monocytogenes ab	16	20	25	0	.00
86727	Lymph choriomeningitis ab	48	59	73	0	.00
86727-26	Lymph choriomeningitis ab	15	19	23	0	.00
86729	Lympho venereum antibody	45	55	69	0	.00
86729-26	Lympho venereum antibody	15	18	23	0	.00
86732	Mucormycosis antibody	46	56	70	0	.00
86732-26	Mucormycosis antibody	16	20	25	0	.00
86735	Mumps antibody	87	108	134	0	.00
86735-26	Mumps antibody	30	38	47	0	.00
86738	Mycoplasma antibody	68	85	105	0	.00
86738-26	Mycoplasma antibody	24	30	37	0	.00

CPT	SHORT DESCRIPTION	50th	75th	90th	MFS	RVU
86741	Neisseria meningitidis	46	56	70	0	.00
86741-26	Neisseria meningitidis	16	20	25	0	.00
86744	Nocardia antibody	46	56	70	0	.00
86744-26	Nocardia antibody	16	20	25	0	.00
86747	Parvovirus antibody	84	104	130	0	.00
86747-26	Parvovirus antibody	27	33	42	0	.00
86750	Malaria antibody	46	56	70	0	.00
86750-26	Malaria antibody	16	20	25	0	.00
86753	Protozoa antibody nos	86	107	133	0	.00
86753-26	Protozoa antibody nos	28	34	43	0	.00
86756	Respiratory virus antibody	49	61	76	0	.00
86756-26	Respiratory virus antibody	16	20	24	0	.00
86757	Rickettsia antibody	0	0	0	0	.00
86759	Rotavirus antibody	41	51	63	0	.00
86759-26	Rotavirus antibody	14	18	22	0	.00
86762	Rubella antibody	37	46	57	0	.00
86762-26	Rubella antibody	12	15	19	0	.00
86765	Rubeola antibody	105	130	161	0	.00
86765-26	Rubeola antibody	33	42	52	0	.00
86768	Salmonella antibody	46	56	70	0	.00
86768-26	Salmonella antibody	16	20	25	0	.00
86771	Shigella antibody	46	56	70	0	.00
86771-26	Shigella antibody	16	20	25	0	.00
86774	Tetanus antibody	85	105	131	0	.00
86774-26	Tetanus antibody	27	34	42	0	.00
86777	Toxoplasma antibody	70	87	108	0	.00

NEW CODE CPT 2002 •

CPT	SHORT DESCRIPTION	50th	75th	90th	MFS	RVU
86777-26	Toxoplasma antibody	23	29	36	0	.00
86778	Toxoplasma antibody, igm	94	116	144	0	.00
86778-26	Toxoplasma antibody, igm	30	37	46	0	.00
86781	Treponema pallidum, confirm	68	84	104	0	.00
86781-26	Treponema pallidum, confirm	22	28	34	0	.00
86784	Trichinella antibody	46	56	70	0	.00
86784-26	Trichinella antibody	16	20	25	0	.00
86787	Varicella-zoster antibody	91	113	141	0	.00
86787-26	Varicella-zoster antibody	29	36	45	0	.00
86790	Virus antibody nos	87	108	134	0	.00
86790-26	Virus antibody nos	30	38	47	0	.00
86793	Yersinia antibody	46	56	70	0	.00
86793-26	Yersinia antibody	16	20	25	0	.00
86800	Thyroglobulin antibody	74	92	114	0	.00
86800-26	Thyroglobulin antibody	24	29	36	0	.00
86803	Hepatitis C ab test	84	104	129	0	.00
86803-26	Hepatitis C ab test	29	36	45	0	.00
86804	Hepatitis C ab test, confirm	193	239	298	0	.00
86804-26	Hepatitis C ab test, confirm	62	77	95	0	.00
86805	Lymphocytotoxicity assay	162	201	250	0	.00
86805-26	Lymphocytotoxicity assay	55	68	85	0	.00
86806	Lymphocytotoxicity assay	54	68	84	0	.00
86806-26	Lymphocytotoxicity assay	18	22	28	0	.00
86807	Cytotoxic antibody screening	63	78	97	0	.00
86807-26	Cytotoxic antibody screening	19	23	29	0	.00
86808	Cytotoxic antibody screening	63	78	97	0	.00

CPT	SHORT DESCRIPTION	50th	75th	90th	MFS	RVU
86808-26	Cytotoxic antibody screening	18	23	28	0	.00
86812	Hla typing, a, b, or c	134	167	207	0	.00
86812-26	Hla typing, a, b, or c	40	50	62	0	.00
86813	Hla typing, a, b, or c	137	170	212	0	.00
86813-26	Hla typing, a, b, or c	41	51	63	0	.00
86816	Hla typing, dr/dq	113	140	174	0	.00
86816-26	Hla typing, dr/dq	33	41	51	0	.00
86817	Hla typing, dr/dq	388	481	598	0	.00
86817-26	Hla typing, dr/dq	116	144	179	0	.00
86821	Lymphocyte culture, mixed	345	429	533	0	.00
86821-26	Lymphocyte culture, mixed	104	129	160	0	.00
86822	Lymphocyte culture, primed	82	102	127	0	.00
86822-26	Lymphocyte culture, primed	27	34	42	0	.00
86849	Immunology procedure	0	0	0	0	.00

TRANSFUSION MEDICINE

CPT	SHORT DESCRIPTION	50th	75th	90th	MFS	RVU
86850	Rbc antibody screen	30	44	61	0	.00
86850-26	Rbc antibody screen	11	16	22	0	.00
86860	Rbc antibody elution	46	67	93	0	.00
86860-26	Rbc antibody elution	16	23	32	0	.00
86870	Rbc antibody identification	52	76	106	0	.00
86870-26	Rbc antibody identification	20	29	40	0	.00
86880	Coombs test	32	46	65	0	.00
86880-26	Coombs test	10	15	21	0	.00
86885	Coombs test	54	79	111	0	.00
86885-26	Coombs test	16	23	32	0	.00
86886	Coombs test	35	51	71	0	.00

  NEW CODE CPT 2002 •

CPT	SHORT DESCRIPTION	50th	75th	90th	MFS	RVU
86886-26	Coombs test	11	16	22	0	.00
86890	Autologous blood process	165	240	334	0	.00
86890-26	Autologous blood process	28	41	57	0	.00
86891	Autologous blood, op salvage	165	241	335	0	.00
86891-26	Autologous blood, op salvage	50	72	100	0	.00
86900	Blood typing, abo	14	20	28	0	.00
86900-26	Blood typing, abo	4	6	8	0	.00
86901	Blood typing, rh (d)	19	28	39	0	.00
86901-26	Blood typing, rh (d)	7	10	14	0	.00
86903	Blood typing, antigen screen	34	49	68	0	.00
86903-26	Blood typing, antigen screen	12	18	25	0	.00
86904	Blood typing, patient serum	71	103	144	0	.00
86904-26	Blood typing, patient serum	23	34	47	0	.00
86905	Blood typing, rbc antigens	36	52	72	0	.00
86905-26	Blood typing, rbc antigens	9	13	18	0	.00
86906	Blood typing, rh phenotype	16	23	32	0	.00
86906-26	Blood typing, rh phenotype	5	7	9	0	.00
86910	Blood typing, paternity test	193	281	392	0	.00
86910-26	Blood typing, paternity test	58	84	118	0	.00
86911	Blood typing, antigen system	22	32	45	0	.00
86911-26	Blood typing, antigen system	7	11	15	0	.00
86915	Bone marrow/stem cell prep	599	873	1215	0	.00
86915-26	Bone marrow/stem cell prep	239	349	486	0	.00
86920	Compatibility test	79	115	160	0	.00
86920-26	Compatibility test	17	24	34	0	.00
86921	Compatibility test	78	114	159	0	.00

CPT	SHORT DESCRIPTION	50th	75th	90th	MFS	RVU
86921-26	Compatibility test	25	37	51	0	.00
86922	Compatibility test	63	92	128	0	.00
86922-26	Compatibility test	20	29	41	0	.00
86927	Plasma, fresh frozen	55	80	111	0	.00
86927-26	Plasma, fresh frozen	14	20	28	0	.00
86930	Frozen blood prep	143	209	291	0	.00
86930-26	Frozen blood prep	43	63	87	0	.00
86931	Frozen blood thaw	143	209	291	0	.00
86931-26	Frozen blood thaw	43	63	87	0	.00
86932	Frozen blood freeze/thaw	148	216	300	0	.00
86932-26	Frozen blood freeze/thaw	44	65	90	0	.00
86940	Hemolysins/agglutinins, auto	25	36	51	0	.00
86940-26	Hemolysins/agglutinins, auto	7	11	15	0	.00
86941	Hemolysins/agglutinins	36	53	74	0	.00
86941-26	Hemolysins/agglutinins	11	15	21	0	.00
86945	Blood product/irradiation	46	67	93	0	.00
86945-26	Blood product/irradiation	14	21	29	0	.00
86950	Leukacyte transfuse	414	604	841	0	.00
86950-26	Leukacyte transfuse	124	181	252	0	.00
86965	Pooling blood platelets	54	79	110	0	.00
86965-26	Pooling blood platelets	16	23	32	0	.00
86970	Rbc pretreat	96	140	194	0	.00
86970-26	Rbc pretreat	28	40	56	0	.00
86971	Rbc pretreat	20	29	41	0	.00
86971-26	Rbc pretreat	5	8	11	0	.00
86972	Rbc pretreat	20	30	41	0	.00

   NEW CODE CPT 2002 •

CPT	SHORT DESCRIPTION	50th	75th	90th	MFS	RVU
86972-26	Rbc pretreat	7	10	13	0	.00
86975	Rbc pretreat, serum	117	170	237	0	.00
86975-26	Rbc pretreat, serum	36	53	74	0	.00
86976	Rbc pretreat, serum	117	170	237	0	.00
86976-26	Rbc pretreat, serum	36	53	74	0	.00
86977	Rbc pretreat, serum	117	170	237	0	.00
86977-26	Rbc pretreat, serum	36	53	74	0	.00
86978	Rbc pretreat, serum	150	219	305	0	.00
86978-26	Rbc pretreat, serum	47	68	95	0	.00
86985	Split blood or products	36	52	73	0	.00
86985-26	Split blood or products	12	17	24	0	.00
86999	Transfuse procedure	0	0	0	0	.00

MICROBIOLOGY

CPT	SHORT DESCRIPTION	50th	75th	90th	MFS	RVU
87001	Small animal inoculation	36	47	59	0	.00
87001-26	Small animal inoculation	11	14	18	0	.00
87003	Small animal inoculation	58	75	95	0	.00
87003-26	Small animal inoculation	18	24	31	0	.00
87015	Specimen concentration	34	44	56	0	.00
87015-26	Specimen concentration	11	15	18	0	.00
87040	Blood culture for bacteria	49	64	81	0	.00
87040-26	Blood culture for bacteria	17	22	28	0	.00
87045	Fecesculture, bacteria	50	66	83	0	.00
87045-26	Fecesculture, bacteria	17	22	28	0	.00
87046	Stool culture, bacteria, each	17	22	28	0	.00
87070	Culture bacteria, other	45	59	75	0	.00
87070-26	Culture bacteria, other	14	18	23	0	.00

CPT	SHORT DESCRIPTION	50th	75th	90th	MFS	RVU
87071	Culture bacteri aerobic other	21	28	35	0	.00
87073	Culture bacteria anaerobic	0	0	0	0	.00
87075	Culture bacteria anaerobic	44	57	72	0	.00
87075-26	Culture bacteria anaerobic	15	20	25	0	.00
87076	Culture anaerobe ident, each	44	58	73	0	.00
87076-26	Culture anaerobe ident, each	16	20	26	0	.00
87077	Culture aerobic identify	26	33	42	0	.00
87081	Culture screen only	28	36	46	0	.00
87081-26	Culture screen only	7	10	12	0	.00
87084	Culture specimen by kit	23	30	38	0	.00
87084-26	Culture specimen by kit	7	10	12	0	.00
87086	Urine culture/colony count	44	57	73	0	.00
87086-26	Urine culture/colony count	10	13	17	0	.00
87088	Urine bacteria culture	31	40	51	0	.00
87088-26	Urine bacteria culture	11	14	18	0	.00
87101	Skin fungi culture	35	45	57	0	.00
87101-26	Skin fungi culture	11	14	18	0	.00
87102	Fungus isolation culture	46	60	76	0	.00
87102-26	Fungus isolation culture	15	19	24	0	.00
87103	Blood fungus culture	35	45	58	0	.00
87103-26	Blood fungus culture	12	15	20	0	.00
87106	Fungi identification, yeast	37	47	60	0	.00
87106-26	Fungi identification, yeast	11	14	17	0	.00
87107	Fungi identification, mold	48	63	80	0	.00
87109	Mycoplasma	115	150	191	0	.00
87109-26	Mycoplasma	37	48	61	0	.00

NEW CODE CPT 2002 •

CPT	SHORT DESCRIPTION	50th	75th	90th	MFS	RVU
87110	Chlamydia culture	58	75	95	0	.00
87110-26	Chlamydia culture	17	23	29	0	.00
87116	Mycobacteria culture	62	80	102	0	.00
87116-26	Mycobacteria culture	18	23	30	0	.00
87118	Mycobacteric identification	39	51	65	0	.00
87118-26	Mycobacteric identification	11	15	19	0	.00
87140	Cultur type immunofluoresc	22	28	36	0	.00
87140-26	Cultur type immunofluoresc	7	9	11	0	.00
87143	Culture typing, glc/hplc	55	72	92	0	.00
87143-26	Culture typing, glc/hplc	18	23	29	0	.00
87147	Culture type, immunologic	35	45	58	0	.00
87147-26	Culture type, immunologic	11	14	18	0	.00
87149	Culture type, nucleic acid	56	72	92	0	.00
87152	Culture type pulse field gel	0	0	0	0	.00
87158	Culture typing, added method	18	23	29	0	.00
87158-26	Culture typing, added method	4	5	6	0	.00
87164	Dark field examination	91	118	150	0	.00
87164-26	Dark field examination	32	41	52	18	.50
87166	Dark field examination	36	47	59	0	.00
87166-26	Dark field examination	11	14	18	0	.00
87168	Macroscopic exam arthropod	0	0	0	0	.00
87169	Macacroscopic exam parasite	0	0	0	0	.00
87172	Pinworm exam	0	0	0	0	.00
87176	Tissue homogenization, culture	27	35	45	0	.00
87176-26	Tissue homogenization, culture	9	12	15	0	.00
87177	Ova and parasites smears	42	55	70	0	.00

CPT	SHORT DESCRIPTION	50th	75th	90th	MFS	RVU
87177-26	Ova and parasites smears	15	19	24	0	.00
87181	Microbe susceptible, diffuse	21	28	35	0	.00
87181-26	Microbe susceptible, diffuse	7	9	12	0	.00
87184	Microbe susceptible, disk	28	37	47	0	.00
87184-26	Microbe susceptible, disk	7	9	12	0	.00
87185	Microbe susceptible, enzyme	26	34	43	0	.00
87186	Microbe susceptible, mic	38	50	64	0	.00
87186-26	Microbe susceptible, mic	10	14	17	0	.00
87187	Microbe susceptible, mlc	34	44	56	0	.00
87187-26	Microbe susceptible, mlc	5	7	9	0	.00
87188	Microbe suscept, macrobroth	29	38	48	0	.00
87188-26	Microbe suscept, macrobroth	8	11	14	0	.00
87190	Microbe suscept, mycobacteri	27	35	45	0	.00
87190-26	Microbe suscept, mycobacteri	8	10	13	0	.00
87197	Bactericidal level, serum	48	62	79	0	.00
87197-26	Bactericidal level, serum	16	20	26	0	.00
• 87198	Cytomegalovirus antibody dfa	0	0	0	0	.00
• 87199	Enterovirus antibody, dfa	0	0	0	0	.00
87205	Smear, gram stain	20	26	33	0	.00
87205-26	Smear, gram stain	6	8	10	0	.00
87206	Smear, fluorescent/acid stai	32	41	53	0	.00
87206-26	Smear, fluorescent/acid stai	7	9	11	0	.00
87207	Smear, special stain	42	55	70	0	.00
87207-26	Smear, special stain	14	18	23	20	.56
87210	Smear, wet mount, saline/ink	19	25	32	0	.00
87210-26	Smear, wet mount, saline/ink	5	6	8	0	.00

  NEW CODE CPT 2002 •

CPT	SHORT DESCRIPTION	50th	75th	90th	MFS	RVU
87220	Tissue exam for fungi	22	28	36	0	.00
87220-26	Tissue exam for fungi	8	10	13	0	.00
87230	Assay toxin or antitoxin	74	96	122	0	.00
87230-26	Assay toxin or antitoxin	23	30	38	0	.00
87250	Virus inoculate, eggs/animal	77	100	127	0	.00
87250-26	Virus inoculate, eggs/animal	31	40	51	0	.00
87252	Virus inoculation, tissue	78	101	129	0	.00
87252-26	Virus inoculation, tissue	25	32	41	0	.00
87253	Virus inoculate tissue, addl	59	77	98	0	.00
87253-26	Virus inoculate tissue, addl	18	23	29	0	.00
87254	Virus inoculation, shell via	118	154	195	0	.00
87260	Adenovirus ag, if	59	77	98	0	.00
87260-26	Adenovirus ag, if	19	25	31	0	.00
87265	Pertussis ag, if	53	69	87	0	.00
87265-26	Pertussis ag, if	17	22	28	0	.00
87270	Chlamydia trachomatis ag, if	50	66	83	0	.00
87270-26	Chlamydia trachomatis ag, if	16	21	27	0	.00
87272	Cryptosporidum/gardia ag, if	47	61	78	0	.00
87272-26	Cryptosporidum/gardia ag, if	15	20	25	0	.00
87273	Herpes simplex 2, ag, if	0	0	0	0	.00
87274	Herpes simplex 1, ag, if	64	84	106	0	.00
87274-26	Herpes simplex 1, ag, if	21	27	34	0	.00
87275	Influenza B, ag, if	0	0	0	0	.00
87276	Influenza A, ag, if	42	55	70	0	.00
87276-26	Influenza A, ag, if	13	18	22	0	.00
87277	Legionella micdadei, ag, if	0	0	0	0	.00

CPT	SHORT DESCRIPTION	50th	75th	90th	MFS	RVU
87278	Legion pneumophilia ag, if	57	75	95	0	.00
87278-26	Legion pneumophilia ag, if	18	24	30	0	.00
87279	Parainfluenza, ag, if	0	0	0	0	.00
87280	Respiratory syncytial ag, if	60	78	100	0	.00
87280-26	Respiratory syncytial ag, if	19	25	32	0	.00
87281	Pneumocystis carinii, ag, if	0	0	0	0	.00
87283	Rubeola, ag, if	0	0	0	0	.00
87285	Treponema pallidum, ag, if	57	75	95	0	.00
87285-26	Treponema pallidum, ag, if	18	24	30	0	.00
87290	Varicella zoster, ag, if	62	80	102	0	.00
87290-26	Varicella zoster, ag, if	20	26	33	0	.00
87299	Antibody detection, nos, if	0	0	0	0	.00
87300	Ag detection, polyval, if	0	0	0	0	.00
87301	Adenovirus ag, eia	33	43	54	0	.00
87301-26	Adenovirus ag, eia	11	14	17	0	.00
87320	Chylmd trach ag, eia	42	54	69	0	.00
87320-26	Chylmd trach ag, eia	13	17	22	0	.00
87324	Clostridium ag, eia	76	99	126	0	.00
87324-26	Clostridium ag, eia	24	32	40	0	.00
87327	Cryptococcus neoform ag, eia	0	0	0	0	.00
87328	Cryptospor ag, eia	59	77	98	0	.00
87328-26	Cryptospor ag, eia	19	25	31	0	.00
87332	Cytomegalovirus ag, eia	33	43	54	0	.00
87332-26	Cytomegalovirus ag, eia	11	14	17	0	.00
87335	E coli 0157 ag, eia	86	111	142	0	.00
87335-26	E coli 0157 ag, eia	27	36	45	0	.00

NEW CODE CPT 2002 •

CPT	SHORT DESCRIPTION	50th	75th	90th	MFS	RVU
87336	Entamoeb hist dispr, ag, eia	0	0	0	0	.00
87337	Entamoeb hist group, ag, eia	0	0	0	0	.00
87338	Hpylori, stool, eia	88	114	145	0	.00
87338-26	Hpylori, stool, eia	24	31	39	0	.00
87339	H pylori ag, eia	0	0	0	0	.00
87340	Hepatitis b surface ag, eia	42	55	70	0	.00
87340-26	Hepatitis b surface ag, eia	14	18	22	0	.00
87341	Hepatitis b surface, ag, eia	64	83	106	0	.00
87350	Hepatitis be ag, eia	52	67	86	0	.00
87350-26	Hepatitis be ag, eia	17	22	27	0	.00
87380	Hepatitis delta ag, eia	44	58	73	0	.00
87380-26	Hepatitis delta ag, eia	14	18	23	0	.00
87385	Histoplasma capsul ag, eia	33	43	54	0	.00
87385-26	Histoplasma capsul ag, eia	11	14	17	0	.00
87390	HIV-1 ag, eia	61	79	100	0	.00
87390-26	HIV-1 ag, eia	21	27	34	0	.00
87391	HIV-2 ag, eia	59	76	97	0	.00
87391-26	HIV-2 ag, eia	20	26	33	0	.00
87400	Influenza a/b, ag, eia	37	48	61	0	.00
87420	Resp syncytial ag, eia	60	78	100	0	.00
87420-26	Resp syncytial ag, eia	19	25	32	0	.00
87425	Rotavirus ag, eia	100	130	165	0	.00
87425-26	Rotavirus ag, eia	32	42	53	0	.00
87427	Shiga-like toxin ag, eia	0	0	0	0	.00
87430	Strep A ag, eia	27	35	45	0	.00
87430-26	Strep A ag, eia	9	11	14	0	.00

CPT	SHORT DESCRIPTION	50th	75th	90th	MFS	RVU
87449	Ag detect nos, eia, mult	0	0	0	0	.00
87450	Ag detect nos, eia, single	32	41	53	0	.00
87450-26	Ag detect nos, eia, single	10	12	16	0	.00
87451	Ag detect polyval, eia, mult	0	0	0	0	.00
87470	Bartonella, dna, dir probe	57	75	95	0	.00
87470-26	Bartonella, dna, dir probe	18	24	30	0	.00
87471	Bartonella, dna, amp probe	100	130	165	0	.00
87471-26	Bartonella, dna, amp probe	33	43	54	0	.00
87472	Bartonella, dna, quant	121	157	200	0	.00
87472-26	Bartonella, dna, quant	39	50	64	0	.00
87475	Lyme dis, dna, dir probe	56	73	93	0	.00
87475-26	Lyme dis, dna, dir probe	18	23	30	0	.00
87476	Lyme dis, dna, amp probe	128	166	212	0	.00
87476-26	Lyme dis, dna, amp probe	42	55	70	0	.00
87477	Lyme dis, dna, quant	121	157	200	0	.00
87477-26	Lyme dis, dna, quant	39	50	64	0	.00
87480	Candida, dna, dir probe	63	82	104	0	.00
87480-26	Candida, dna, dir probe	20	26	33	0	.00
87481	Candida, dna, amp probe	100	130	165	0	.00
87481-26	Candida, dna, amp probe	33	43	54	0	.00
87482	Candida, dna, quant	118	154	195	0	.00
87482-26	Candida, dna, quant	39	51	64	0	.00
87485	Chylmd pneum, dna, dir probe	58	75	96	0	.00
87485-26	Chylmd pneum, dna, dir probe	19	24	31	0	.00
87486	Chylmd pneum, dna, amp probe	100	130	165	0	.00
87486-26	Chylmd pneum, dna, amp probe	33	43	54	0	.00

  NEW CODE CPT 2002 •

CPT	SHORT DESCRIPTION	50th	75th	90th	MFS	RVU
87487	Chylmd pneum, dna, quant	121	157	200	0	.00
87487-26	Chylmd pneum, dna, quant	39	50	64	0	.00
87490	Chylmd trach, dna, dir probe	54	70	89	0	.00
87490-26	Chylmd trach, dna, dir probe	17	22	29	0	.00
87491	Chylmd trach, dna, amp probe	305	396	504	0	.00
87491-26	Chylmd trach, dna, amp probe	101	131	166	0	.00
87492	Chylmd trach, dna, quant	100	130	165	0	.00
87492-26	Chylmd trach, dna, quant	33	43	54	0	.00
87495	Cytomeg, dna, dir probe	57	75	95	0	.00
87495-26	Cytomeg, dna, dir probe	18	24	30	0	.00
87496	Cytomeg, dna, amp probe	271	353	449	0	.00
87496-26	Cytomeg, dna, amp probe	90	116	148	0	.00
87497	Cytomeg, dna, quant	121	157	200	0	.00
87497-26	Cytomeg, dna, quant	39	50	64	0	.00
87510	Gardner vag, dna, dir probe	63	82	104	0	.00
87510-26	Gardner vag, dna, dir probe	20	26	33	0	.00
87511	Gardner vag, dna, amp probe	100	130	165	0	.00
87511-26	Gardner vag, dna, amp probe	33	43	54	0	.00
87512	Gardner vag, dna, quant	118	154	195	0	.00
87512-26	Gardner vag, dna, quant	39	51	64	0	.00
87515	Hepatitis B, dna, dir probe	57	75	95	0	.00
87515-26	Hepatitis B, dna, dir probe	18	24	30	0	.00
87516	Hepatitis B, dna, amp probe	200	260	331	0	.00
87516-26	Hepatitis B, dna, amp probe	66	86	109	0	.00
87517	Hepatitis B, dna, quant	202	263	334	0	.00
87517-26	Hepatitis B, dna, quant	65	84	107	0	.00

• NEW CODE CPT 2002　　CPT codes and descriptions only copyright AMA

CPT	SHORT DESCRIPTION	50th	75th	90th	MFS	RVU
87520	Hepatitis C, rna, dir probe	57	75	95	0	.00
87520-26	Hepatitis C, rna, dir probe	18	24	30	0	.00
87521	Hepatitis C, rna, amp probe	239	310	394	0	.00
87521-26	Hepatitis C, rna, amp probe	79	102	130	0	.00
87522	Hepatitis C, rna, quant	307	398	507	0	.00
87522-26	Hepatitis C, rna, quant	98	128	162	0	.00
87525	Hepatitis G, dna, dir probe	57	75	95	0	.00
87525-26	Hepatitis G, dna, dir probe	18	24	30	0	.00
87526	Hepatitis G, dna, amp probe	100	130	165	0	.00
87526-26	Hepatitis G, dna, amp probe	33	43	54	0	.00
87527	Hepatitis G, dna, quant	118	154	195	0	.00
87527-26	Hepatitis G, dna, quant	39	51	64	0	.00
87528	Hsv, dna, dir probe	57	75	95	0	.00
87528-26	Hsv, dna, dir probe	18	24	30	0	.00
87529	Hsv, dna, amp probe	100	130	165	0	.00
87529-26	Hsv, dna, amp probe	33	43	54	0	.00
87530	Hsv, dna, quant	121	157	200	0	.00
87530-26	Hsv, dna, quant	39	50	64	0	.00
87531	Hhv-6, dna, dir probe	57	75	95	0	.00
87531-26	Hhv-6, dna, dir probe	18	24	30	0	.00
87532	Hhv-6, dna, amp probe	100	130	165	0	.00
87532-26	Hhv-6, dna, amp probe	33	43	54	0	.00
87533	Hhv-6, dna, quant	118	154	195	0	.00
87533-26	Hhv-6, dna, quant	39	51	64	0	.00
87534	HIV-1, dna, dir probe	57	75	95	0	.00
87534-26	HIV-1, dna, dir probe	18	24	30	0	.00

 NEW CODE CPT 2002 •

CPT	SHORT DESCRIPTION	50th	75th	90th	MFS	RVU
87535	HIV-1, dna, amp probe	233	303	385	0	.00
87535-26	HIV-1, dna, amp probe	77	100	127	0	.00
87536	HIV-1, dna, quant	308	400	508	0	.00
87536-26	HIV-1, dna, quant	102	132	168	0	.00
87537	HIV-2, dna, dir probe	57	75	95	0	.00
87537-26	HIV-2, dna, dir probe	18	24	30	0	.00
87538	HIV-2, dna, amp probe	100	130	165	0	.00
87538-26	HIV-2, dna, amp probe	33	43	54	0	.00
87539	HIV-2, dna, quant	121	157	200	0	.00
87539-26	HIV-2, dna, quant	39	50	64	0	.00
87540	Legion pneumo, dna, dir prob	57	75	95	0	.00
87540-26	Legion pneumo, dna, dir prob	18	24	30	0	.00
87541	Legion pneumo, dna, amp prob	100	130	165	0	.00
87541-26	Legion pneumo, dna, amp prob	33	43	54	0	.00
87542	Legion pneumo, dna, quant	118	154	195	0	.00
87542-26	Legion pneumo, dna, quant	39	51	64	0	.00
87550	Mycobacteria, dna, dir probe	57	75	95	0	.00
87550-26	Mycobacteria, dna, dir probe	18	24	30	0	.00
87551	Mycobacteria, dna, amp probe	100	130	165	0	.00
87551-26	Mycobacteria, dna, amp probe	33	43	54	0	.00
87552	Mycobacteria, dna, quant	121	157	200	0	.00
87552-26	Mycobacteria, dna, quant	39	50	64	0	.00
87555	M.Tuberculo, dna, dir probe	57	75	95	0	.00
87555-26	M.Tuberculo, dna, dir probe	18	24	30	0	.00
87556	M.Tuberculo, dna, amp probe	100	130	165	0	.00
87556-26	M.Tuberculo, dna, amp probe	33	43	54	0	.00

CPT	SHORT DESCRIPTION	50th	75th	90th	MFS	RVU
87557	M.Tuberculo, dna, quant	121	157	200	0	.00
87557-26	M.Tuberculo, dna, quant	39	50	64	0	.00
87560	M.Avium-intra, dna, dir prob	57	75	95	0	.00
87560-26	M.Avium-intra, dna, dir prob	18	24	30	0	.00
87561	M.Avium-intra, dna, amp prob	100	130	165	0	.00
87561-26	M.Avium-intra, dna, amp prob	33	43	54	0	.00
87562	M.Avium-intra, dna, quant	121	157	200	0	.00
87562-26	M.Avium-intra, dna, quant	39	50	64	0	.00
87580	M.Pneumon, dna, dir probe	57	75	95	0	.00
87580-26	M.Pneumon, dna, dir probe	18	24	30	0	.00
87581	M.Pneumon, dna, amp probe	100	130	165	0	.00
87581-26	M.Pneumon, dna, amp probe	33	43	54	0	.00
87582	M.Pneumon, dna, quant	118	154	195	0	.00
87582-26	M.Pneumon, dna, quant	39	51	64	0	.00
87590	N.Gonorrhoeae, dna, dir prob	53	69	88	0	.00
87590-26	N.Gonorrhoeae, dna, dir prob	17	22	28	0	.00
87591	N.Gonorrhoeae, dna, amp prob	305	396	504	0	.00
87591-26	N.Gonorrhoeae, dna, amp prob	101	131	166	0	.00
87592	N.Gonorrhoeae, dna, quant	121	157	200	0	.00
87592-26	N.Gonorrhoeae, dna, quant	39	50	64	0	.00
87620	Hpv, dna, dir probe	106	137	174	0	.00
87620-26	Hpv, dna, dir probe	34	44	56	0	.00
87621	Hpv, dna, amp probe	305	396	504	0	.00
87621-26	Hpv, dna, amp probe	101	131	166	0	.00
87622	Hpv, dna, quant	118	154	195	0	.00
87622-26	Hpv, dna, quant	39	51	64	0	.00

NEW CODE CPT 2002 •

CPT	SHORT DESCRIPTION	50th	75th	90th	MFS	RVU
87650	Strep A, dna, dir probe	175	228	290	0	.00
87650-26	Strep A, dna, dir probe	56	73	93	0	.00
87651	Strep A, dna, amp probe	100	130	165	0	.00
87651-26	Strep A, dna, amp probe	33	43	54	0	.00
87652	Strep A, dna, quant	118	154	195	0	.00
87652-26	Strep A, dna, quant	39	51	64	0	.00
87797	Detect agent nos, dna, dir	58	75	95	0	.00
87797-26	Detect agent nos, dna, dir	18	24	31	0	.00
87798	Detect agent nos, dna, amp	305	396	504	0	.00
87798-26	Detect agent nos, dna, amp	101	131	166	0	.00
87799	Detect agent nos, dna, quant	0	0	0	0	.00
87800	Detect agent mult, dna, direc	122	159	202	0	.00
87801	Detect agent mult, dna, ampli	0	0	0	0	.00
• 87802	Strep B assay w/optic	0	0	0	0	.00
• 87803	Clostridium toxin a w/optic	0	0	0	0	.00
• 87804	Influenza assay w/optic	0	0	0	0	.00
87810	Chylmd trach assay w/optic	44	57	72	0	.00
87810-26	Chylmd trach assay w/optic	14	18	23	0	.00
87850	N. Gonorrhoeae assay w/optic	49	63	81	0	.00
87850-26	N. Gonorrhoeae assay w/optic	16	20	26	0	.00
87880	Strep A assay w/optic	42	55	70	0	.00
87880-26	Strep A assay w/optic	13	18	22	0	.00
87899	Agent nos assay w/optic	45	59	75	0	.00
87899-26	Agent nos assay w/optic	14	19	24	0	.00
87901	Genotype, dna, hiv reverse t	507	659	838	0	.00
• 87902	Genotype, dna, hepatitis c	0	0	0	0	.00

CPT	SHORT DESCRIPTION	50th	75th	90th	MFS	RVU
87903	Phenotype, dna hiv w/culture	0	0	0	0	.00
87904	Phenotype, dna hiv w/clt add	43	56	72	0	.00
87999	Microbiology procedure	0	0	0	0	.00

ANATOMIC PATHOLOGY

CPT	SHORT DESCRIPTION	50th	75th	90th	MFS	RVU
88000	Autopsy (necropsy), gross	454	550	675	0	.00
88005	Autopsy (necropsy), gross	511	619	759	0	.00
88007	Autopsy (necropsy), gross	568	688	844	0	.00
88012	Autopsy (necropsy), gross	476	577	708	0	.00
88014	Autopsy (necropsy), gross	476	577	708	0	.00
88016	Autopsy (necropsy), gross	585	709	870	0	.00
88020	Autopsy (necropsy), complete	732	886	1088	0	.00
88025	Autopsy (necropsy), complete	804	974	1195	0	.00
88027	Autopsy (necropsy), complete	878	1064	1305	0	.00
88028	Autopsy (necropsy), complete	822	995	1221	0	.00
88029	Autopsy (necropsy), complete	822	995	1221	0	.00
88036	Limited autopsy	680	824	1011	0	.00
88037	Limited autopsy	553	669	821	0	.00
88040	Forensic autopsy (necropsy)	2056	2490	3055	0	.00
88045	Coroner's autopsy (necropsy)	0	0	0	0	.00
88099	Necropsy (autopsy) procedure	0	0	0	0	.00

CYTOPATHOLOGY

CPT	SHORT DESCRIPTION	50th	75th	90th	MFS	RVU
88104	Cytopathology, fluids	107	130	160	48	1.32
88104-26	Cytopathology, fluids	73	89	109	30	.84
88106	Cytopathology, fluids	229	277	340	48	1.32
88106-26	Cytopathology, fluids	69	83	102	30	.84

          NEW CODE CPT 2002 •

CPT	SHORT DESCRIPTION	50th	75th	90th	MFS	RVU
88107	Cytopathology, fluids	103	125	153	66	1.82
88107-26	Cytopathology, fluids	81	98	121	41	1.14
88108	Cytopath, concentrate tech	109	132	162	56	1.54
88108-26	Cytopath, concentrate tech	87	106	130	30	.84
88125	Forensic cytopathology	68	83	102	21	.58
88125-26	Forensic cytopathology	21	25	30	14	.39
88130	Sex chromatin identification	45	54	66	0	.00
88130-26	Sex chromatin identification	13	16	19	0	.00
88140	Sex chromatin identification	35	42	51	0	.00
88140-26	Sex chromatin identification	10	12	15	0	.00
88141	Cytopath, c/v, interpret	36	44	54	22	.62
88142	Cytopath, c/v, thin layer	62	75	92	0	.00
88142-26	Cytopath, c/v, thin layer	17	20	25	0	.00
88143	Cytopath, c/v, thin lyr redo	60	72	89	0	.00
88143-26	Cytopath, c/v, thin lyr redo	21	25	31	0	.00
88144	Cytopath, c/v, thin lyr redo	94	114	139	0	.00
88144-26	Cytopath, c/v, thin lyr redo	20	24	29	0	.00
88145	Cytopath, c/v, thin lyr sel	99	120	147	0	.00
88145-26	Cytopath, c/v, thin lyr sel	25	30	37	0	.00
88147	Cytopath, c/v, automated	73	88	108	0	.00
88148	Cytopath, c/v, auto rescreen	62	75	91	0	.00
88148-26	Cytopath, c/v, auto rescreen	13	16	19	0	.00
88150	Cytopath, c/v, manual	27	32	40	0	.00
88150-26	Cytopath, c/v, manual	7	9	11	0	.00
88152	Cytopath, c/v, auto redo	38	47	57	0	.00
88152-26	Cytopath, c/v, auto redo	7	9	11	0	.00

CPT	SHORT DESCRIPTION	50th	75th	90th	MFS	RVU
88153	Cytopath, c/v, redo	75	91	111	0	.00
88153-26	Cytopath, c/v, redo	20	24	30	0	.00
88154	Cytopath, c/v, select	94	114	139	0	.00
88154-26	Cytopath, c/v, select	20	24	29	0	.00
88155	Cytopath, c/v, index add-on	28	34	41	0	.00
88155-26	Cytopath, c/v, index add-on	7	9	11	0	.00
88160	Cytopath smear, other source	55	67	82	56	1.55
88160-26	Cytopath smear, other source	27	32	39	27	.75
88161	Cytopath smear, other source	79	96	118	64	1.76
88161-26	Cytopath smear, other source	32	39	48	27	.75
88162	Cytopath smear, other source	127	154	189	56	1.54
88162-26	Cytopath smear, other source	38	46	57	41	1.14
88164	Cytopath tbs, c/v, manual	35	43	52	0	.00
88164-26	Cytopath tbs, c/v, manual	14	17	21	0	.00
88165	Cytopath tbs, c/v, redo	61	73	90	0	.00
88165-26	Cytopath tbs, c/v, redo	28	34	41	0	.00
88166	Cytopath tbs, c/v, auto redo	38	46	57	0	.00
88166-26	Cytopath tbs, c/v, auto redo	10	12	15	0	.00
88167	Cytopath tbs, c/v, select	80	97	119	0	.00
88167-26	Cytopath tbs, c/v, select	25	30	37	0	.00
88172	Cytopathology eval fna	153	185	227	48	1.32
88172-26	Cytopathology eval fna	121	146	180	33	.90
88173	Cytopath eval, fna, report	199	241	295	118	3.26
88173-26	Cytopath eval, fna, report	159	192	236	75	2.08
88180	Cell marker study	174	211	259	36	.99
88180-26	Cell marker study	66	80	98	20	.54

  NEW CODE CPT 2002 •

CPT	SHORT DESCRIPTION	50th	75th	90th	MFS	RVU
88182	Cell marker study	342	414	508	96	2.64
88182-26	Cell marker study	130	157	193	42	1.16
88199	Cytopathology procedure	0	0	0	0	.00

CYTOGENETIC STUDIES

CPT	SHORT DESCRIPTION	50th	75th	90th	MFS	RVU
88230	Tissue culture, lymphocyte	280	339	416	0	.00
88230-26	Tissue culture, lymphocyte	84	102	125	0	.00
88233	Tissue culture, skin/biopsy	307	372	456	0	.00
88233-26	Tissue culture, skin/biopsy	92	111	137	0	.00
88235	Tissue culture, placenta	301	364	447	0	.00
88235-26	Tissue culture, placenta	90	109	134	0	.00
88237	Tissue culture, bone marrow	330	399	490	0	.00
88237-26	Tissue culture, bone marrow	99	120	147	0	.00
88239	Tissue culture, tumor	219	265	325	0	.00
88239-26	Tissue culture, tumor	66	79	97	0	.00
88240	Cell cryopreserve/storage	120	146	179	0	.00
88240-26	Cell cryopreserve/storage	36	44	54	0	.00
88241	Frozen cell preparation	135	164	201	0	.00
88241-26	Frozen cell preparation	41	49	60	0	.00
88245	Chromosome analysis, 20-25	206	250	307	0	.00
88245-26	Chromosome analysis, 20-25	62	75	92	0	.00
88248	Chromosome analysis, 50-100	338	409	502	0	.00
88248-26	Chromosome analysis, 50-100	111	135	166	0	.00
88249	Chromosome analysis, 100	483	585	717	0	.00
88249-26	Chromosome analysis, 100	159	193	237	0	.00
88261	Chromosome analysis, 5	305	370	454	0	.00
88261-26	Chromosome analysis, 5	92	111	136	0	.00

CPT	SHORT DESCRIPTION	50th	75th	90th	MFS	RVU
88262	Chromosome analysis, 15-20	367	444	545	0	.00
88262-26	Chromosome analysis, 15-20	110	133	163	0	.00
88263	Chromosome analysis, 45	385	466	572	0	.00
88263-26	Chromosome analysis, 45	115	140	172	0	.00
88264	Chromosome analysis, 20-25	395	478	587	0	.00
88264-26	Chromosome analysis, 20-25	182	220	270	0	.00
88267	Chromosome analys, placenta	431	522	640	0	.00
88267-26	Chromosome analys, placenta	129	157	192	0	.00
88269	Chromosome analys, amniotic	418	506	621	0	.00
88269-26	Chromosome analys, amniotic	138	167	205	0	.00
88271	Cytogenetics, dna probe	52	64	78	0	.00
88272	Cytogenetics, 3-5	0	0	0	0	.00
88273	Cytogenetics, 10-30	142	172	211	0	.00
88274	Cytogenetics, 25-99	105	127	156	0	.00
88275	Cytogenetics, 100-300	166	201	247	0	.00
88280	Chromosome karyotype study	90	109	134	0	.00
88280-26	Chromosome karyotype study	27	33	40	0	.00
88283	Chromosome banding study	105	127	155	0	.00
88283-26	Chromosome banding study	31	38	47	0	.00
88285	Chromosome count, additional	132	160	196	0	.00
88285-26	Chromosome count, additional	40	48	59	0	.00
88289	Chromosome study, additional	108	131	160	0	.00
88289-26	Chromosome study, additional	32	39	48	0	.00
88291	Cyto/molecular report	97	117	144	28	.77
88291-26	Cyto/molecular report	29	35	43	0	.00
88299	Cytogenetic study	0	0	0	0	.00

  NEW CODE CPT 2002 •

CPT	SHORT DESCRIPTION	50th	75th	90th	MFS	RVU

SURGICAL PATHOLOGY

CPT	SHORT DESCRIPTION	50th	75th	90th	MFS	RVU
88300	Surgical path, gross	50	65	82	16	.44
88300-26	Surgical path, gross	39	51	64	5	.13
88302	Tissue exam by pathologist	88	115	144	32	.89
88302-26	Tissue exam by pathologist	70	92	115	7	.20
88304	Tissue exam by pathologist	129	170	213	43	1.20
88304-26	Tissue exam by pathologist	102	134	168	12	.33
88305	Tissue exam by pathologist	174	228	287	93	2.58
88305-26	Tissue exam by pathologist	139	183	229	41	1.12
88307	Tissue exam by pathologist	312	409	514	160	4.41
88307-26	Tissue exam by pathologist	250	327	411	87	2.39
88309	Tissue exam by pathologist	446	585	734	210	5.81
88309-26	Tissue exam by pathologist	357	468	588	123	3.41
88311	Decalcify tissue	43	56	70	17	.47
88311-26	Decalcify tissue	35	46	58	13	.36
88312	Special stains	176	231	290	82	2.26
88312-26	Special stains	56	74	93	29	.81
88313	Special stains	135	177	222	63	1.73
88313-26	Special stains	43	57	71	13	.36
88314	Histochemical stain	98	129	161	49	1.35
88314-26	Histochemical stain	29	39	48	24	.67
88318	Chemical histochemistry	143	187	235	37	1.03
88318-26	Chemical histochemistry	61	80	101	23	.63
88319	Enzyme histochemistry	140	184	231	109	3.02
88319-26	Enzyme histochemistry	67	88	111	29	.79
88321	Microslide consultation	146	191	240	71	1.96

CPT	SHORT DESCRIPTION	50th	75th	90th	MFS	RVU
88323	Microslide consultation	164	215	270	101	2.79
88325	Comprehensive review data	252	331	415	119	3.28
88329	Path consult introp	108	141	177	39	1.08
88331	Path consult intraop, 1 bloc	254	334	419	77	2.13
88331-26	Path consult intraop, 1 bloc	173	227	285	64	1.78
88332	Path consult intraop, addl	128	168	210	40	1.10
88332-26	Path consult intraop, addl	86	112	141	32	.88
88342	Immunocytochemistry	147	193	242	84	2.33
88342-26	Immunocytochemistry	98	129	162	46	1.27
88346	Immunofluorescent study	107	140	175	76	2.11
88346-26	Immunofluorescent study	75	98	123	46	1.28
88347	Immunofluorescent study	131	172	216	102	2.81
88347-26	Immunofluorescent study	98	129	162	46	1.27
88348	Electron microscopy	480	629	790	311	8.58
88348-26	Electron microscopy	365	478	600	81	2.25
88349	Scanning electron microscopy	326	428	537	338	9.35
88349-26	Scanning electron microscopy	248	325	408	41	1.14
88355	Analysis, skeletal muscle	342	448	562	159	4.38
88355-26	Analysis, skeletal muscle	253	332	416	101	2.78
88356	Analysis, nerve	332	436	547	295	8.14
88356-26	Analysis, nerve	246	323	405	163	4.49
88358	Analysis, tumor	213	280	351	172	4.74
88358-26	Analysis, tumor	158	207	260	153	4.22
88362	Nerve teasing preparations	224	294	368	205	5.65
88362-26	Nerve teasing preparations	128	167	210	117	3.23
88365	Tissue hybridization	129	170	213	109	3.01

NEW CODE CPT 2002 •

CPT	SHORT DESCRIPTION	50th	75th	90th	MFS	RVU
88371	Protein, western blot tissue	83	109	137	0	.00
88371-26	Protein, western blot tissue	27	36	45	19	.53
88372	Protein analysis w/probe	114	149	187	0	.00
88372-26	Protein analysis w/probe	37	49	62	20	.55
• **88380**	Microdissection	0	0	0	0	.00
88399	Surgical pathology procedure	0	0	0	0	.00

OTHER PROCEDURES

CPT	SHORT DESCRIPTION	50th	75th	90th	MFS	RVU
88400	Bilirubin total transcut	0	0	0	0	.00
89050	Body fluid cell count	25	34	45	0	.00
89050-26	Body fluid cell count	8	11	15	0	.00
89051	Body fluid cell count	28	39	51	0	.00
89051-26	Body fluid cell count	9	13	17	0	.00
89060	Exam synovial fluid crystals	38	51	68	0	.00
89060-26	Exam synovial fluid crystals	12	17	22	20	.56
89100	Sample intestinal contents	626	852	1134	105	2.91
89100-26	Sample intestinal contents	188	256	340	0	.00
89105	Sample intestinal contents	596	812	1080	100	2.77
89105-26	Sample intestinal contents	185	252	335	0	.00
89125	Specimen fat stain	29	39	52	0	.00
89125-26	Specimen fat stain	9	12	16	0	.00
89130	Sample stomach contents	577	785	1045	97	2.68
89130-26	Sample stomach contents	167	228	303	0	.00
89132	Sample stomach contents	291	395	526	49	1.35
89132-26	Sample stomach contents	93	127	168	0	.00
89135	Sample stomach contents	721	981	1305	121	3.35
89135-26	Sample stomach contents	209	285	379	0	.00

CPT	SHORT DESCRIPTION	50th	75th	90th	MFS	RVU
89136	Sample stomach contents	489	665	885	82	2.27
89136-26	Sample stomach contents	156	213	283	0	.00
89140	Sample stomach contents	717	975	1297	121	3.33
89140-26	Sample stomach contents	237	322	428	0	.00
89141	Sample stomach contents	865	1177	1566	146	4.02
89141-26	Sample stomach contents	303	412	548	0	.00
89160	Exam feces for meat fibers	11	15	20	0	.00
89160-26	Exam feces for meat fibers	4	5	7	0	.00
89190	Nasal smear for eosinophils	55	74	99	0	.00
89190-26	Nasal smear for eosinophils	18	25	33	0	.00
89250	Fertilization oocyte	1116	1519	2021	0	.00
89251	Culture oocyte w/embryos	0	0	0	0	.00
89252	Assist oocyte fertilization	2094	2849	3790	0	.00
89253	Embryo hatching	1061	1443	1921	0	.00
89254	Oocyte identification	579	788	1048	0	.00
89255	Prepare embryo for transfer	345	470	625	0	.00
89256	Prepare cryopreserved embryo	0	0	0	0	.00
89257	Sperm identification	0	0	0	0	.00
89258	Cryopreservation, embryo	666	906	1205	0	.00
89259	Cryopreservation, sperm	181	246	328	0	.00
89260	Sperm isolation, simple	99	134	179	0	.00
89261	Sperm isolation, complex	165	224	298	0	.00
89264	Identify sperm tissue	0	0	0	0	.00
89300	Semen analysis	55	74	99	0	.00
89300-26	Semen analysis	18	25	33	0	.00
89310	Semen analysis	45	62	82	0	.00

  NEW CODE CPT 2002 •

CPT	SHORT DESCRIPTION	50th	75th	90th	MFS	RVU
89310-26	Semen analysis	13	17	23	0	.00
89320	Semen analysis	91	123	164	0	.00
89320-26	Semen analysis	26	36	48	0	.00
89321	Semen analysis	43	58	77	0	.00
89325	Sperm antibody test	86	117	156	0	.00
89325-26	Sperm antibody test	24	33	44	0	.00
89329	Sperm evaluation test	75	102	136	0	.00
89329-26	Sperm evaluation test	28	38	50	0	.00
89330	Evaluation cervical mucus	85	116	154	0	.00
89330-26	Evaluation cervical mucus	24	32	43	0	.00
89350	Sputum specimen collection	21	29	39	15	.41
89350-26	Sputum specimen collection	7	10	14	0	.00
89355	Exam feces for starch	10	14	18	0	.00
89355-26	Exam feces for starch	3	4	6	0	.00
89360	Collect sweat for test	45	62	82	16	.45
89360-26	Collect sweat for test	13	18	24	0	.00
89365	Water load test	25	34	46	0	.00
89365-26	Water load test	8	10	14	0	.00
89399	Pathology lab procedure	0	0	0	0	.00

CPT	SHORT DESCRIPTION	50th	75th	90th	MFS	RVU

NEW CODE CPT 2002 •

CPT	SHORT DESCRIPTION	50th	75th	90th	MFS	RVU
IMMUNE GLOBULINS						
90281	Human ig, IM	38	46	55	0	.00
90283	Human ig, IV	67	80	97	0	.00
90287	Botulinum antitoxin	0	0	0	0	.00
90288	Botulism ig, IV	0	0	0	0	.00
90291	Cmv ig, IV	0	0	0	0	.00
90296	Diphtheria antitoxin	0	0	0	0	.00
90371	Hepatitis B ig, IM	82	99	119	0	.00
90375	Rabies ig, IM/sc	0	0	0	0	.00
90376	Rabies ig, heat treated	0	0	0	0	.00
90378	Rsv ig, IM, 50mg	1360	1636	1973	0	.00
90379	Rsv ig, IV	0	0	0	0	.00
90384	Rh ig, full-dose, IM	133	161	194	0	.00
90385	Rh ig, minidose, IM	0	0	0	0	.00
90386	Rh ig, IV	0	0	0	0	.00
90389	Tetanus ig, IM	0	0	0	0	.00
90393	Vaccina ig, IM	0	0	0	0	.00
90396	Varicella-zoster ig, IM	0	0	0	0	.00
90399	Immune globulin	0	0	0	0	.00
IMMUNIZATION ADMINISTRATION FOR VACCINES/TOXOIDS						
90471	Immunization admin	14	17	21	4	.11
90472	Immunization admin, each add	15	18	21	4	.11

CPT	SHORT DESCRIPTION	50th	75th	90th	MFS	RVU
• **90473**	Immune admin oral/nasal	0	0	0	0	.00
• **90474**	Immune admin oral/nasal addl	0	0	0	0	.00

VACCINES, TOXOIDS

CPT	SHORT DESCRIPTION	50th	75th	90th	MFS	RVU
90476	Adenovirus vaccine, type 4	0	0	0	0	.00
90477	Adenovirus vaccine, type 7	0	0	0	0	.00
90581	Anthrax vaccine, sc	0	0	0	0	.00
90585	Bcg vaccine, percut	27	32	39	0	.00
90586	Bcg vaccine, intravesical	0	0	0	0	.00
90632	Hepatitis A vaccine, adult IM	82	99	119	0	.00
90633	Hepatitis A vacc, ped/adol, 2 dose	56	68	82	0	.00
90634	Hepatitis A vacc, ped/adol, 3 dose	60	72	87	0	.00
90636	Hepatitis A/hep b vacc, adult IM	84	101	121	0	.00
90645	Hib vaccine, hboc, IM	37	45	54	0	.00
90646	Hib vaccine, prp-d, IM	39	47	57	0	.00
90647	Hib vaccine, prp-omp, IM	35	42	50	0	.00
90648	Hib vaccine, prp-t, IM	37	44	53	0	.00
90657	Flu vaccine, 6-35 mo, IM	17	20	24	0	.00
90658	Flu vaccine, 3 yrs, IM	15	19	22	0	.00
90659	Flu vaccine, whole, IM	17	20	24	0	.00
90660	Flu vaccine, nasal	13	16	19	0	.00
90665	Lyme disease vaccine, IM	81	97	117	0	.00
90669	Pneumococcal vacc, ped<5	87	104	126	0	.00
90675	Rabies vaccine, IM	174	210	253	0	.00
90676	Rabies vaccine, id	116	140	169	0	.00
90680	Rotovirus vaccine, oral	66	79	96	0	.00

NEW CODE CPT 2002 •

CPT	SHORT DESCRIPTION	50th	75th	90th	MFS	RVU
90690	Typhoid vaccine, oral	49	59	71	0	.00
90691	Typhoid vaccine, IM	57	68	82	0	.00
90692	Typhoid vaccine, h-p, sc/id	33	40	48	0	.00
90693	Typhoid vaccine, akd, sc	0	0	0	0	.00
90700	Dtap vaccine, IM	39	47	57	0	.00
90701	Dtp vaccine, IM	32	39	47	0	.00
90702	Dt vaccine < 7, IM	33	40	49	0	.00
90703	Tetanus vaccine, IM	30	36	43	0	.00
90704	Mumps vaccine, sc	37	45	54	0	.00
90705	Measles vaccine, sc	36	43	52	0	.00
90706	Rubella vaccine, sc	36	43	52	0	.00
90707	Mmr vaccine, sc	54	65	79	0	.00
90708	Measles-rubella vaccine, sc	48	58	70	0	.00
90709	Rubella & mumps vaccine, sc	40	48	58	0	.00
90710	Mmrv vaccine, sc	53	64	77	0	.00
90712	Oral poliovirus vaccine	31	37	45	0	.00
90713	Poliovirus, ipv, sc	37	45	54	0	.00
90716	Chicken pox vaccine, sc	72	87	105	0	.00
90717	Yellow fever vaccine, sc	83	99	120	0	.00
90718	Td vaccine > 7, IM	22	26	32	0	.00
90719	Diphtheria vaccine, IM	22	26	31	0	.00
90720	Dtp/hib vaccine, IM	56	67	81	0	.00
90721	Dtap/hib vaccine, IM	64	77	93	0	.00
90725	Cholera vaccine, injectable	26	32	38	0	.00
90727	Plague vaccine, IM	24	29	35	0	.00
90732	Pneumococcal vaccine	45	54	65	0	.00

CPT	SHORT DESCRIPTION	50th	75th	90th	MFS	RVU
90733	Meningococcal vaccine, sc	87	105	127	0	.00
90735	Encephalitis vaccine, sc	94	114	137	0	.00
90744	Hepatitis B vacc ped/adol 3 dose IM	63	76	92	0	.00
90746	Hepatitis B vaccine, adult, IM	79	95	114	0	.00
90747	Hepatitis B vacc, ill pat 4 dose IM	75	90	109	0	.00
90748	Hepatitis B/hib vaccine, IM	68	82	98	0	.00
90749	Vaccine toxoid	0	0	0	0	.00

THERAPEUTIC OR DIAGNOSTIC INFUSIONS (EXCLUDES CHEMOTHERAPY)

CPT	SHORT DESCRIPTION	50th	75th	90th	MFS	RVU
90780	IV infuse therapy, 1 hour	118	163	217	41	1.12
90781	IV infuse, additional hour	81	113	150	20	.56

THERAPEUTIC, PROPHYLACTIC OR DIAGNOSTIC INJECTIONS

CPT	SHORT DESCRIPTION	50th	75th	90th	MFS	RVU
90782	Injection, SC/IM	16	22	30	4	.11
90783	Injection, IA	17	24	32	15	.41
90784	Injection, IV	54	75	100	17	.48
90788	Injectiion antibiotic	17	23	31	4	.12
90799	Ther/prophylactic/dx inject	0	0	0	0	.00

PSYCHIATRY

CPT	SHORT DESCRIPTION	50th	75th	90th	MFS	RVU
90801	Psych dx interview	164	193	225	145	4.00
90802	Intac psych dx interview	190	224	261	154	4.25
90804	Psych, office, 20-30 min	76	90	105	64	1.77
90805	Psych, office, 20-30 min w/e&m	99	117	136	72	1.99
90806	Psych, office, 45-50 min	111	130	152	96	2.65
90807	Psych, office, 45-50 min w/e&m	151	178	208	104	2.86
90808	Psych, office, 75-80 min	167	197	230	142	3.92

NEW CODE CPT 2002 •

CPT	SHORT DESCRIPTION	50th	75th	90th	MFS	RVU
90809	Psych, office, 75-80, w/e&m	224	264	308	150	4.13
90810	Intac psych, off, 20-30 min	84	99	115	69	1.91
90811	Intac psych, 20-30, w/e&m	94	111	129	77	2.14
90812	Intac psych, off, 45-50 min	118	139	162	102	2.82
90813	Intac psych, 45-50 min w/e&m	179	211	246	110	3.05
90814	Intac psych, off, 75-80 min	181	214	249	149	4.12
90815	Intac psych, 75-80 w/e&m	188	222	259	155	4.28
90816	Psych, hosp, 20-30 min	106	125	146	67	1.85
90817	Psych, hosp, 20-30 min w/e&m	107	126	147	75	2.06
90818	Psych, hosp, 45-50 min	152	180	209	99	2.73
90819	Psych, hosp, 45-50 min w/e&m	166	195	228	106	2.93
90821	Psych, hosp, 75-80 min	167	197	230	145	4.00
90822	Psych, hosp, 75-80 min w/e&m	234	275	321	158	4.36
90823	Intac psych, hosp, 20-30 min	105	124	145	74	2.04
90824	Intac psych, hsp 20-30 w/e&m	115	135	158	81	2.25
90826	Intac psych, hosp, 45-50 min	129	153	178	106	2.94
90827	Intac psych, hsp 45-50 w/e&m	137	162	189	113	3.12
90828	Intac psych, hosp, 75-80 min	199	235	274	178	4.91
90829	Intac psych, hsp 75-80 w/e&m	194	228	266	159	4.40
90845	Psychoanalysis	121	150	192	92	2.54
90846	Family psych w/o patient	123	153	196	94	2.60
90847	Family psych w/patient	115	142	182	113	3.12
90849	Multiple family group psych	78	97	123	33	.91
90853	Group psychotherapy	64	80	102	34	.95
90857	Intac group psych	72	90	115	37	1.02
90862	Medication management	80	94	107	51	1.41

CPT	SHORT DESCRIPTION	50th	75th	90th	MFS	RVU
90865	Narcosynthesis	285	336	385	167	4.61
90870	Electroconvulsive therapy	194	228	262	96	2.66
90871	Electroconvulsive therapy	159	188	219	138	3.82
90875	Psychophysiological therapy	80	94	108	77	2.13
90876	Psychophysiological therapy	127	150	172	113	3.12
90880	Hypnotherapy	117	137	158	114	3.15
90882	Environmental manipulate	61	72	83	0	.00
90885	Psych evaluation records	59	70	80	50	1.38
90887	Consult with family	104	122	140	85	2.34
90889	Prepare report	57	67	77	0	.00
90899	Psychiatric service/therapy	0	0	0	0	.00

BIOFEEDBACK

CPT	SHORT DESCRIPTION	50th	75th	90th	MFS	RVU
90901	Biofeedback train, any meth	105	135	164	45	1.25
90911	Biofeedback peri/uro/rectal	207	266	323	65	1.80

DIALYSIS

CPT	SHORT DESCRIPTION	50th	75th	90th	MFS	RVU
90918	ESRD related services, month	787	1056	1458	616	17.01
90919	ESRD related services, month	619	831	1147	482	13.31
90920	ESRD related services, month	748	1004	1386	416	11.48
90921	ESRD related services, month	480	644	889	273	7.55
90922	ESRD related services, day	31	41	57	20	.55
90923	ESRD related services, day	36	49	67	16	.44
90924	ESRD related services, day	36	49	67	14	.38
90925	ESRD related services, day	17	23	32	9	.26
90935	Hemodialysis, one evaluation	273	367	507	76	2.11
90937	Hemodialysis, repeated eval	496	666	920	122	3.37

NEW CODE CPT 2002 •

CPT	SHORT DESCRIPTION	50th	75th	90th	MFS	RVU
• 90939	Hemodialysis study, transcut	0	0	0	0	.00
90940	Hemodialysis access study	0	0	0	0	.00
90945	Dialysis, one evaluation	263	353	488	80	2.21
90947	Dialysis, repeated eval	437	587	810	125	3.46
90989	Dialysis training, complete	715	961	1326	0	.00
90993	Dialysis training, incompl	125	167	231	0	.00
90997	Hemoperfuse	286	385	531	108	2.99
90999	Dialysis procedure	0	0	0	0	.00

GASTROENTEROLOGY

CPT	SHORT DESCRIPTION	50th	75th	90th	MFS	RVU
91000	Esophageal intubation	95	128	181	39	1.09
91000-26	Esophageal intubation	77	104	146	37	1.01
91010	Esophagus motility study	420	568	803	143	3.95
91010-26	Esophagus motility study	265	358	506	64	1.76
91011	Esophagus motility study	417	564	797	156	4.31
91011-26	Esophagus motility study	263	355	502	76	2.10
91012	Esophagus motility study	427	577	816	142	3.93
91012-26	Esophagus motility study	269	363	514	75	2.06
91020	Gastric motility	399	540	763	163	4.51
91020-26	Gastric motility	259	351	496	73	2.01
91030	Acid perfuse esophagus	167	226	319	117	3.23
91030-26	Acid perfuse esophagus	107	144	204	46	1.28
91032	Esophagus, acid reflux test	358	484	684	129	3.57
91032-26	Esophagus, acid reflux test	229	310	438	62	1.70
91033	Prolonged acid reflux test	569	770	1088	148	4.08
91033-26	Prolonged acid reflux test	313	423	599	66	1.83
91052	Gastric analysis test	183	247	349	110	3.03

CPT	SHORT DESCRIPTION	50th	75th	90th	MFS	RVU
91052-26	Gastric analysis test	106	143	203	40	1.11
91055	Gastric intubation for smear	129	175	247	117	3.22
91055-26	Gastric intubation for smear	86	117	165	46	1.26
91060	Gastric saline load test	100	135	191	28	.77
91060-26	Gastric saline load test	59	80	113	22	.62
91065	Breath hydrogen test	216	293	414	173	4.78
91065-26	Breath hydrogen test	132	178	252	10	.28
91100	Pass intestine bleeding tube	108	147	207	59	1.62
91105	Gastric intubation treat	119	161	227	22	.60
91122	Anal pressure record	283	382	541	170	4.71
91122-26	Anal pressure record	167	226	319	90	2.50
• **91123**	Irrigate fecal impaction	0	0	0	0	.00
91132	Electrogastrography	0	0	0	0	.00
91133	Electrogastrography w/test	0	0	0	0	.00
91299	Gastroenterology procedure	0	0	0	0	.00

OPHTHALMOLOGY

CPT	SHORT DESCRIPTION	50th	75th	90th	MFS	RVU
92002	Eye exam, new patient	76	89	105	67	1.86
92004	Eye exam, new patient	140	163	193	123	3.41
92012	Eye exam established pat	72	85	101	61	1.69
92014	Eye exam & treat	97	114	135	91	2.52
92015	Refraction	91	118	149	69	1.90
92018	New eye exam & treat	274	354	447	133	3.67
92019	Eye exam & treat	89	115	145	71	1.95
92020	Special eye evaluation	49	63	80	48	1.33
92060	Special eye evaluation	64	83	105	52	1.45
92060-26	Special eye evaluation	48	62	79	37	1.01

NEW CODE CPT 2002 •

CPT	SHORT DESCRIPTION	50th	75th	90th	MFS	RVU
92065	Orthoptic/pleoptic training	64	83	105	57	1.58
92065-26	Orthoptic/pleoptic training	43	56	70	19	.53
92070	Fitting contact lens	126	163	205	66	1.83
92081	Visual field exam(s)	106	138	174	80	2.22
92081-26	Visual field exam(s)	78	100	127	19	.53
92082	Visual field exam(s)	69	89	112	47	1.31
92082-26	Visual field exam(s)	54	70	89	24	.65
92083	Visual field exam(s)	103	133	168	73	2.03
92083-26	Visual field exam(s)	82	107	135	27	.74
92100	Serial tonometry exam(s)	81	105	132	61	1.69
92120	Tonography & eye evaluation	79	101	128	59	1.64
92130	Water provocation tonography	84	109	137	63	1.75
92135	Opthalmic dx imaging	97	125	158	67	1.85
92135-26	Opthalmic dx imaging	58	75	95	19	.53
• **92136**	Ophthalmic biometry	102	132	167	77	2.13
• **92136-26**	Ophthalmic biometry	37	48	60	28	.77
92140	Glaucoma provocative tests	58	75	95	55	1.52
92225	Special eye exam, initial	82	99	119	22	.62
92226	Special eye exam, subsequent	73	88	106	20	.56
92230	Eye exam with photos	232	279	337	85	2.35
92235	Eye exam with photos	214	258	311	127	3.50
92235-26	Eye exam with photos	126	152	183	44	1.22
92240	Icg angiography	277	334	402	232	6.41
92240-26	Icg angiography	169	203	245	60	1.65
92250	Eye exam with photos	81	97	117	66	1.83
92250-26	Eye exam with photos	64	77	93	24	.65

• NEW CODE CPT 2002   CPT codes and descriptions only copyright AMA

CPT	SHORT DESCRIPTION	50th	75th	90th	MFS	RVU
92260	Ophthalmoscopy/dynamometry	91	109	131	16	.45
92265	Eye muscle evaluation	205	247	298	75	2.08
92265-26	Eye muscle evaluation	177	213	256	44	1.21
92270	Electro-oculography	98	119	143	73	2.01
92270-26	Electro-oculography	85	102	123	44	1.21
92275	Electroretinography	213	257	309	83	2.30
92275-26	Electroretinography	183	221	266	54	1.49
92283	Color vision examination	34	41	49	34	.93
92283-26	Color vision examination	24	29	34	9	.25
92284	Dark adaptation eye exam	108	130	156	73	2.01
92284-26	Dark adaptation eye exam	76	92	111	12	.34
92285	Eye photography	52	63	76	37	1.02
92285-26	Eye photography	37	45	54	11	.30
92286	Internal eye photography	186	224	270	134	3.69
92286-26	Internal eye photography	162	195	235	36	.99
92287	Internal eye photography	362	436	525	144	3.99
92310	Contact lens fitting	179	269	375	83	2.30
92311	Contact lens fitting	145	218	305	83	2.28
92312	Contact lens fitting	191	287	401	89	2.46
92313	Contact lens fitting	216	324	452	78	2.15
92314	Prescribe contact lens	125	188	263	58	1.61
92315	Prescribe contact lens	146	219	306	51	1.41
92316	Prescribe contact lens	232	349	487	62	1.72
92317	Prescribe contact lens	151	226	316	52	1.43
92325	Modify contact lens	22	33	45	14	.39
92326	Replace contact lens	125	187	261	58	1.60

  NEW CODE CPT 2002 •

CPT	SHORT DESCRIPTION	50th	75th	90th	MFS	RVU
92330	Fitting artificial eye	151	227	317	77	2.13
92335	Fitting artificial eye	112	168	234	52	1.45
92340	Fitting spectacles	42	64	89	38	1.06
92341	Fitting spectacles	46	69	96	43	1.20
92342	Fitting spectacles	134	201	281	46	1.28
92352	Special spectacles fitting	47	71	99	38	1.06
92353	Special spectacles fitting	97	146	204	45	1.25
92354	Special spectacles fitting	618	929	1296	307	8.49
92355	Special spectacles fitting	301	452	631	149	4.12
92358	Eye prosthesis service	70	105	146	35	.96
92370	Repair & adjust spectacles	131	198	276	32	.88
92371	Repair & adjust spectacles	163	244	341	22	.61
92390	Supply spectacles	0	0	0	0	.00
92391	Supply contact lenses	0	0	0	0	.00
92392	Supply low vision aids	284	349	437	140	3.86
92393	Supply artificial eye	911	1118	1401	449	12.39
92395	Supply spectacles	101	125	156	50	1.38
92396	Supply contact lenses	164	202	253	81	2.25
92499	Eye service or procedure	0	0	0	0	.00

SPECIAL OTORHINOLARYNGOLOGIC SERVICES

CPT	SHORT DESCRIPTION	50th	75th	90th	MFS	RVU
92502	Ear and throat examination	244	328	445	103	2.85
92504	Ear microscopy examination	102	138	186	47	1.29
92506	Speech/hearing evaluation	110	148	200	95	2.62
92507	Speech/hearing therapy	164	221	300	75	2.08
92508	Speech/hearing therapy	161	217	294	74	2.04
92510	Rehab for ear implant	158	213	289	133	3.67

CPT	SHORT DESCRIPTION	50th	75th	90th	MFS	RVU
92511	Nasopharyngoscopy	168	226	306	81	2.23
92512	Nasal function studies	0	0	0	62	1.70
92516	Facial nerve function test	134	181	245	50	1.39
92520	Laryngeal function studies	0	0	0	47	1.31
92525	Oral function evaluation	220	296	401	118	3.26
92526	Oral function therapy	168	226	306	77	2.12
92531	Spontaneous nystagmus study	53	71	97	0	.00
92532	Positional nystagmus test	52	70	95	0	.00
92533	Caloric vestibular test	61	82	111	0	.00
92534	Optokinetic nystagmus test	32	43	58	0	.00
92541	Spontaneous nystagmus test	87	118	161	68	1.89
92541-26	Spontaneous nystagmus test	31	41	56	22	.62
92542	Positional nystagmus test	84	113	154	63	1.75
92542-26	Positional nystagmus test	28	37	51	18	.51
92543	Caloric vestibular test	96	129	177	18	.51
92543-26	Caloric vestibular test	29	39	53	6	.16
92544	Optokinetic nystagmus test	224	301	413	59	1.64
92544-26	Optokinetic nystagmus test	40	54	74	14	.40
92545	Oscillating tracking test	127	171	235	57	1.58
92545-26	Oscillating tracking test	37	50	68	13	.36
92546	Sinusoidal rotational test	152	205	281	92	2.54
92546-26	Sinusoidal rotational test	90	121	166	16	.44
92547	Supplemental electrical test	49	66	91	46	1.26
92548	Posturography	245	330	452	98	2.72
92548-26	Posturography	100	135	185	29	.80
92551	Pure tone hearing test, air	25	30	37	0	.00

  CPT codes and descriptions only copyright AMA NEW CODE CPT 2002 •

CPT	SHORT DESCRIPTION	50th	75th	90th	MFS	RVU
92552	Pure tone audiometry, air	31	38	46	16	.45
92553	Audiometry, air & bone	51	62	76	24	.67
92555	Speech threshold audiometry	30	36	44	14	.39
92556	Speech audiometry, complete	48	58	71	21	.59
92557	Comprehensive hearing test	91	110	135	45	1.23
92559	Group audiometric testing	61	74	91	0	.00
92560	Bekesy audiometry, screen	25	30	37	0	.00
92561	Bekesy audiometry, diagnosis	32	39	48	26	.73
92562	Loudness balance test	22	27	33	15	.42
92563	Tone decay hearing test	36	43	53	14	.39
92564	Sisi hearing test	43	52	64	18	.49
92565	Stenger test, pure tone	38	46	56	15	.41
92567	Tympanometry	35	42	52	20	.55
92568	Acoustic reflex testing	30	36	44	14	.39
92569	Acoustic reflex decay test	33	40	49	15	.42
92571	Filtered speech hearing test	23	28	34	14	.40
92572	Staggered spondaic word test	25	31	38	3	.09
92573	Lombard test	22	27	33	13	.36
92575	Sensorineural acuity test	32	38	47	11	.30
92576	Synthetic sentence test	31	38	46	17	.46
92577	Stenger test, speech	30	36	44	27	.74
92579	Visual audiometry (vra)	60	73	90	27	.74
92582	Conditioning play audiometry	60	73	89	27	.74
92583	Select picture audiometry	48	58	71	33	.91
92584	Electrocochleography	217	262	322	91	2.52
92585	Auditor evoke potent, compre	317	384	471	95	2.62

CPT	SHORT DESCRIPTION	50th	75th	90th	MFS	RVU
92585-26	Auditor evoke potent, compre	63	77	94	27	.75
92586	Auditor evoke potent, limit	127	154	189	68	1.87
92587	Evoked auditory test	86	104	128	56	1.54
92587-26	Evoked auditory test	22	26	32	8	.21
92588	Evoked auditory test	129	156	191	75	2.06
92588-26	Evoked auditory test	37	45	56	20	.55
92589	Auditory function test(s)	41	50	62	20	.56
92590	Hearing aid exam, one ear	89	108	133	0	.00
92591	Hearing aid exam, both ears	125	152	186	0	.00
92592	Hearing aid check, one ear	43	52	64	0	.00
92593	Hearing aid check, both ears	65	79	97	0	.00
92594	Electro hearing aid test, one	34	41	51	0	.00
92595	Electro hearing aid test, both	50	60	74	0	.00
92596	Ear protector evaluation	41	50	61	22	.61
92597	Oral speech device eval	190	229	282	0	.00
92598	Modify oral speech device	121	146	180	0	.00
92599	Ent procedure/service	0	0	0	0	.00

CARDIOVASCULAR SERVICES

CPT	SHORT DESCRIPTION	50th	75th	90th	MFS	RVU
92950	Heart/lung resuscitation cpr	503	596	708	203	5.60
92953	Temporary external pacing	124	147	174	17	.47
92960	Cardioversion electric, ext	394	466	554	165	4.56
92961	Cardioversion, electric, int	462	547	650	240	6.62
92970	Cardioassist, internal	435	515	612	180	4.96
92971	Cardioassist, external	197	234	277	97	2.69
• **92973**	Percut coronary thrombectomy	696	824	979	174	4.82
• **92974**	Cath place, cardio brachytx	786	931	1105	197	5.44

     NEW CODE CPT 2002 •

CPT	SHORT DESCRIPTION	50th	75th	90th	MFS	RVU
92975	Dissolve clot, heart vessel	1125	1333	1583	379	10.48
92977	Dissolve clot, heart vessel	666	789	937	291	8.03
92978	Intravasc us, heart add-on	367	434	516	259	7.15
92978-26	Intravasc us, heart add-on	260	308	366	95	2.62
92979	Intravasc us, heart add-on	711	842	1000	157	4.35
92979-26	Intravasc us, heart add-on	476	564	670	75	2.06
92980	Insert intracoronary stent	3365	3986	4733	791	21.84
92981	Insert intracoronary stent	1115	1321	1568	222	6.13
92982	Coronary artery dilation	2959	3504	4161	584	16.14
92984	Coronary artery dilation	1070	1267	1504	158	4.37
92986	Revise aortic valve	2772	3283	3899	1208	33.37
92987	Revise mitral valve	3317	3929	4665	1257	34.73
92990	Revise pulmonary valve	2232	2644	3140	965	26.65
92992	Revise heart chamber	4309	5103	6060	0	.00
92993	Revise heart chamber	2860	3387	4023	0	.00
92995	Coronary atherectomy	3206	3797	4510	644	17.78
92996	Coronary atherectomy add-on	1388	1643	1952	174	4.80
92997	Pul art balloon repair, percut	2497	2957	3512	622	17.18
92998	Pul art balloon repair, percut	1332	1578	1874	303	8.37
93000	ECG, complete	70	83	100	25	.70
93005	ECG, tracing	50	60	73	16	.45
93010	ECG, report	37	44	54	9	.25
93012	Transmission ECG	323	385	465	87	2.39
93014	Report on transmitted ECG	71	85	103	26	.73
93015	Cardiovascular stress test	332	396	478	100	2.76
93016	Cardiovascular stress test	92	110	132	23	.64

CPT	SHORT DESCRIPTION	50th	75th	90th	MFS	RVU
93017	Cardiovascular stress test	172	205	248	61	1.69
93018	Cardiovascular stress test	132	157	190	16	.43
93024	Cardiac drug stress test	360	430	519	102	2.83
93024-26	Cardiac drug stress test	169	202	244	61	1.69
• 93025	Microvolt t-wave assess	927	1105	1335	264	7.28
93040	Rhythm ECG with report	43	52	62	13	.37
93041	Rhythm ECG, tracing	21	25	30	5	.15
93042	Rhythm ECG, report	27	32	39	8	.22
93224	ECG monitor/report, 24 hrs	388	463	559	152	4.20
93225	ECG monitor/record, 24 hrs	109	130	157	45	1.25
93226	ECG monitor/report, 24 hrs	210	251	303	80	2.20
93227	ECG monitor/review, 24 hrs	154	183	221	27	.75
93230	ECG monitor/report, 24 hrs	390	465	562	161	4.46
93231	ECG monitor/record, 24 hrs	114	136	164	55	1.53
93232	ECG monitor/report, 24 hrs	156	187	225	79	2.18
93233	ECG monitor/review, 24 hrs	154	183	221	27	.75
93235	ECG monitor/report, 24 hrs	321	383	462	117	3.24
93236	ECG monitor/report, 24 hrs	109	130	157	94	2.61
93237	ECG monitor/review, 24 hrs	136	162	195	23	.63
93268	ECG record/review	399	476	574	159	4.38
93268-26	ECG record/review	80	95	115	0	.00
93270	ECG recording	102	122	148	45	1.25
93271	ECG monitoring and analysis	746	890	1075	87	2.39
93272	ECG review, interpret only	90	108	130	27	.74
93278	ECG signal-averaged	214	255	308	56	1.54
93278-26	ECG signal-averaged	68	82	98	13	.36

    NEW CODE CPT 2002 •

CPT	SHORT DESCRIPTION	50th	75th	90th	MFS	RVU
93303	Echo transthoracic	420	501	605	206	5.69
93303-26	Echo transthoracic	151	180	218	67	1.84
93304	Echo transthoracic	393	468	566	110	3.03
93304-26	Echo transthoracic	169	201	243	39	1.07
93307	Echo exam heart	502	649	863	188	5.18
93307-26	Echo exam heart	171	221	293	48	1.33
93308	Echo exam heart	435	562	747	99	2.73
93308-26	Echo exam heart	170	219	291	28	.77
93312	Echo transesophageal	1070	1382	1837	252	6.97
93312-26	Echo transesophageal	471	608	808	114	3.14
93313	Echo transesophageal	293	379	504	228	6.29
93314	Echo transesophageal	951	1228	1633	204	5.63
93314-26	Echo transesophageal	285	368	490	65	1.80
93315	Echo transesophageal	1060	1370	1821	283	7.82
93315-26	Echo transesophageal	509	657	874	144	3.99
93316	Echo transesophageal	766	990	1316	268	7.39
93317	Echo transesophageal	799	1032	1371	233	6.44
93317-26	Echo transesophageal	319	413	549	94	2.61
93318	Echo transesophageal intraop	0	0	0	0	.00
93320	Doppler echo exam, heart	278	359	477	83	2.28
93320-26	Doppler echo exam, heart	105	136	181	20	.55
93321	Doppler echo exam, heart	184	238	317	49	1.35
93321-26	Doppler echo exam, heart	46	60	79	8	.22
93325	Doppler color flow add-on	227	293	389	110	3.03
93325-26	Doppler color flow add-on	116	149	198	4	.11
93350	Echo transthoracic	707	914	1215	141	3.89

CPT	SHORT DESCRIPTION	50th	75th	90th	MFS	RVU
93350-26	Echo transthoracic	361	466	619	76	2.11
93501	Right heart catheterization	3066	4271	5661	770	21.28
93501-26	Right heart catheterization	889	1239	1642	160	4.42
93503	Insert/place heart catheter	585	815	1080	137	3.78
93505	Biopsy heart lining	1132	1576	2089	304	8.41
93505-26	Biopsy heart lining	815	1135	1504	232	6.41
93508	Cath placement, angiography	1994	2777	3681	669	18.49
93508-26	Cath placement, angiography	698	972	1288	218	6.02
93510	Left heart catheterization	5861	8163	10820	1565	43.23
93510-26	Left heart catheterization	879	1224	1623	231	6.37
93511	Left heart catheterization	9864	13738	18209	1566	43.26
93511-26	Left heart catheterization	1480	2061	2731	268	7.39
93514	Left heart catheterization	2431	3386	4488	1667	46.06
93514-26	Left heart catheterization	608	847	1122	369	10.19
93524	Left heart catheterization	2338	3257	4317	2066	57.06
93524-26	Left heart catheterization	468	651	863	368	10.17
93526	Rt & lt heart catheters	7310	10181	13495	2063	56.98
93526-26	Rt & lt heart catheters	1389	1934	2564	319	8.80
93527	Rt & lt heart catheters	7208	10039	13307	2084	57.58
93527-26	Rt & lt heart catheters	1586	2209	2928	387	10.69
93528	Rt & lt heart catheters	2451	3413	4524	2178	60.17
93528-26	Rt & lt heart catheters	515	717	950	481	13.28
93529	Rt & lt heart catheterization	2205	3070	4070	1953	53.94
93529-26	Rt & lt heart catheterization	309	430	570	255	7.05
93530	Rt heart cath, congenital	1224	1704	2259	830	22.93
93530-26	Rt heart cath, congenital	392	545	723	220	6.07

NEW CODE CPT 2002 •

CPT	SHORT DESCRIPTION	50th	75th	90th	MFS	RVU
93531	Rt & lt heart cath, congenital	3636	5063	6712	2180	60.23
93531-26	Rt & lt heart cath, congenital	800	1114	1477	436	12.05
93532	Rt & lt heart cath, congenital	3251	4527	6001	2227	61.53
93532-26	Rt & lt heart cath, congenital	878	1222	1620	530	14.64
93533	Rt & lt heart cath, congenital	2965	4129	5473	2048	56.57
93533-26	Rt & lt heart cath, congenital	504	702	930	350	9.68
93539	Inject for cardiac cath	250	349	462	45	1.25
93540	Inject for cardiac cath	268	373	495	47	1.30
93541	Inject for lung angiogram	285	397	526	15	.42
93542	Inject for heart x-rays	306	427	565	15	.42
93543	Inject for heart x-rays	262	364	483	31	.85
93544	Inject for aortography	240	334	443	29	.79
93545	Inject for coronary x-rays	411	573	760	46	1.26
93555	Imaging, cardiac cath	844	1175	1557	268	7.39
93555-26	Imaging, cardiac cath	135	188	249	43	1.18
93556	Imaging, cardiac cath	1314	1830	2426	398	10.99
93556-26	Imaging, cardiac cath	158	220	291	44	1.21
93561	Cardiac output measurement	181	253	335	45	1.24
93561-26	Cardiac output measurement	140	195	258	25	.68
93562	Cardiac output measurement	106	148	196	20	.54
93562-26	Cardiac output measurement	71	99	131	8	.22
93571	Heart flow reserve measure	526	732	970	260	7.17
93571-26	Heart flow reserve measure	194	271	359	96	2.64
93572	Heart flow reserve measure	327	455	603	160	4.42
93572-26	Heart flow reserve measure	105	146	193	77	2.13
93600	Bundle his recording	585	760	1015	184	5.08

CPT	SHORT DESCRIPTION	50th	75th	90th	MFS	RVU
93600-26	Bundle his recording	251	327	436	113	3.12
93602	Intra-atrial recording	319	415	554	153	4.24
93602-26	Intra-atrial recording	198	257	344	113	3.12
93603-26	Right ventricular recording	188	245	327	112	3.09
93609	Map tachycardia, add-on	4421	5749	7676	364	10.06
93609-26	Map tachycardia, add-on	1326	1725	2303	266	7.34
93610	Intra-atrial pacing	434	565	754	210	5.79
93610-26	Intra-atrial pacing	204	265	354	160	4.42
93612	Intraventricular pacing	454	590	788	219	6.04
93612-26	Intraventricular pacing	195	254	339	160	4.42
• **93613**	Electrophys map, 3D, add-on	0	0	0	0	.00
93615	Esophageal recording	301	391	522	62	1.70
93615-26	Esophageal recording	144	188	251	50	1.38
93616	Esophageal recording	251	327	437	86	2.37
93616-26	Esophageal recording	116	150	201	74	2.05
93618	Heart rhythm pacing	2449	3184	4251	370	10.22
93618-26	Heart rhythm pacing	979	1274	1701	227	6.26
93619	Electrophysiology evaluation	3241	4215	5628	666	18.41
93619-26	Electrophysiology evaluation	2172	2824	3771	387	10.70
93620	Electrophysiology evaluation	4307	5601	7477	940	25.96
93620-26	Electrophysiology evaluation	2885	3753	5010	616	17.01
93621-26	Electrophysiology evaluation	3244	4219	5632	113	3.13
93622-26	Electrophysiology evaluation	2368	3079	4111	184	5.07
93623-26	Stimulation, pacing heart	1052	1368	1826	152	4.19
93624	Electrophysiologic study	1624	2112	2820	327	9.04
93624-26	Electrophysiologic study	1445	1880	2510	255	7.05

          NEW CODE CPT 2002 •

CPT	SHORT DESCRIPTION	50th	75th	90th	MFS	RVU
93631	Heart pacing, mapping	1337	1739	2322	631	17.42
93631-26	Heart pacing, mapping	869	1130	1509	401	11.07
93640	Evaluation heart device	1551	2017	2693	446	12.32
93640-26	Evaluation heart device	776	1009	1347	187	5.16
93641	Electrophysiology evaluation	2178	2833	3782	574	15.87
93641-26	Electrophysiology evaluation	1503	1955	2610	315	8.71
93642	Electrophysiology evaluation	1992	2591	3459	516	14.25
93642-26	Electrophysiology evaluation	1096	1425	1902	257	7.09
93650	Ablate heart dysrhythm focus	2852	3709	4952	557	15.38
93651	Ablate heart dysrhythm focus	3776	4911	6557	864	23.88
93652	Ablate heart dysrhythm focus	3678	4783	6385	940	25.96
93660	Tilt table evaluation	607	790	1055	158	4.36
93660-26	Tilt table evaluation	279	363	485	99	2.74
93662	Intracardiac ECG (ice)	579	754	1006	0	.00
93668	Peripheral vascular rehab	1	1	1	0	.00
• **93701**	Bioimpedance, thoracic	96	120	156	35	.97
• **93701-26**	Bioimpedance, thoracic	25	31	41	9	.25
93720	Total body plethysmography	107	134	174	35	.96
93721	Plethysmography tracing	83	104	135	26	.72
93722	Plethysmography report	46	58	75	9	.24
93724	Analyze pacemaker system	942	1178	1526	401	11.07
93724-26	Analyze pacemaker system	631	789	1022	257	7.11
93727	Analyze ilr system	55	69	89	28	.78
93731	Analyze pacemaker system	99	124	160	42	1.16
93731-26	Analyze pacemaker system	57	72	93	24	.66
93732	Analyze pacemaker system	144	181	234	67	1.85

CPT	SHORT DESCRIPTION	50th	75th	90th	MFS	RVU
93732-26	Analyze pacemaker system	92	116	150	48	1.33
93733	Telephone analy, pacemaker	85	106	137	36	.99
93733-26	Telephone analy, pacemaker	25	32	41	9	.25
93734	Analyze pacemaker system	83	103	134	33	.90
93734-26	Analyze pacemaker system	52	65	84	20	.55
93735	Analyze pacemaker system	127	159	206	55	1.52
93735-26	Analyze pacemaker system	74	92	119	39	1.07
93736	Telephone analy, pacemaker	77	96	124	31	.87
93736-26	Telephone analy, pacemaker	20	25	32	8	.22
93740	Temperature gradient studies	38	48	62	14	.39
93740-26	Temperature gradient studies	26	33	42	8	.23
93741	Analyze ht pace device sngl	135	168	218	66	1.81
93741-26	Analyze ht pace device sngl	85	106	137	42	1.15
93742	Analyze ht pace device sngl	161	202	261	71	1.97
93742-26	Analyze ht pace device sngl	94	117	152	47	1.31
93743	Analyze ht pace device dual	163	204	264	80	2.22
93743-26	Analyze ht pace device dual	95	118	153	54	1.49
93744	Analyze ht pace device dual	209	261	338	85	2.36
93744-26	Analyze ht pace device dual	134	167	217	62	1.70
93760	Cephalic thermogram	215	269	348	0	.00
93760-26	Cephalic thermogram	178	223	289	0	.00
93762	Peripheral thermogram	287	359	465	0	.00
93762-26	Peripheral thermogram	238	298	386	0	.00
93770	Measure venous pressure	17	21	27	10	.27
93770-26	Measure venous pressure	10	13	17	8	.23
93784	Ambulatory bp monitoring	284	355	459	0	.00

NEW CODE CPT 2002 •

CPT	SHORT DESCRIPTION	50th	75th	90th	MFS	RVU
93786	Ambulatory bp recording	53	66	85	0	.00
93788	Ambulatory bp analysis	152	190	246	0	.00
93790	Review/report bp recording	215	269	349	0	.00
93797	Cardiac rehab	69	86	112	19	.52
93798	Cardiac rehab/monitor	88	110	143	26	.73
93799	Cardiovascular procedure	0	0	0	0	.00

NON-INVASIVE VASCULAR DIAGNOSTIC STUDIES

CPT	SHORT DESCRIPTION	50th	75th	90th	MFS	RVU
93875	Extracranial study	194	263	364	52	1.45
93875-26	Extracranial study	78	105	145	11	.31
93880	Extracranial study	426	578	798	170	4.69
93880-26	Extracranial study	102	139	192	31	.86
93882	Extracranial study	267	362	500	113	3.12
93882-26	Extracranial study	101	138	190	21	.59
93886	Intracranial study	498	675	932	207	5.71
93886-26	Intracranial study	124	169	233	50	1.39
93888	Intracranial study	531	720	995	137	3.79
93888-26	Intracranial study	111	151	209	33	.90
93922	Extremity study	266	361	499	56	1.56
93922-26	Extremity study	152	206	284	13	.36
93923	Extremity study	301	408	564	105	2.91
93923-26	Extremity study	183	249	344	24	.65
93924	Extremity study	345	468	646	115	3.19
93924-26	Extremity study	214	290	401	26	.73
93925	Lower extremity study	407	552	762	169	4.67
93925-26	Lower extremity study	102	138	191	30	.83
93926	Lower extremity study	279	379	524	113	3.12

CPT	SHORT DESCRIPTION	50th	75th	90th	MFS	RVU
93926-26	Lower extremity study	48	64	89	20	.56
93930	Upper extremity study	371	503	695	171	4.73
93930-26	Upper extremity study	67	91	125	24	.65
93931	Upper extremity study	280	380	525	114	3.15
93931-26	Upper extremity study	36	49	68	16	.44
93965	Extremity study	239	324	448	59	1.64
93965-26	Extremity study	105	143	197	18	.50
93970	Extremity study	543	737	1018	189	5.22
93970-26	Extremity study	152	206	285	35	.97
93971	Extremity study	490	665	918	126	3.47
93971-26	Extremity study	93	126	174	23	.64
93975	Vascular study	426	578	799	267	7.37
93975-26	Vascular study	170	231	319	92	2.55
93976	Vascular study	491	666	920	178	4.93
93976-26	Vascular study	138	187	258	62	1.70
93978	Vascular study	379	514	710	177	4.89
93978-26	Vascular study	87	118	163	34	.93
93979	Vascular study	256	347	480	118	3.27
93979-26	Vascular study	41	56	77	23	.64
93980	Penile vascular study	456	618	854	194	5.35
93980-26	Penile vascular study	191	260	359	64	1.76
93981	Penile vascular study	212	288	398	142	3.93
93981-26	Penile vascular study	64	86	119	22	.61
93990	Doppler flow testing	186	252	348	106	2.92
93990-26	Doppler flow testing	26	35	49	13	.36

NEW CODE CPT 2002 •

CPT	SHORT DESCRIPTION	50th	75th	90th	MFS	RVU
PULMONARY SERVICES						
94010	Breathing capacity test	76	100	132	37	1.02
94010-26	Breathing capacity test	44	57	75	9	.24
94014	Patient recorded spirometry	75	98	130	37	1.01
94014-26	Patient recorded spirometry	44	58	77	0	.00
94015	Patient recorded spirometry	25	32	42	11	.30
94015-26	Patient recorded spirometry	12	16	21	0	.00
94016	Review patient spirometry	52	68	90	26	.71
94060	Evaluation wheezing	129	169	223	63	1.73
94060-26	Evaluation wheezing	39	51	67	15	.42
94070	Evaluation wheezing	181	237	312	148	4.08
94070-26	Evaluation wheezing	59	72	90	29	.81
94150	Vital capacity test	28	36	48	26	.72
94150-26	Vital capacity test	11	15	20	4	.11
94200	Lung function test (mbc/mvv)	38	50	66	17	.47
94200-26	Lung function test (mbc/mvv)	23	30	39	6	.16
94240	Residual lung capacity	103	135	178	57	1.57
94240-26	Residual lung capacity	28	36	48	13	.35
94250	Expired gas collection	33	44	58	27	.74
94250-26	Expired gas collection	11	15	20	6	.16
94260	Thoracic gas volume	88	115	152	20	.55
94260-26	Thoracic gas volume	29	38	50	7	.18
94350	Lung nitrogen washout curve	82	108	143	47	1.31
94350-26	Lung nitrogen washout curve	27	36	47	13	.35
94360	Measure airflow resistance	90	118	155	30	.82
94360-26	Measure airflow resistance	32	42	56	13	.35

CPT	SHORT DESCRIPTION	50th	75th	90th	MFS	RVU
94370	Breath airway closing volume	189	248	327	84	2.32
94370-26	Breath airway closing volume	40	52	69	13	.35
94375	Respiratory flow volume loop	74	97	129	29	.80
94375-26	Respiratory flow volume loop	25	32	42	15	.42
94400	Co2 breathing response curve	160	210	277	42	1.16
94400-26	Co2 breathing response curve	147	193	255	20	.54
94450	Hypoxia response curve	151	198	261	47	1.29
94450-26	Hypoxia response curve	139	182	240	20	.54
94620	Pulmonary stress test/simple	197	258	340	87	2.40
94620-26	Pulmonary stress test/simple	79	103	136	31	.87
94621	Pulm stress test/complex	335	440	580	101	2.80
94621-26	Pulm stress test/complex	94	123	162	70	1.94
94640	Airway inhalation treat	37	49	64	28	.76
94642	Aerosol inhalation treat	305	400	528	0	.00
94650	Pressure breathing (ippb)	38	49	65	25	.69
94651	Pressure breathing (ippb)	30	40	52	23	.64
94652	Pressure breathing (ippb)	49	65	86	30	.83
94656	Initial ventilator mgmt	338	443	585	58	1.61
94657	Continued ventilator mgmt	137	180	237	41	1.12
94660	Pos airway pressure, cpap	160	209	276	53	1.46
94662	Neg press ventilation, cnp	119	157	206	37	1.02
94664	Aerosol or vapor inhalations	41	54	72	20	.56
94665	Aerosol or vapor inhalations	35	45	60	21	.57
94667	Chest wall manipulate	53	70	92	38	1.05
94668	Chest wall manipulate	39	52	68	28	.77
94680	Exhaled air analysis, O_2	139	183	241	54	1.49

NEW CODE CPT 2002 •

CPT	SHORT DESCRIPTION	50th	75th	90th	MFS	RVU
94680-26	Exhaled air analysis, O_2	70	91	120	13	.36
94681	Exhaled air analysis, O_2/CO_2	178	234	308	59	1.63
94681-26	Exhaled air analysis, O_2/CO_2	89	117	154	10	.28
94690	Exhaled air analysis	199	261	344	62	1.70
94690-26	Exhaled air analysis	30	39	52	4	.10
94720	Monoxide diffusing capacity	114	150	198	59	1.64
94720-26	Monoxide diffusing capacity	43	57	75	13	.35
94725	Membrane diffuse capacity	137	180	237	39	1.08
94725-26	Membrane diffuse capacity	52	68	90	13	.35
94750	Pulmonary compliance study	77	101	133	48	1.33
94750-26	Pulmonary compliance study	33	43	57	11	.31
94760	Measure blood oxygen level	31	41	54	4	.12
94761	Measure blood oxygen level	59	78	102	7	.19
94762	Measure blood oxygen level	128	167	220	30	.82
94770	Exhaled carbon dioxide test	102	133	176	41	1.13
94770-26	Exhaled carbon dioxide test	57	75	98	7	.20
94772	Breath recording, infant	0	0	0	0	.00
94799	Pulmonary service/procedure	0	0	0	0	.00

ALLERGY AND CLINICAL IMMUNOLOGY

CPT	SHORT DESCRIPTION	50th	75th	90th	MFS	RVU
95004	Allergy skin tests	6	7	9	4	.10
95010	Sensitivity skin tests	35	42	52	22	.61
95015	Sensitivity skin tests	31	38	47	20	.55
95024	Allergy skin tests	8	10	12	5	.15
95027	Skin end point titration	10	12	15	5	.15
95028	Allergy skin tests	12	15	18	8	.23
95044	Allergy patch tests	10	12	15	7	.20

CPT	SHORT DESCRIPTION	50th	75th	90th	MFS	RVU
95052	Photo patch test	12	14	18	9	.25
95056	Photosensitivity tests	10	12	15	7	.18
95060	Eye allergy tests	25	30	37	13	.35
95065	Nose allergy test	15	18	22	7	.20
95070	Bronchial allergy tests	149	180	223	79	2.19
95071	Bronchial allergy tests	159	191	237	101	2.79
95075	Ingestion challenge test	143	173	214	64	1.78
95078	Provocative testing	15	18	22	9	.26
95115	Immunotherapy, one inject	16	20	25	14	.39
95117	Immunotherapy, injections	21	27	34	18	.50
95120	Immunotherapy, one inject	39	49	62	0	.00
95125	Immunotherapy, many antigens	51	64	81	0	.00
95130	Immunotherapy, insect venom	27	33	42	0	.00
95131	Immunotherapy, insect venoms	49	61	78	0	.00
95132	Immunotherapy, insect venoms	48	60	76	0	.00
95133	Immunotherapy, insect venoms	77	96	122	0	.00
95134	Immunotherapy, insect venoms	83	103	131	0	.00
95144	Antigen therapy services	14	17	22	12	.32
95145	Antigen therapy services	22	27	34	20	.54
95146	Antigen therapy services	34	42	53	25	.69
95147	Antigen therapy services	52	65	82	35	.98
95148	Antigen therapy services	52	65	82	32	.88
95149	Antigen therapy services	62	77	98	40	1.11
95165	Antigen therapy services	12	15	19	10	.28
95170	Antigen therapy services	24	30	37	12	.33
95180	Rapid desensitization	159	199	253	134	3.71

   NEW CODE CPT 2002 •

CPT	SHORT DESCRIPTION	50th	75th	90th	MFS	RVU
95199	Allergy immunology services	0	0	0	0	.00
• 95250	Glucose monitoring, cont	61	76	97	52	1.45

NEUROLOGY AND NEUROMUSCULAR PROCEDURES

CPT	SHORT DESCRIPTION	50th	75th	90th	MFS	RVU
95805	Multiple sleep latency test	826	1083	1408	294	8.11
95805-26	Multiple sleep latency test	264	347	450	96	2.64
95806	Sleep study, unattended	630	826	1074	228	6.29
95806-26	Sleep study, unattended	271	355	462	83	2.29
95807	Sleep study, attended	1391	1825	2372	462	12.76
95807-26	Sleep study, attended	320	420	546	82	2.27
95808	Polysomnography, 1-3	765	1003	1304	457	12.63
95808-26	Polysomnography, 1-3	398	522	678	135	3.73
95810	Polysomnography, 4 or more	987	1295	1684	757	20.92
95810-26	Polysomnography, 4 or more	444	583	758	178	4.91
95811	Polysomnography w/cpap	990	1299	1688	778	21.48
95811-26	Polysomnography w/cpap	495	649	844	191	5.27
95812	Electroencephalogram (EEG)	358	469	610	187	5.17
95812-26	Electroencephalogram (EEG)	175	230	299	58	1.60
95813	Electroencephalogram (EEG)	351	460	598	268	7.41
95813-26	Electroencephalogram (EEG)	165	216	281	91	2.52
95816	Electroencephalogram (EEG)	565	741	963	167	4.62
95816-26	Electroencephalogram (EEG)	136	178	231	58	1.61
95819	Electroencephalogram (EEG)	641	841	1093	201	5.54
95819-26	Electroencephalogram (EEG)	141	185	241	58	1.61
95822	Sleep electroencephalogram	360	473	615	109	3.01
95822-26	Sleep electroencephalogram	76	99	129	58	1.61
95824	Electroencephalography	254	333	433	0	.00

CPT	SHORT DESCRIPTION	50th	75th	90th	MFS	RVU
95824-26	Electroencephalography	71	93	121	39	1.09
95827	Night electroencephalogram	284	349	437	140	3.87
95829	Surgery electrocorticogram	3524	4624	6009	1373	37.93
95829-26	Surgery electrocorticogram	3242	4254	5529	341	9.42
95830	Insert electrodes for EEG	263	345	449	200	5.53
95831	Limb muscle testing, manual	57	74	97	29	.81
95832	Hand muscle testing, manual	58	77	99	28	.78
95833	Body muscle testing, manual	53	70	91	37	1.02
95834	Body muscle testing, manual	70	92	120	44	1.21
95851	Range motion measurements	51	66	86	26	.72
95852	Range motion measurements	45	59	76	22	.61
95857	Tensilon test	111	146	189	44	1.21
95858	Tensilon test & myogram	306	402	522	99	2.73
95858-26	Tensilon test & myogram	184	241	313	84	2.32
95860	Muscle test, one limb	211	277	360	79	2.19
95860-26	Muscle test, one limb	156	205	267	52	1.44
95861	Muscle test, two limbs	316	415	539	111	3.06
95861-26	Muscle test, two limbs	231	303	394	84	2.31
95863	Muscle test, 3 limbs	401	526	683	135	3.74
95863-26	Muscle test, 3 limbs	289	379	492	101	2.80
95864	Muscle test, 4 limbs	508	666	866	173	4.77
95864-26	Muscle test, 4 limbs	360	473	615	108	2.98
95867	Muscle test, head or neck	235	309	401	64	1.77
95867-26	Muscle test, head or neck	172	225	293	43	1.19
95868	Muscle test, head or neck	408	535	695	90	2.49
95868-26	Muscle test, head or neck	322	422	549	65	1.79

  NEW CODE CPT 2002 •

CPT	SHORT DESCRIPTION	50th	75th	90th	MFS	RVU
95869	Muscle test, thor paraspinal	138	181	235	28	.77
95869-26	Muscle test, thor paraspinal	84	110	143	20	.55
95870	Muscle test, nonparaspinal	112	147	191	28	.77
95870-26	Muscle test, nonparaspinal	82	108	140	20	.55
95872	Muscle test, one fiber	369	484	629	102	2.83
95872-26	Muscle test, one fiber	269	354	460	80	2.22
95875	Limb exercise test	101	133	172	93	2.57
95875-26	Limb exercise test	76	100	129	59	1.63
95900	Motor nerve conduction test	93	122	158	43	1.18
95900-26	Motor nerve conduction test	57	75	98	23	.63
95903	Motor nerve conduction test	132	173	225	42	1.15
95903-26	Motor nerve conduction test	92	121	157	32	.89
95904	Sense nerve conduction test	94	123	160	37	1.01
95904-26	Sense nerve conduction test	56	74	96	18	.51
95920	Intraop nerve test add-on	422	554	720	164	4.54
95920-26	Intraop nerve test add-on	308	404	525	117	3.24
95921	Autonomic nerv function test	153	201	261	60	1.65
95921-26	Autonomic nerv function test	104	137	177	46	1.27
95922	Autonomic nerv function test	142	186	242	65	1.80
95922-26	Autonomic nerv function test	95	125	162	51	1.42
95923	Autonomic nerv function test	157	206	268	127	3.52
95923-26	Autonomic nerv function test	107	140	182	48	1.33
95925	Somatosensory testing	326	428	556	62	1.71
95925-26	Somatosensory testing	85	111	145	29	.80
95926	Somatosensory testing	318	418	543	62	1.72
95926-26	Somatosensory testing	83	109	141	29	.81

CPT	SHORT DESCRIPTION	50th	75th	90th	MFS	RVU
95927	Somatosensory testing	178	234	304	63	1.75
95927-26	Somatosensory testing	46	61	79	30	.84
95930	Visual evoked potential test	239	314	408	44	1.21
95930-26	Visual evoked potential test	103	135	175	19	.52
95933	Blink reflex test	197	259	336	60	1.67
95933-26	Blink reflex test	122	160	208	32	.88
95934	H-reflex test	100	131	171	36	.99
95934-26	H-reflex test	68	89	116	28	.77
95936	H-reflex test	90	119	154	38	1.04
95936-26	H-reflex test	63	83	108	30	.82
95937	Neuromuscular junction test	94	124	161	47	1.29
95937-26	Neuromuscular junction test	59	77	100	34	.95
95950	Ambulatory EEG monitoring	704	924	1200	249	6.88
95950-26	Ambulatory EEG monitoring	232	305	396	83	2.29
95951	EEG monitoring/videorecord	2077	2725	3542	831	22.96
95951-26	EEG monitoring/videorecord	769	1008	1311	323	8.92
95953	EEG monitoring/computer	977	1281	1665	396	10.93
95953-26	EEG monitoring/computer	371	487	633	165	4.56
95954	EEG monitoring/giving drugs	653	857	1114	254	7.03
95954-26	EEG monitoring/giving drugs	562	737	958	131	3.62
95955	EEG during surgery	361	474	616	125	3.46
95955-26	EEG during surgery	181	237	308	53	1.46
95956	EEG monitoring, cable/radio	836	1097	1426	577	15.94
95956-26	EEG monitoring, cable/radio	226	296	385	164	4.54
95957	EEG digital analysis	333	437	567	169	4.67
95957-26	EEG digital analysis	146	192	250	107	2.95

NEW CODE CPT 2002 •

CPT	SHORT DESCRIPTION	50th	75th	90th	MFS	RVU
95958	EEG monitoring/function test	508	666	866	291	8.05
95958-26	EEG monitoring/function test	345	453	589	228	6.29
95961	Electrode stimulation, brain	546	717	932	213	5.88
95961-26	Electrode stimulation, brain	410	538	699	166	4.58
95962	Electrode stim, brain add-on	364	478	621	223	6.16
95962-26	Electrode stim, brain add-on	273	358	466	176	4.86
• 95965	Meg, spontaneous	4810	6311	8203	0	.00
• 95965-26	Meg, spontaneous	1058	1388	1805	412	11.39
• 95966	Meg, evoked, single	2441	3202	4162	0	.00
• 95966-26	Meg, evoked, single	537	704	916	209	5.78
• 95967	Meg, evoked, each addl	2142	2810	3652	0	.00
• 95967-26	Meg, evoked, each addl	471	618	803	184	5.07
95970	Analyze neurostim, no prog	94	123	160	24	.66
95971	Analyze neurostim, simple	178	234	304	41	1.12
95972	Analyze neurostim, complex	242	318	413	83	2.29
95973	Analyze neurostim, complex	155	204	265	51	1.41
95974	Cranial neurostim, complex	326	428	556	164	4.52
95975	Cranial neurostim, complex	323	424	551	92	2.55
95999	Neurological procedure	0	0	0	0	.00
• 96000	Motion analysis, video/3d	236	310	402	92	2.54
• 96001	Motion test w/ft press meas	281	369	480	110	3.03
• 96002	Dynamic surface emg	55	72	94	21	.59
• 96003	Dynamic fine wire emg	51	67	87	20	.55
• 96004	Phys review motion tests	242	317	412	94	2.60
96100	Psychological testing	140	183	238	66	1.82
96105	Assessment aphasia	194	254	331	66	1.82

CPT	SHORT DESCRIPTION	50th	75th	90th	MFS	RVU
96110	Developmental test, lim	194	255	331	0	.00
96111	Developmental test, extend	160	211	274	66	1.82
96115	Neurobehavior status exam	147	193	251	66	1.82
96117	Neuropsych test battery	175	230	299	66	1.82

HEALTH AND BEHAVIOR ASSESSMENT INTERVENTION

CPT	SHORT DESCRIPTION	50th	75th	90th	MFS	RVU
• **96150**	Assess health/behave, init	68	89	116	26	.73
• **96151**	Assess health/behave, subseq	66	87	113	26	.71
• **96152**	Intervene health/behave, indiv	63	83	107	25	.68
• **96153**	Intervene health/behave, group	14	18	24	5	.15
• **96154**	Interv health/behav, fam w/pt	61	80	105	24	.66
• **96155**	Interv health/behav fam no pt	59	78	101	23	.64

CHEMOTHERAPY ADMINISTRATION

CPT	SHORT DESCRIPTION	50th	75th	90th	MFS	RVU
96400	Chemotherapy, sc/im	34	45	59	5	.14
96405	Intralesional chemo admin	101	135	175	88	2.42
96406	Intralesional chemo admin	141	188	245	136	3.76
96408	Chemotherapy, push technique	98	131	170	35	.97
96410	Chemotherapy, infuse method	156	209	272	56	1.54
96412	Chemo, infuse method add-on	109	146	190	42	1.15
96414	Chemo, infuse method add-on	176	235	306	49	1.34
96420	Chemotherapy, push technique	90	120	156	45	1.25
96422	Chemotherapy, infuse method	155	207	269	45	1.24
96423	Chemo, infuse method add-on	56	75	98	17	.48
96425	Chemotherapy, infuse method	95	127	165	52	1.43
96440	Chemotherapy, intracavitary	1103	1477	1919	379	10.48
96445	Chemotherapy, intracavitary	1159	1552	2016	399	11.01

NEW CODE CPT 2002 •

CPT	SHORT DESCRIPTION	50th	75th	90th	MFS	RVU
96450	Chemotherapy, into CNS	918	1170	1520	316	8.74
96520	Pump refilling, maintenance	78	105	136	32	.89
96530	Pump refilling, maintenance	82	110	143	38	1.06
96542	Chemotherapy inject	650	870	1130	223	6.17
96545	Provide chemotherapy agent	63	85	110	0	.00
96549	Chemotherapy, unspecified	0	0	0	0	.00

PHOTODYNAMIC THERAPY

CPT	SHORT DESCRIPTION	50th	75th	90th	MFS	RVU
• **96567**	Photodynamic tx, skin	175	234	304	60	1.66
96570	Photodynamic tx, 30 min	109	145	189	58	1.60
96571	Photodynamic tx, addl 15 min	54	73	95	29	.79

SPECIAL DERMATOLOGICAL PROCEDURES

CPT	SHORT DESCRIPTION	50th	75th	90th	MFS	RVU
96900	Ultraviolet light therapy	32	40	52	17	.47
96902	Trichogram	47	59	76	24	.67
96910	Photochemotherapy with UV-b	108	134	172	51	1.40
96912	Photochemotherapy with UV-a	122	151	195	57	1.58
96913	Photochemotherapy, UV-a or b	182	225	291	85	2.34
96999	Dermatological procedure	0	0	0	0	.00

PHYSICAL MEDICINE AND REHABILITATION

CPT	SHORT DESCRIPTION	50th	75th	90th	MFS	RVU
97001	Physical therapy evaluation	90	113	137	67	1.86
97002	Physical therapy re-evaluation	57	72	87	36	.99
97003	Occupational therapy evaluation	87	110	133	70	1.94
97004	Occupational therapy re-evaluation	52	65	79	47	1.31
• **97005**	Athletic train eval	0	0	0	0	.00
• **97006**	Athletic train reevaluation	0	0	0	0	.00
97010	Hot or cold packs therapy	22	28	34	4	.11

CPT	SHORT DESCRIPTION	50th	75th	90th	MFS	RVU
97012	Mechanical traction therapy	26	33	40	13	.37
97014	Electric stimulation therapy	27	34	41	14	.38
97016	Vasopneumatic device therapy	33	41	50	12	.33
97018	Paraffin bath therapy	33	41	50	7	.19
97020	Microwave therapy	27	34	42	4	.12
97022	Whirlpool therapy	36	45	54	16	.44
97024	Diathermy treat	27	34	41	4	.12
97026	Infrared therapy	31	39	48	4	.12
97028	Ultraviolet therapy	22	27	33	5	.15
97032	Electrical stimulation	31	39	47	17	.47
97033	Electric current therapy	41	51	62	14	.40
97034	Contrast bath therapy	33	41	50	13	.36
97035	Ultrasound therapy	31	39	47	11	.30
97036	Hydrotherapy	35	44	54	23	.63
97039	Physical therapy treat	28	35	43	10	.28
97110	Therapeutic exercises	39	47	55	26	.73
97112	Neuromuscular reeducation	39	47	55	28	.76
97113	Aquatic therapy/exercises	44	52	62	29	.80
97116	Gait training therapy	36	43	51	23	.63
97124	Massage therapy	32	38	45	21	.57
97139	Physical medicine procedure	24	29	34	16	.43
97140	Manual therapy	46	55	65	25	.68
97150	Group therapeutic procedures	40	48	56	18	.49
97504	Orthotic training	40	48	56	26	.73
97520	Prosthetic training	43	52	61	25	.68
97530	Therapeutic activities	40	48	56	33	.91

 CPT codes and descriptions only copyright AMA NEW CODE CPT 2002 •

CPT	SHORT DESCRIPTION	50th	75th	90th	MFS	RVU
97532	Cognitive skills development	41	50	58	22	.62
97533	Sensory integration	45	54	63	24	.66
97535	Self care management training	37	44	51	30	.82
97537	Community/work reintegration	40	48	57	24	.66
97542	Wheelchair management training	27	32	38	25	.68
97545	Work hardening	147	176	208	0	.00
97546	Work hardening add-on	57	68	80	0	.00
97601	Wound(s) care, selective	132	157	186	88	2.44
97602	Wound(s) care non-selective	0	0	0	0	.00
97703	Prosthetic checkout	40	48	57	26	.71
97750	Physical performance test	50	59	70	26	.71
97780	Acupuncture w/o stimulation	0	0	0	0	.00
97781	Acupuncture w/stimulation	0	0	0	0	.00
97799	Physical medicine procedure	0	0	0	0	.00

MEDICAL NUTRITION THERAPY

CPT	SHORT DESCRIPTION	50th	75th	90th	MFS	RVU
97802	Medical nutrition, indiv, in	222	265	313	17	.46
97803	Med nutrition, indiv, subseq	142	170	201	17	.46
97804	Medical nutrition, group	127	152	179	7	.18

OSTEOPATHIC MANIPULATIVE TREATMENT

CPT	SHORT DESCRIPTION	50th	75th	90th	MFS	RVU
98925	Osteopathic manipulation	46	55	65	30	.84
98926	Osteopathic manipulation	62	74	87	40	1.11
98927	Osteopathic manipulation	83	99	117	51	1.42
98928	Osteopathic manipulation	94	112	132	60	1.65
98929	Osteopathic manipulation	109	130	153	68	1.88

CPT	SHORT DESCRIPTION	50th	75th	90th	MFS	RVU

CHIROPRACTIC MANIPULATIVE TREATMENT

CPT	SHORT DESCRIPTION	50th	75th	90th	MFS	RVU
98940	Chiropractic manipulation	38	46	54	26	.71
98941	Chiropractic manipulation	46	55	64	35	.98
98942	Chiropractic manipulation	54	65	77	46	1.27
98943	Chiropractic manipulation	37	44	52	27	.75

SPECIAL SERVICES, PROCEDURES AND REPORTS

CPT	SHORT DESCRIPTION	50th	75th	90th	MFS	RVU
99000	Specimen handling	16	21	27	0	.00
99001	Specimen handling	23	31	40	0	.00
99002	Device handling	10	13	17	0	.00
99024	Postop follow-up visit	0	0	0	0	.00
99025	Initial surgical evaluation	63	83	107	0	.00
99050	Medical services after hrs	25	33	43	0	.00
99052	Medical services at night	44	58	75	0	.00
99054	Medical services, unusual hrs	44	58	75	0	.00
99056	Non-office medical services	22	29	38	0	.00
99058	Office emergency care	38	51	65	0	.00
99070	Special supplies	0	0	0	0	.00
99071	Patient education materials	0	0	0	0	.00
99075	Medical testimony	232	306	395	0	.00
99078	Group health education	0	0	0	0	.00
99080	Special reports or forms	0	0	0	0	.00
99082	Unusual physician travel	0	0	0	0	.00
99090	Computer data analysis	121	160	207	0	.00
• 99091	Collect/review data from pt	0	0	0	0	.00

NEW CODE CPT 2002 •

CPT	SHORT DESCRIPTION	50th	75th	90th	MFS	RVU

QUALIFYING CIRCUMSTANCES FOR ANESTHESIA

CPT	SHORT DESCRIPTION	50th	75th	90th	MFS	RVU
99100	Special anesthesia service	67	88	114	0	.00
99116	Anesthesia with hypothermia	217	287	370	0	.00
99135	Special anesthesia procedure	75	100	129	0	.00
99140	Emergency anesthesia	116	154	199	0	.00

SEDATION WITH OR WITHOUT ANALGESIA CONSCIOUS SEDATION

CPT	SHORT DESCRIPTION	50th	75th	90th	MFS	RVU
99141	Sedation, IV/IM or inhalant	135	178	230	107	2.96
99142	Sedation, oral/rectal/nasal	130	171	221	68	1.87

OTHER SERVICES AND PROCEDURES

CPT	SHORT DESCRIPTION	50th	75th	90th	MFS	RVU
99170	Anogenital exam, child	254	330	468	139	3.84
99172	Ocular function screen	0	0	0	0	.00
99173	Visual acuity screen	21	27	39	0	.00
99175	Induction vomiting	73	94	134	51	1.40
99183	Hyperbaric oxygen therapy	260	338	480	117	3.23
99185	Regional hypothermia	54	70	99	23	.64
99186	Total body hypothermia	216	280	398	75	2.06
99190	Special pump services	438	567	806	0	.00
99191	Special pump services	807	1046	1487	0	.00
99192	Special pump services	537	697	990	0	.00
99195	Phlebotomy	50	65	92	16	.44
99199	Special service/proc/report	0	0	0	0	.00

CPT	SHORT DESCRIPTION	50th	75th	90th	MFS	RVU

NEW CODE CPT 2002 •

GEOGRAPHIC ADJUSTMENTS

GEOGRAPHIC VARIABILITY OF MEDICAL FEES

The percentile fees presented in this book are based on national fee data; however, medical fees vary substantially by geographic area. In rural areas and smaller towns and cities, medical fees may be significantly lower than the percentiles presented in this book. Likewise, in larger cities, medical fees may be significantly higher than the fees presented. There are two primary reasons for the geographic variation in medical fees; namely, the cost of running a medical practice and the cost of medical malpractice insurance.

The cost of practice includes rent, employee costs, and other overhead costs, but not medical malpractice costs. According to the cost of practice indexes published in the *Medicare Physicians Fee Schedule*, New York City has the highest cost of practice and small eastern cities of Missouri have the lowest cost of practice. The cost of running a medical practice in New York City is almost 68% higher than running a medical practice in a small eastern city of Missouri.

The second reason for the geographic variation in medical fees is the cost of medical malpractice insurance. According to the malpractice expense indexes published in the Medicare Fee Schedule, New York City has the highest cost of medical malpractice insurance and South Dakota has the lowest cost of medical malpractice insurance. Medical malpractice insurance costs are just over 248% higher in New York City than they are in South Dakota.

These differences in the cost of practice and medical malpractice insurance are reflected in the wide range of fees charged by doctors for identical services provided in different geographic locations.

THE GEOGRAPHIC ADJUSTMENT FACTOR

In order to help you improve the accuracy of the percentile medical fees in the area where you practice, we have included this appendix of the Medicare Fee Schedule geographic cost of practice indexes (GPCI) and a simple geographic adjustment factor. A geographic adjustment factor (GAF) is a multiplier used to determine a more accurate fee for a specific location of medical practice. This appendix includes a list of geographic adjustment factors for cities, counties, areas, regions and states which can be used to "fine tune" the medical fees listed in this book. The geographic adjustment factors listed below are from the 2002 *Medicare Physician's Fee Schedule*.

The GAF listed on the following page is a simple average of the work, practice expense and malpractice expense components of the most current Medicare Fee Schedule. The GAF is used to calculate the approximate variations of geographic location on both the UCR and Medicare fees listed in this publication.

STATE/LOCALITY

The geographic region included in the geographic adjustment factor. Note that most geographic adjustment factors correspond to entire states or specific cities. But others correspond to specific counties, or terms such as urban, metropolitan, rural, large, small, north west, south west, etc.

CARRIER

The Medicare carrier code assigned by CMS. The carrier code is included so that you can clearly identify the specific geographic regions represented by the geographic adjustment factors.

LOC

The Medicare location code assigned by CMS. The location code is included so that you can clearly identify the specific geographic regions represented by the geographic adjustment factors.

WORK

The Medicare geographic cost of practice index for the work component of the procedure or service.

PE

The Medicare geographic cost of practice index for the practice expense component of the procedure or service.

MPE

The Medicare geographic cost of practice index for the malpractice expense component of the procedure or service.

GAF

The geographic adjustment factor (GAF). The GAF is a simple average of the GPCI factors for work, practice expense and malpractice expense. Multiplying the GAF times the fees listed in this book results in a fee adjusted for the work, practice expense, and malpractice values of a particular geographic area.

HOW TO USE THE GAF TO ADJUST MEDICAL FEES

To use the geographic adjustment factor, first look up the CPT codes in the book that you want to compare to your doctor's fees or health insurance carrier allowances. Write down the 50th, 75th and 90th percentile fees for each CPT code. Then look up the geographic adjustment factor for your city, county, area, region or state in this appendix. Finally, multiply the percentile fees times the geographic adjustment factor to determine the adjusted fee.

In order to clearly illustrate the process, let's look at two medical services provided in Phoenix, New York City, or anywhere in South Carolina. We first look up and write down the percentile fees for each service. Then, looking up these locations in this appendix, we find that the GAF for Phoenix is 1.028, the GAF for New York City is 1.371 and the GAF for South Carolina is .719. Finally, we multiply the percentile fees times the GAF for each location to determine the adjusted fee.

Code	Short Description		50th	75th	90th	MC
99205	Office visit, new patient; 60 minutes		206	240	285	166
	Phoenix	(multiply by 1.028)	212	247	293	170
	New York City	(multiply by 1.371)	282	329	391	228
	South Carolina	(multiply by 0.719)	148	172	205	119

Code	Short Description		50th	75th	90th	MC
33513	CABG, vein, four		7848	9650	11663	1910
	Phoenix	(multiply by 1.028)	8068	9920	11990	1963
	New York City	(multiply by 1.371)	10760	13230	15990	2619
	South Carolina	(multiply by .719)	5642	6938	8386	1373

As these examples clearly illustrate, medical fees in Phoenix are very close to the national average, medical fees in New York are almost 37% higher than the national average and medical fees in South Carolina are a little over 28% lower than the national average. As previously explained, these variations are due to the cost of practice and cost of medical malpractice insurance.

GEOGRAPHIC ADJUSTMENT FACTORS BY STATE OR TERRITORY

STATE/LOCALITY	CARR	LOC	WORK	PE	MPE	GAF
ALABAMA						
Statewide (all counties)	00510	00	0.978	0.870	0.807	**0.885**
ALASKA						
Statewide (all counties)	00831	01	1.064	1.172	1.223	**1.153**
ARIZONA						
Statewide (all counties)	00832	00	0.994	0.978	1.111	**1.028**
ARKANSAS						
Statewide (all counties)	00520	13	0.953	0.847	0.340	**0.713**
CALIFORNIA						
Anaheim/Santa Ana	02050	26	1.037	1.184	0.955	**1.059**
Los Angeles	02050	18	1.056	1.139	0.955	**1.050**
Marin/napa/Solano	31140	03	1.015	1.248	0.687	**0.984**
Oakland/Berkeley	31140	07	1.041	1.235	0.687	**0.988**
San Francisco	31140	05	1.068	1.458	0.687	**1.071**
San Mateo	31140	06	1.048	1.432	0.687	**1.056**
Santa Clara	31140	09	1.063	1.380	0.639	**1.028**
Ventura	02050	17	1.028	1.125	0.783	**0.979**
Rest of State[1]	02050	99	1.007	1.034	0.748	**0.930**
Rest of State[1]	31140	99	1.007	1.034	0.748	**0.930**
COLORADO						
Statewide (all counties)	00824	01	0.985	0.992	0.840	**0.939**
CONNECTICUT						
Statewide (all counties)	10230	00	1.050	1.156	0.966	**1.057**
DELAWARE						
Statewide (all counties)	00902	01	1.019	1.035	0.712	**0.922**
DISTRICT OF COLUMBIA						
DC + MD/VA SUBURBS	00903	01	1.050	1.166	0.909	**1.042**

STATE/LOCALITY	CARR	LOC	WORK	PE	MPE	GAF
FLORIDA						
Fort Lauderdale	00590	03	0.996	1.018	1.877	**1.297**
Miami	00590	04	1.015	1.052	2.528	**1.532**
Rest of state	00590	99	0.975	0.946	1.265	**1.062**
GEORGIA						
Atlanta	00511	01	1.006	1.059	0.935	**1.000**
Rest of state	00511	99	0.970	0.892	0.935	**0.932**
HAWAII AND GUAM						
Statewide (all counties)	00833	01	0.997	1.124	0.834	**0.985**
IDAHO						
Statewide (all counties)	05130	00	0.960	0.881	0.497	**0.779**
ILLINOIS						
Chicago	00952	16	1.028	1.092	1.797	**1.305**
East St. Louis	00952	12	0.988	0.924	1.691	**1.201**
Suburban Chicago	00952	15	1.006	1.071	1.645	**1.240**
Rest of state	00952	99	0.964	0.889	1.157	**1.004**
INDIANA						
Statewide (all counties)	00630	00	0.981	0.922	0.481	**0.795**
IOWA						
Statewide (all counties)	00826	00	0.959	0.876	0.596	**0.811**
KANSAS						
Kansas[1]	00650	00	0.963	0.895	0.756	**0.871**
Kansas[1]	00740	04	0.963	0.895	0.756	**0.871**
KENTUCKY						
Statewide (all counties)	00660	00	0.970	0.866	0.877	**0.904**
LOUISIANA						
New Orleans	00528	01	0.998	0.945	1.283	**1.075**
Rest of state	00528	99	0.968	0.870	1.073	**0.971**

STATE/LOCALITY	CARR	LOC	WORK	PE	MPE	GAF
MAINE						
Southern Maine	31142	03	0.979	0.999	0.666	**0.882**
Rest of state	31142	99	0.961	0.910	0.666	**0.846**
MARYLAND						
Baltimore and surrounding counties	00901	01	1.021	1.038	0.916	**0.992**
Rest of state	00901	99	0.984	0.972	0.774	**0.910**
MASSACHUSETTS						
Metropolitan Boston	31143	01	1.041	1.239	0.784	**1.021**
Rest of state	31143	99	1.010	1.129	0.784	**0.974**
MICHIGAN						
Detroit	00953	01	1.043	1.038	2.738	**1.606**
Rest of state	00953	99	0.997	0.938	1.571	**1.169**
MINNESOTA						
Statewide (all counties)	10240	00	0.990	0.974	0.452	**0.805**
MISSISSIPPI						
Statewide (all counties)	10250	00	0.957	0.837	0.779	**0.857**
MISSOURI						
Metropolitan Kansas City	00740	02	0.988	0.967	0.846	**0.933**
Metropolitan St. Louis	00523	01	0.994	0.938	0.846	**0.926**
Rest of state[1]	00740	99	0.946	0.825	0.793	**0.854**
Rest of state[1]	00523	99	0.946	0.825	0.793	**0.854**
MONTANA						
Statewide (all counties)	00751	01	0.950	0.876	0.727	**0.851**
NEBRASKA						
Statewide (all counties)	00655	00	0.948	0.877	0.430	**0.752**
NEVADA						
Statewide (all counties)	00834	00	1.005	1.039	1.209	**1.084**

STATE/LOCALITY	CARR	LOC	WORK	PE	MPE	GAF
NEW HAMPSHIRE						
Statewide (all counties)	31144	40	0.986	1.030	0.825	**0.947**
NEW JERSEY						
Northern New Jersey	00805	01	1.058	1.193	0.860	**1.037**
Rest of state	00805	99	1.029	1.110	0.860	**1.000**
NEW MEXICO						
Statewide (all counties)	00521	05	0.973	0.900	0.902	**0.925**
NEW YORK						
Manhattan	00803	01	1.094	1.351	1.668	**1.371**
NYC suburbs/Long Island	00803	02	1.068	1.251	1.952	**1.424**
Poughkipsie/N NYC suburbs	00803	03	1.011	1.075	1.275	**1.120**
Queens	14330	04	1.058	1.228	1.871	**1.385**
Rest of state	00801	99	0.998	0.944	0.764	**0.902**
NORTH CAROLINA						
Statewide (all counties)	05535	00	0.970	0.931	0.595	**0.832**
NORTH DAKOTA						
Statewide (all counties)	00820	01	0.950	0.880	0.657	**0.829**
OHIO						
Statewide (all counties)	16360	00	0.988	0.944	0.957	**0.963**
OKLAHOMA						
Statewide (all counties)	00522	00	0.968	0.876	0.444	**0.763**
OREGON						
Portland	00835	01	0.996	1.049	0.436	**0.827**
Rest of state	00835	99	0.961	0.933	0.436	**0.777**
PENNSYLVANIA						
Metropolitan Philadelphia	00865	01	1.023	1.092	1.413	**1.176**
Rest of state	00865	99	0.989	0.929	0.774	**0.897**

STATE/LOCALITY	CARR	LOC	WORK	PE	MPE	GAF
PUERTO RICO						
Statewide (all counties)	00973	20	0.881	0.712	0.275	**0.622**
RHODE ISLAND						
Statewide (all counties)	00870	01	1.017	1.065	0.883	**0.988**
SOUTH CAROLINA						
Statewide (all counties)	00880	01	0.974	0.904	0.279	**0.719**
SOUTH DAKOTA						
Statewide (all counties)	00820	02	0.935	0.878	0.406	**0.740**
TENNESSEE						
Statewide (all counties)	05440	35	0.975	0.900	0.592	**0.822**
TEXAS						
Austin	00900	31	0.986	0.996	0.859	**0.947**
Beaumont	00900	20	0.992	0.890	1.338	**1.073**
Brazoria	00900	09	0.992	0.978	1.338	**1.103**
Dallas	00900	11	1.010	1.065	0.931	**1.002**
Fort Worth	00900	28	0.987	0.981	0.931	**0.966**
Galveston	00900	15	0.988	0.969	1.338	**1.098**
Houston	00900	18	1.020	1.007	1.336	**1.121**
Rest of state	00900	99	0.966	0.880	0.956	**0.934**
UTAH						
Statewide (all counties)	00910	09	0.976	0.941	0.644	**0.854**
VERMONT						
Statewide (all counties)	31145	50	0.973	0.986	0.539	**0.833**
VIRGIN ISLANDS						
Statewide (all counties)	00973	50	0.965	1.023	1.002	**0.997**
VIRGINIA						
Statewide (all counties)	10490	00	0.984	0.938	0.500	**0.807**

STATE/LOCALITY	CARR	LOC	WORK	PE	MPE	GAF
WASHINGTON						
Seattle (King County)	00836	02	1.005	1.100	0.788	**0.964**
Rest of state	00836	99	0.981	0.972	0.788	**0.913**
WEST VIRGINIA						
Statewide (all counties)	16510	16	0.963	0.850	1.378	**1.064**
WISCONSIN						
Statewide (all counties)	00951	00	0.981	0.929	0.939	**0.950**
WYOMING						
Statewide (all counties)	00825	21	0.967	0.895	1.005	**0.956**

[1]Payment locality is serviced by two Medicare carriers

INDEX

A

abdomen, peritoneum and
      omentum 176
ability to pay 17
accessory sinuses 111
adenoids 155
adjusted historical payment
      basis (AHPB) 1, 2, 435
adrenal glands 213, 275
allergen immunotherapy 353
allergy and clinical
      immunology 419
allowables 2-4
anatomic pathology 23, 382
ankle joint 92-94, 96
anterior segment 234
anus 169-172
aorta and arteries 272
arteries and veins 129, 220, 272
arthroscopy 105-108
artificial eye 403
auditory system 245, 406

B

back and flank 59
biliary tract 173
biofeedback 398
bladder 165, 168, 184-
                        191, 195, 203,
                        270-271, 304
bone marrow 143, 281, 296,
                        347, 367, 385
brain 215-221, 251,
                        253, 255, 302-
                        303, 425
breast 45-47, 279-
                        280, 283
bronchi 114, 256

C

cardiovascular 121, 301, 406-
                        408, 415
cardiovascular system 121
care plan oversight services 31
carotid body 213, 214
case management services 31
casts and strapping 103
Center for Medicare and Medicaid
      Services (*see also*
      CMS) 8, 25
cervix 12, 204, 209
chemistry 313, 345
chemotherapy administration 426
chest 10, 46, 49, 58-59,
                104, 116-119, 130, 136,
                141, 147, 255-257,
                259-260, 274-
                275, 283, 418
chiropractic manipulative
      treatment 430
clinical pathology . 292, 312, 345, 419
CMS (*see also* Centers for
      Medicare and
      Medicaid Services) . . 8, 10,
                23, 25, 434
computerized fee schedules 14
conjunctiva 242
consultations 7, 28, 312
contract fee schedules . . . 15, 19, 209
conversion factor (CF) . . . 11-13, 24
corpus uteri 205
cost benefit analysis 2
CPT (Current Procedural
      Terminology) . 3-11, 13, 16,
                23-25, 27, 33, 251,
                307, 393, 435
critical care services 29
custodial care 30
cytopathology 382-385

D

dentoalveolar structures 152
dermatological procedures 427
determining fees for new
       procedures 13
diagnostic radiology 251
diagnostic ultrasound 283
dialysis 398, 399
diaphragm 12, 147, 202, 229
digestive system 149
discount business 21, 22
discussing fees 17-19
drug testing 308

E

elbow 66-70, 104, 106,
       229, 262
emergency department services . . 29
endocrine system 213
epididymis 196
esophagus 156, 157, 159-
       160, 268, 399
ESRD (end stage renal disease) . . 398
evaluation and management services
       (E/M) 16
evocative/suppression testing 310
explanation of benefits (EOB) 9
external ear 128, 140, 169,
       245, 290, 406
extracranial nerves 226
eye and ocular adnexa 233
eyeball 233

f

fee comparison 16
fee consistency 16
fee schedule 1-4, 7-9, 14-17,
       23-25, 433, 434
fee schedule review 2, 9, 14
female genital system 201
femur 84, 85, 87, 88
fibula 51, 92-95
fingers 76

foot and toes 97, 100
forearm and wrist 70

G

GAF (*see also* geographic adjustment
       factor) 4, 433-441
gastroenterology 399, 400
gastrointestinal tract 267
genitalia 285
geographic adjustment factor (*see also*
       GAF) 433-434
geographic cost of practice indexes
       (GCPI) 8, 433
geographic variability 4, 433
going rate, the 19

H

hand and fingers 76
harvard study 17
HCPCS (Health Care Procedural
       Coding System) . . . 7-10, 13
head 41, 50, 52, 58,
       63, 66-68, 85, 219-
       220, 229, 231, 251,
       253-255, 272-
       273, 283, 422
head and neck 251, 283
heart 117, 121-126, 128,
       271, 285, 286, 300-301,
       406-407, 409-413
heart and pericardium 121
hematology and coagulation 345
hemic and lymphatic systems . . . 143
hemodialysis 398, 399
hip joint 83-85, 87
home services 30
hospital discharge 7, 9, 23,
       27-28, 32
how to implement your new fee
       schedule 16
how to review your fee schedule . . 7
humerus 63, 65-69, 262

INDEX

IJ

ICD-9-CM (International Classification
of Diseases) . . . 7, 8, 10, 13
immune globulins 393
immunization administration 393
immunology 353, 366, 419, 421
injection(s) 10, 17, 396, 420
inner ear 248, 249
insurance carrier 1, 9, 13, 435
integumentary system 33
intensive care 29
intersex surgery 199
intestines 162

KL

kidney 140, 181-184, 189,
271, 273, 275,
284, 303-304
knee joint 87-90, 92, 265
laboratory services 4
larynx 112-114, 253
leg 41, 87-88, 90, 92-97,
104-105, 129-130, 141,
229, 231, 232,
265, 272-275
lips 149
lower extremities 264
lungs and pleura 116
lymph nodes 143-144

M

male genital system 193
managed care 3
market driven procedures 20
maternity care and delivery 209
meckel's diverticulum 166, 299
mediastinum and diaphragm 147
Medicare fee schedule . 1, 4-5, 7-10,
14-15, 17, 22-25,
433-434, 441
medicine services . . . 10-11, 31, 295,
305-306, 366,
393, 427-429

meninges 215
microbiology 369, 382
middle ear 246-248, 251
modifier 23
molecular diagnostics 334, 335
mouth 57, 110, 149-153, 252
multiple fee schedules 14, 177,
295-296, 299-302,
341, 397, 421
musculoskeletal system 49

N

nails 36
neonatal intensive care 29, 342
nerves 58, 224, 226, 230-231
nervous system . . 215, 226, 232, 303
neuromuscular procedures 421
newborn care 32
nose 55-56, 109-110,
153, 155-156,
278, 420
nuclear medicine 295, 305, 306

O

ocular adnexa 233, 239
office or other outpatient 5, 27
omentum 176, 177
organ or disease oriented panels . 307
osteopathic manipulative
treatment 429
otorhinolaryngologic services . . . 403
ovary 12, 206-207
oviduct 206-207

P

palate and uvula 152
pelvis 50, 83-85, 87,
144, 204-205, 230, 257,
260-261, 264, 271,
273-274, 284
pelvis and hip joint 83
penis 141, 193-195, 270

percentile 2-7, 11, 12,
24, 433, 435
pericardium 121
pharynx 113, 153, 155
physical medicine . . . 8, 21, 427-429
pleura 116
posterior segment 237
practice management
    applications . . . 2-4, 7-11, 14,
17-18, 20-22, 433-435
preventive medicine services 31
price sensitivity 20
professional component 23
prolonged services 30
promotional pricing 21
prosthesis 47, 52-53, 72,
84, 90, 114, 153, 165,
191, 195, 237, 403
psychiatry 396
pulmonary services 417

QR
radiation oncology 289
radius/ulna 74
RBRVS (*see also* relative based
    resource value system) . . . 1,
4, 8, 25
rectum 278, 162, 166-169, 203
rehabilitation 427
relationship building 20
relationship to payer allowables . . . 3
relative value 1, 3-4, 8,
11-17, 24, 25
repair 9, 12, 17, 36-39,
42, 57-58, 64, 67-68,
72-74, 78, 80-81, 85,
88-90, 93-95, 99-103,
105, 110, 115-116,
117-119, 122-133,
136, 140, 143, 147,
149-154, 156-157,
159-162, 165-166,
168-172, 178-179, 182,

185-188, 190-192,
194-197, 201-207,
209, 219-221,
226, 231, 233-234,
236-238, 240-241,
243, 247-248,
276-277, 286,
403, 407
resource based relative value system
    (*see also* RBRVS) . . 1, 3, 7,
8, 17, 25
respiratory system 109
rest home or custodial care 30

S
salivary gland . . . 153-154, 253, 298
scrotum 196, 197, 285
sedation 431
seminal vesicles 198
setting fees 1
shoulder 62-66, 104,
106, 262
skin, subcutaneous and accessory
    structures 33
sources of the data 3
spermatic cord 197, 198
spinal canal 222, 284
spine 59-62, 176, 221-223,
226, 228, 257-261,
273, 278
spine and pelvis 257
spine and spinal cord 221
spleen 131, 140, 143,
274, 297, 298
stomach 159-162, 230,
270, 389, 390
strategic pricing concepts 20
subsequent hospital care 27, 28
surgical pathology . . . 9, 18-19, 112,
116, 118-119, 156,
159, 160, 165, 168,
198, 387, 389, 430

_T_

technical component 23
temporal bone . . . 141, 246, 248, 249
testis 195, 196
therapeutic drug assays 308
therapeutic or diagnostic
        infusions 396
thorax 58-60, 137,
        223, 257, 261
thymus 213, 214
thyroid gland 213
tibia 92-95, 97
toes 97, 100, 103, 105
tongue and floor of mouth 150
tonsils 155
trachea and bronchi 114
transfusion medicine 366
tunica vaginalis 197

_U_

upper extremities 262
ureter 181-186, 188-189

_V_

vaccines, toxoids 394
vas deferens 197
veins and lymphatics 274
vestibule of mouth 149
volume consideration 21
vulva, perineum and introitus . . . 201

_W_

worker's compensation 1, 14, 15
wrist 70-77, 104, 106,
        229, 262-263

urethra 187-188, 190-192,
        194-195, 203,
        270-271
urinalysis 10, 312, 313
urinary system 181
urinary tract 187, 270
usual, customary and reasonable
        (UCR) 2-5, 23-24, 434